T0265268

Rheumatology in Clinical Practice

Rheumatology in Clinical Practice

Editor: Sullivan Princeton

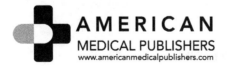

AMERICAN
MEDICAL PUBLISHERS
www.americanmedicalpublishers.com

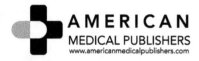

Cataloging-in-Publication Data

Rheumatology in clinical practice / edited by Sullivan Princeton.
    p. cm.
Includes bibliographical references and index.
ISBN 979-8-88740-441-7
1. Rheumatology. 2. Rheumatism--Diagnosis. 3. Rheumatism--Treatment.
4. Connective tissues--Diseases. 5. Joints--Diseases. I. Princeton, Sullivan.
RC927 .R44 2023
616.723--dc23

American Medical Publishers,
41 Flatbush Avenue,
1st Floor, New York,
NY 11217, USA

ISBN 979-8-88740-441-7 (Hardback)

Contents

Permissions

List of Contributors

Index

Preface

Rheumatology refers to a subspecialty of pediatrics and internal medicine that focuses on the joints, soft tissues and heritable connective tissue disorders. This discipline is also concerned with the diagnosis and treatment of systemic autoimmune diseases, musculoskeletal diseases, gout, polymyositis, Sjogren's syndrome, polychondritis and polymyalgia rheumatica. Physical examination including multiple joint examination and musculoskeletal inspection along with specialized tests such as general musculoskeletal exam (GMSE) and screening musculoskeletal exam (SMSE) can be utilized for diagnosing rheumatic diseases. Nonsteroidal anti-inflammatory drugs (NSAIDs), disease-modifying antirheumatic drugs (DMARDs), analgesics, methotrexate, steroids, as well as monoclonal antibodies like adalimumab and infliximab are used to treat the majority of rheumatic diseases. This book explores all the important aspects of clinical rheumatology in the modern day. It strives to provide a fair idea about rheumatic diseases and to help develop a better understanding of the latest advances in their clinical management. Those in search of information to further their knowledge will be greatly assisted by this book.

Various studies have approached the subject by analyzing it with a single perspective, but the present book provides diverse methodologies and techniques to address this field. This book contains theories and applications needed for understanding the subject from different perspectives. The aim is to keep the readers informed about the progresses in the field; therefore, the contributions were carefully examined to compile novel researches by specialists from across the globe.

Indeed, the job of the editor is the most crucial and challenging in compiling all chapters into a single book. In the end, I would extend my sincere thanks to the chapter authors for their profound work. I am also thankful for the support provided by my family and colleagues during the compilation of this book.

Editor

A case-control study about bite force, symptoms and signs of temporomandibular disorders in patients with idiopathic musculoskeletal pain syndromes

Liete Zwir*[iD], Melissa Fraga, Monique Sanches, Carmen Hoyuela, Claudio Len and Maria Teresa Terreri

Abstract

Background: The purposes of this study were to assess the prevalence of temporomandibular disorders symptoms and signs and the bite force in pediatric patients with idiopathic musculoskeletal pain syndrome and to compare to healthy control individuals paired by gender and age.

Methods: Forty consecutive patients (32 girls) from our outpatient pediatric rheumatology pain clinic with diagnosis of idiopathic musculoskeletal pain syndrome were included in this study. Twenty healthy subjects (16 girls) were considered the control group. All individuals were interviewed according to a standardized questionnaire concerning the presence of orofacial pain and functional impairment, and were submitted to a clinical evaluation following a structured protocol. After that the bite force was measured.

Results: Twelve patients met the ACR criteria for fibromyalgia, and 28 presented the diagnosis of pain amplification syndrome. The mean age of patients was 13.1 years (range, 6–18 years) and of controls was 12.8 years (range, 6–18 years) with no significant difference. Orofacial symptoms occurred in 25 patients (62.5%) and in 3 controls (15%) ($p = 0.0014$). Sixteen (40%) patients and four (20%) controls presented pain during mandibular function with no significant difference. Although both pain groups presented separately more frequently orofacial symptoms and pain on palpation than the controls, maximal voluntary bite force was similar between patients and controls, between both patient groups and between the two pain groups and controls.

Conclusions: Our findings indicate that temporomandibular disorders symptoms were more prevalent in patients with idiopathic musculoskeletal pain syndrome than in healthy controls. However the bite force was not different among the groups.

Background

Chronic musculoskeletal pain in children is common, affecting 10–20% of schoolchildren [1]. Although a serious underlying disease is not the cause in most cases, some may be life-threatening or potentially crippling [2]. A number of children may develop an idiopathic chronic musculoskeletal pain syndrome (IMPS) and become

disabled [3]. This syndrome includes three entities: growing pains (limb pain), pain amplification syndrome and fibromyalgia.

Pain amplification syndrome is a condition where patients develop an abnormal pain sensitivity [4]. Fibromyalgia (FM) is currently defined as chronic widespread pain with allodynia or hyperalgesia to pressure pain [5]. FM may coexist with other clinical conditions such as temporomandibular disorders (TMD).

* Correspondence: lfzwir@gmail.com
Universidade Federal de São Paulo (UNIFESP), Rua Guilherme Moura, São Paulo 95, Brazil

TMD is a term that includes clinical disorders involving the masticatory muscles, the temporomandibular joints (TMJ), and associated structures [6]. The most prevalent reported TMD's symptoms in children and adolescents are headaches, TMJ sounds, difficulty in mouth opening, jaw and facial pain, impaired chewing ability and the most common clinical signs of TMD are TMJ and muscle tenderness, limitation of mandibular movements, and TMJ sounds [7].

It has been shown that adult patients with FM have a high prevalence of orofacial signs and symptoms, ranging from 33 to 97% [8–11].

Bite force (BF) is an indicator of the functional state of the masticatory system in children, and can be considered one of the key determinants of the masticatory performance [12, 13]. Signs and symptoms of TMD have been suggested to affect BF measurements [14]. It has been reported that pain in the masticatory muscles and TMJ can cause significant changes in the maximal BF when compared to individuals without such pain [15]. To the best of our knowledge, there is no study addressing BF in pediatric IMPS patients.

The objectives of the present study were to assess the prevalence of TMD symptoms and signs in pediatric patients with IMPS and controls, and to measure the BF in those patients and to compare them to healthy control individuals paired by gender and age.

Methods
Patients
This was a cross-sectional study where sixty-three consecutive patients with diagnosis of IMPS from our outpatient pain clinic in the pediatric rheumatology division were evaluated and forty were included in the final sample. IMPS was defined by the presence of generalized musculoskeletal pain in 3 or more areas of the body for at least 3 months, and these symptoms are not explained by other causes or diseases [3]. FM was characterized by widespread musculoskeletal pain associated with fatigue, sleep, memory and mood issues [5] and pain amplification syndrome was defined as by the presence of musculoskeletal pain without a well-defined organic basis.

Twenty healthy subjects were considered as control group.

The inclusion criteria were patients with IMPS (FM and pain amplification syndrome) as defined in the literature [3, 5]. Healthy subjects who were referred for control orthodontic evaluation were included as control group and were gender and age matched to the patients. Other inclusion criteria for both groups were the presence of the permanent central incisors completed erupted, first permanent molars in occlusion, and the absence of dental related pain. Twenty-three patients

were excluded because they presented problems with their teeth in the areas where the BF was measured.

After informed consent was obtained, demographic and clinical data were collected from the patients' medical records.

Methods
All patients underwent a rheumatologic examination performed by a single pediatric rheumatologist, and an orofacial examination performed by a single dentist. These examinations were scheduled for the same week.

Assessment of subjective symptoms of the TMJ
The subjects were interviewed according to a standardized questionnaire concerning the presence of pain and functional impairment. Patients and their parents answered questions regarding the presence of headaches, abdominal pain, TMJ or masticatory muscle pain at rest or during functional mandibular movements, impaired maximal mouth opening and impaired chewing ability. The questions were answered by categorical (yes/no) responses.

Clinical examination
Only one blind assessor (dentist) performed the clinical evaluation following a structured protocol. The following registrations were made:

- Maximum mouth opening between the incisal edges of the front teeth (in mm) was measured using a millimeter ruler and adjusted for overbite and open bite as necessary. The subjects were asked to open his or her mouth as widely as possible. The patients performed the movements without any help from the examiner. Limitation of opening was defined as a range of movement in the central incisor region of less than 40 mm from the fully occluded to maximal open position [16, 17].
- Presence of pain on palpation on facial sites (6 sites):
  - Presence of tenderness on lateral digital palpation of the TMJ on either side (2 sites);
  - Presence of tenderness on digital palpation of the masseter and temporalis muscles on either side (4 sites);
- Presence of pain on function: during active mandibular movements (open, laterotrusion and protrusion).

Bite force measurement
The BF registration procedure was carefully explained to all participants. Subjects sat in an upright position without head support. The BF was measured unilaterally in the area of the first permanent molars (right and left sides) and central incisors region, using a calibrated dynamometer (Crown DBC, Oswaldo Filizola, São Paulo,

SP, Brazil). The stainless steel rods were 40 mm long X 12.7 mm wide X 13.5 mm thick. A piece of simple disposable foam tape (15 mm long X 13 mm wide X 4 mm tall) covered the BF application site. The peak force measurements were displayed digitally on its screen and recorded for further analysis. The dynamometer was cleaned with alcohol, a piece of sterile latex encased the device and it was replaced after each subject evaluation. Subjects were instructed to bite as hard as possible. The measurements were repeated three times, with one-minute rest between them. The highest value from the three recordings was considered as the maximal BF. The same operator performed all measurements. BF was not taken if the anterior teeth or the first permanent molars were not completely erupted or if they had had extensive restorations. The measured BF was calculated in Newton (N) and displayed digitally.

Written informed consent was obtained from all participants. This study was reviewed and approved by the local Medical Ethics Committee.

Statistical analysis

In order to verify the association between the variables presence of headaches, abdominal pain, and TMD symptoms and signs in the two patient groups, Pearson's chi-square test and Fisher's exact test were used. These tests were also used to evaluate the association between the TMD symptoms and signs in each patient group and the control group. Student's t-test was used to verify the variation of age, maximal mouth opening capacity, and the BF measurements between each patient group and the control group. The STATISTICA 12.7 (Dell®) program was used for the statistical analysis. The level of significance was set to 5% ($p < 0.05$).

Results

This study included 40 patients with IMPS. Twelve met the ACR criteria for FM (11 girls), and 28 (21 girls) presented the diagnosis of pain amplification syndrome. The mean age of patients was 13.1 years (range, 6–18 years) and of controls was 12.8 years (range, 6–18 years) with no significant difference ($p = 0.464$) (Table 1).

TMD symptoms occurred in 25 patients (62.5%) and in 3 controls (15%) ($p = 0.0014$). Sixteen (40%) patients and four (20%) controls presented pain during mandibular function ($p = 0.2081$). During palpation, 36 (90%) patients and only six (30%) controls complained about pain at least in one site ($p < 0.0001$) (Table 1). In addition, the mean measurement of the vertical range of motion of the mandible during maximum unassisted opening was 48.9 mm (ranging from 37 to 50 mm) in patients and 43.4 mm (ranging from 40 to 64 mm) in control group.

Table 1 Demographic and Temporomandibular Disorders (TMD) symptoms and signs and bite force measurement of patients and controls

	Controls	Patients	p
TOTAL (n)	20	40	
Girls (%)	16 (80.0)	32 (80.0)	0.998
Age (mean)	12.8 years	13.1 years	0.464
TMD symptoms (%)	3 (15.0)	25 (62.5)	0.0014*
Pain on palpation (%)	6 (30.0)	36 (90.0)	< 0.0001*
Pain on function (%)	4 (20.0)	16 (40.0)	0.2081
Bite force (mean), in N			
Anterior	143.3	139.7	0.811
Right side	313.2	337.9	0.386
Left side	314.7	353.0	0.107

N Newton, TMD Temporomandibular Disorders
*-statistically significant difference at $p \leq .05$

When we compared the two pain groups we observed that the FM group complained more frequently of soft tissue swelling over the TMJ ($p = 0.0175$). We did not find any difference in relation to the frequency of the complaint of headaches or abdominal pain between them. Both pain groups presented similar TMD signs, but there was a statistically difference between the frequency of 4 or more painful sites on palpation in FM patients compared with pain amplification syndrome patients ($p = 0.0375$). All other features did not present significant differences between the two patient groups (Table 2).

Each pain group presented more frequently TMD symptoms and pain on palpation than the controls (Table 3).

Maximal voluntary BF was similar between patients and controls (Table 1), between both patient groups (Table 2) and between the two pain groups and controls (Table 3).

Discussion

TMD symptoms and signs in pediatric patients with idiopathic musculoskeletal pain conditions were evaluated in this study. In this pioneer study, we observed that TMD symptoms and pain on palpation were more frequent in patients than in controls.

In relation to gender we found a greater prevalence of girls in our consecutive sample. It is known that chronic pain in females involves several factors such as behavior, hormones, morphological characteristics, and emotion. Pereira et al. showed that female adolescents are more likely to experience TMD than males [18]. It is important to note that females generally have lower pain thresholds than males [19].

FM and pain amplification syndrome patients presented more pain on palpation when compared to controls. The

Table 2 Temporomandibular Disorders (TMD) symptoms and signs and bite force measurement between the two pain groups

	Fibromyalgia	Pain amplification syndrome	Total %	p value
n (40)	12	28	100%	
TMD symptoms (25)	9	16	62.5	p = 0.4774
Pain in the face (13)	6	6	30	NS
Pain during mastication (7)	1	6	17.5	NS
Tiredness during mastication (18)	6	11	42.5	NS
Soft tissue swelling over the TMJ (7)	5	2	17.5	p = 0.0175*
TMJ sounds (8)	2	6	20	NS
TMD signs				
Pain on function (17)	6	10	40	NS
Opening (14)	4	9	32.5	NS
Protrusion (7)	2	5	17.5	NS
Right laterotrusion (12)	5	6	27.5	NS
Left laterotrusion (7)	3	4	17.5	NS
Pain on palpation (36)	12	24	90	NS
Number of painful sites				
0 (4)	0	4	10	
1 (2)	0	2	5	
2 (0)	0	0	0	
3 (3)	0	3	7.5	
4 (11)	4	7	27.5	
5 (3)	2	1	7.5	
6 (17)	6	11	42.5	
Frequency of 4 or more painful sites (31)	100%	67.80%	77.5	p = 0.0375*
Maximal mouth opening capacity (mean)	51.58 mm	47.85 mm		NS
Bite force (Newton)				
Anterior	154.6	133.3		NS
Right side	344.9	334.9		NS
Left side	343.7	357		NS

N Newton, TMJ Temporomandibulat Joint, TMD Temporomandibular Disorders, NS not significant
*statistically significant difference at p ≤ .05

Table 3 Temporomandibular Disorders (TMD) symptoms and signs and bite force measurement of the two patients groups and controls

	Controls	Fibromyalgia	p	Pain Amplification Syndrome	p
TOTAL (n)	20	12		28	
TMD symptoms (%)	3 (15.0)	9(75)	0.001*	16(57.1)	0.003*
Pain on palpation(%)	6 (30.0)	12(100)	0.0001*	24(85.7)	0.0001*
Pain on function(%)	4 (20.0)	6(50)	0.102	10(35.7)	0.252
Bite force (mean) in N					
Anterior	143.3	154.6	0.629	133.3	0.527
Right side	313.2	344.9	0.377	334.9	0.479
Left side	314.7	343.7	0.444	357	0.157

N Newton, TMD Temporomandibular Disorders
*statistically significant difference at p ≤ .05

most important TMD feature is pain, followed by restricted mouth opening capacity and joint sounds as observed by Manfredini [20]. When we compared our findings with this study, we observed a considerable difference, mainly the absence of functional alterations such as restricted mouth opening capacity. Furthermore, we also did not find a difference in BF between patients and controls. These results were unexpected since these patients should have presented the same findings as other patients with TMD symptoms.

BF is an indicator of normal masticatory function, but many factors may influence the values found for this parameter. Facial structure, general muscular force, gender, state of dentition, and signs and symptoms of TMD are some of them [21, 22]. Lower BF was found among adolescents with TMD [23]. Kobayashi et al. did not detect an association between TMD and BF [24]. Similarly, we did not find differences between the pain of patients and controls in relation to BF, even when we compared the two patients groups with the control group and when BF was compared between the two pain conditions.

We found a high prevalence of TMD complaints in our patients with idiopathic musculoskeletal pain, however these complaints did not correspond to the clinical signs. But interestingly, although they presented pain very frequently on palpation they did not present alterations in other clinical parameters such as pain on function, limited mouth opening capacity or lower maximal BF. These findings indicate the need of functional testing for an accurate differential diagnosis with TMD and the appropriate management of those signs and symptoms. One possible explanation for this could be that individuals with idiopathic musculoskeletal pain should be considered as having a somatoform disorder. Somatisation refers to individuals who report symptoms that have no organic cause, or who report symptoms that greatly exceed those expected by the physical condition [2].

The limitations of this study are the small number of patients and the heterogeneity of clinical features that these patients present.

Health professionals who take care of children and adolescents with IMPS should always consider the subjective symptoms related to the orofacial region and the need of an accurate differential diagnosis with TMD; this could provide valuable information for the appropriate conservative management with a multidisciplinary approach.

Conclusions

In conclusion, our findings indicate that TMD symptoms were more prevalent in patients with IMPS than in healthy controls. However, the bite force was not different among the groups.

Authors' contributions
LZ colected the patients data and was the major contributor in writing the manuscript. MF and CL reviewed the manuscript. MS and CH performed the statistical analysis and reviewed the manuscript. MTT analyzed and interpreted the patient data and wrote the manuscript. All authors read and approved the final manuscript.

Ethics approval and consent to participate
Written informed consent was obtained from all participants. This study was reviewed and approved by the local Medical Ethics Committee of Universidade Federal de São Paulo.

References
1. Goodman JE, McGrath PJ. The epidemiology of pain in children and adolescents: a review. Pain. 1991;46:247–64.
2. Malleson PN, Beauchamp RD. Diagnosing musculoskeletal pain in children. CMAJ. 2001;165:183–8.
3. Malleson PN, Al-Matar M, Petty RE. Idiopathic musculoskeletal pain syndromes in children. J Rheumatol. 1992;19:1786–9.
4. Sherry DD, Malleson PN. The idiopathic musculoskeletal pain syndromes in childhood. Rheum Dis Clin North Am. 2002;28:669–85.
5. Wolfe F, Smythe HA, Yunus MB, Bennett RM, Bombardier C, Goldenberg DL, et al. The American College of Rheumatology 1990 Criteria for the Classification of Fibromyalgia. Report of the Multicenter Criteria Committee. Arthritis Rheum. 1990;33:160–72.
6. Thilander B, Rubio G, Pena L, Mayorga C. Prevalence of temporomandibular dysfunction and its association with malocclusion in children and adolescents: an epidemiologic study related to specified stages of dental development. Angle Orthod. 2002;72:146–54.
7. Vierola A, Suominen AL, Ikavalko T, Lintu N, Lindi V, Lakka HM, et al. Clinical signs of temporomandibular disorders and various pain conditions among children 6 to 8 years of age: the PANIC study. J Orofac Pain. 2012;26:17–25.
8. Hedenberg-Magnusson B, Ernberg M, Kopp S. Symptoms and signs of temporomandibular disorders in patients with fibromyalgia and local myalgia of the temporomandibular system. A comparative study. Acta Odontol Scand. 1997;55:344–9.
9. Plesh O, Wolfe F, Lane N. The relationship between fibromyalgia and temporomandibular disorders: prevalence and symptom severity. J Rheumatol. 1996;23:1948–52.
10. Salvetti G, Manfredini D, Bazzichi L, Bosco M. Clinical features of the stomatognathic involvement in fibromyalgia syndrome: a comparison with temporomandibular disorders patients. Cranio. 2007;25:127–33.
11. Gui MS, Pimentel MJ, Rizzatti-Barbosa CM. Temporomandibular disorders in fibromyalgia syndrome: a short-communication. Rev Bras Reumatol. 2015;55:189–94.
12. Hatch JP, Shinkai RS, Sakai S, Rugh JD, Paunovich ED. Determinants of masticatory performance in dentate adults. Arch Oral Biol. 2001;46:641–8.
13. Gavião MB, Raymundo VG, Rentes AM. Masticatory performance and bite force in children with primary dentition. Braz Oral Res. 2007;21:146–52.
14. Pereira LJ, Pastore MG, Bonjardim LR, Castelo PM, Gavião MB. Molar bite force and its correlation with signs of temporomandibular dysfunction in mixed and permanent dentition. J Oral Rehabil. 2007;34:759–66.
15. Svensson P, Graven-Nielsen T. Craniofacial muscle pain: review of mechanisms and clinical manifestations. J Orofac Pain. 2001;15:117–45.
16. Sheppard IM, Sheppard SM. Maximal incisal opening—a diagnostic index? J Dent Med. 1965;20:13–5.
17. Agerberg G. Maximal mandibular movements in children. Acta Odontol Scand. 1974;32:147–59.
18. Pereira LJ, Pereira-Cenci T, Del Bel Cury AA, Pereira SM, Pereira AC, Ambosano GM, et al. Risk indicators of temporomandibular disorder incidences in early adolescence. Pediatr Dent. 2010;32:324–8.
19. Buskila D, Press J, Gedalia A, Klein M, Neumann L, Boehm R, et al. Assessment of nonarticular tenderness and prevalence of FS in children. J Rheumatol. 1993;20:368–70.
20. Manfredini D, Guarda-Nardini L, Winocur E, Piccotti F, Ahlberg J, Lobbezoo F. Research diagnostic criteria for temporo-mandibular disorders: a systematic review of axis I epidemiologic findings. Oral Surg Oral Med Oral Pathol Oral Radiol Endod. 2011;112:453–62.
21. Kiliaridis S, Kjellberg H, Wenneberg B, Engstrom C. The relationship between bite force endurance and facial morphology during growth. A cross-sectional study. Acta Odontol Scand. 1993;51:323–31.

22. Sonnesen L, Bakke M. Molar bite force in relation to occlusion, craniofacial dimensions, and head posture in pre-orthodontic children. Eur J Orthod. 2005;27:58–63.
23. Bonjardim LR, Gaviao MB, Pereira LJ, Castelo PM. Bite force determination in adolescents with and without temporomandibular dysfunction. J Oral Rehabil. 2005;32:577–83.
24. Kobayashi FY, Gavião MB, Montes AB, Marquezin MC, Castelo PM. Evaluation of oro-facial function in young subjects with temporomandibular disorders. J Oral Rehabil. 2014;41:496–506.

2

Cardiac and vascular complications of Behçet disease in the Tunisian context: Clinical characteristics and predictive factors

Melek Kechida[1*], Sana Salah[2], Rim Kahloun[3], Rim Klii[1], Sonia Hammami[1] and Ines Khochtali[1]

Abstract

Background: Cardiac and vascular involvement in Behçet disease (BD), also referred as vasculo BD, is frequent. We aimed to describe clinical characteristics, predictive factors and management of vasculo BD in the Tunisian context.

Methods: We retrospectively studied 213 records of all BD patients followed between January 2004 and May 2016 in the Internal Medicine Department and who fulfilled the ISGBD criteria. We described first clinical features of BD with cardiac and vascular involvement then predictive factors were studied in univariate then multivariate analysis.

Results: Among the 213 patients, 64 (30%) were diagnosed as having vasculo BD. The mean age at diagnosis was 31.5 years. About 81.25% of them were males and 18.75% females. Vascular involvement associated or not with cardiac involvement was found in 64 patients (30%). Deep venous thromboses are most common (62.5%) compared with superficial ones (23.4%), pulmonary arterial thrombosis (14.1%) or aneurysms (9.4%). Cardiac involvement is ranging from pericarditis (1.6%) to intra cardiac thrombosis (3.1%) and myocardial infarction (1.6%). Predictive factors associated with cardiac and vascular involvement in BD are male gender (OR = 3.043, 95% CI = 1.436–6.447, $p = 0.004$), erythema nodosum (OR = 4.134, 95% CI = 1.541–11.091, $p = 0.005$) and neurologic involvement (OR = 2.46, 95% CI = 1.02–5.89, $p = 0.043$).

Conclusion: Cardiac and vascular involvement in BD is frequent in the Tunisian context with a broad spectrum of manifestations ranging from vascular involvement to cardiac one. Male gender, patients with erythema nodosum or neurologic involvement are prone to develop cardiac or vascular features of BD needing therefore a close monitoring.

Keywords: Behcet syndrome, Cardiovascular system, Risk factors

Background

Behçet disease (BD) is a systemic vasculitis of unknown origin with a remitting and relapsing course. It is prevalent along the "silk road" extending from Japan to the Middle Eastern and the Mediterranean countries [1]. BD usually affects patients around the third or fourth decade of life [1]. Sex distribution is roughly equal with some particularities all over the world. In fact, BD would be more prevalent in males in some Middle Eastern and the Mediterranean countries and less frequent in females in Japan and Korea [1].

BD is mainly characterized by recurrent oral and genital aphthosis associated with other cutaneous and ocular manifestations. It may also involve, in a lesser extent, the gastro intestinal tract, joints and the central nervous system. These clinical signs seem to vary in prevalence according to the ethnic groups and geographical regions.

Cardiac and vascular involvement, also referred as vasculo BD, is frequent. It can reach 46% of patients according to the literature [2] affecting all sizes of arteries and veins as well as all the cardiac layers and accounting for the major cause of mortality.

As clinical signs are varying according to the ethnic groups and the geographical regions, and as data regarding prevalence and management of vasculo BD in the North African countries are lacking, we aimed in this

* Correspondence: kechida_mel_lek@hotmail.com
[1]Internal Medicine and Endocrinology Department, Fattouma Bourguiba University Hospital, 1st June Avenue, 5000 Monastir, Tunisia
Full list of author information is available at the end of the article

work to describe clinical characteristics, predictive factors and management of cardiac and vascular involvement in BD in the Tunisian context.

Methods

We retrospectively studied records of Behçet Disease patients followed in Internal Medicine Department of Fattouma Bourguiba University Hospital between January 2004 and May 2016. All patients fulfilled the International Study Group for Behçet Disease criteria [2].

Patients with cardiac involvement are defined as having pericarditis and/or myocarditis and/or intra cardiac thrombosis and/or myocardial infarction associated or not to vascular involvement. Patients with vascular involvement are those having deep venous thrombosis and/or superficial venous thrombosis and/or pulmonary embolism and/or arterial aneurysm without cardiac involvement.

Cardiac and vascular involvement diagnosis was based on clinical examination and imaging techniques including Computed Tomography Angiography, Magnetic Resonance Angiography and Doppler ultrasound. Screening for cardiac and vascular involvement was performed in symptomatic patients only.

We described first clinical features of BD with cardiac and vascular involvement then a comparative study was performed between patients with (group 1) and without cardiac and/or vascular involvement (group2). Predictive factors of cardiac and/or vascular involvement were studied in univariate then multivariate analysis.

The t test was used to analyze the continuous variables. The chi-square test was used to analyze the categorical variables. Multivariate analysis of variables significantly associated with cardiac and vascular involvement in univariate analysis was performed using binary logistic regression. Results are expressed as odds ratios (OR) with accompanying 95% confidence interval (95% CI). A p value < 0.05 was considered significant and if needed Fisher's exact test was used. Only relevant predictive factors highly associated with cardiac and vascular involvement were analyzed according to the goodness of fit of Hosmer-Lemeshow test. All data were assessed on computer using a SPSS 21.0 software package.

Results

Out of 213 BD patients studied, 145 (68.1%) were males and 68 (31.9%) were females. Sex ratio M/F was 2.13. Mean age at diagnosis was 30.6 years. Oral ulcers were found in 210 patients (98.6%) at presentation occurring then in all patients during follow-up. Cutaneous manifestations were present in 190 patients (89.2%). Pathergy test done in 174 patients was positive in 108 of cases (62.06%). Clinical characteristics of the patients are reported in Table 1. HLA 51 done in 113 patients (53.05%) was positive in 18 patients (15.92%).

Among the 213 patients, 64 (30%) were diagnosed as having vasculo BD. The mean age at diagnosis was 31.5 years. About 81.25% of them were males and 18.75% were females.

Vascular involvement was found in 59 patients (27.7%), isolated cardiac involvement in 2 patients (0.9%) and the association of cardiac and vascular involvement was found in 3 patients (1.4%).

Eight patients (12.5%) had cardiac or vascular involvement as a first manifestation of the disease. Deep venous thrombosis were reported in 40 patients (62.5%). Venous thrombosis occurred in more than one site in 3 cases (7.5%).

Superficial venous thrombosis affected 15 patients (23.4%). Arterial involvement was found in 16 patients (25.1%) with pulmonary embolism in 9 patients (14.1%), pulmonary aneurysm in 6 patients (9.4%) and aorta aneurysm in 1 case (1.6%). Cardiac involvement was found in 5 patients (7.9%).

Cardiac and vascular involvement is detailed in Table 2.

Management of cardiac or vascular involvement in BD consisted in colchicine in all patients, corticotherapy in 22 patients (46%) and immunosuppressors in 17 patients (26.6%) which were Cyclophasphamide or Azathioprine. Oral anticoagulation was associated in 44 patients (72.1%). Arterial Embolisation was performed in 2 patients (3.3%).

Table 1 clinical features of patients with Beçet Disease syndrome

Clinical features	Results
Sex	
- Male (n) (%)	145 (68.1)
- Female (n) (%)	68 (31.9)
Age at diagnosis (years)	30.6
Family history of BD (n) (%)	27 (13.8)
Oral ulcers (n) (%)	210 (98.6)
Genital ulceration (n) (%)	178 (83.6)
Pseudofolliculitis (n) (%)	169 (79.3)
Erythema nodosum (n) (%)	21 (9.99)
Positive pathergy reaction (n) (%)	108(62.06)
Joint involvement (n) (%)	94(44.3)
Ophthalmic involvement (n) (%)	67 (31.6)
Neurological manifestations (n) (%)	26 (12.3)
Cardiovascular complications (n) (%)	64 (30)
Gastrointestinal involvement (n) (%)	1(0.5)
Orchitis (n) (%)	12 (5.6)

Table 2 cardiovascular features in Behçet Disease patients

Cardiovascular features	Patients (n)(%)
Vascular involvement (n) (%)	73 (34.27)
Deep venous thrombosis (n) (%)	40 (62.5)
- Upper limb (n) (%)	8(12.5)
- Lower limb (n) (%)	16(25)
- Bilateral lower limb (n) (%)	3 (4.7)
- Inferior vena cava (n) (%)	8(12.5)
- More than one site (n) (%)	3(4.7)
- Budd Chiari syndrome (n) (%)	1(1.55)
- Mesenteric vein (n) (%)	1(1.55)
Superficial venous thrombosis (n) (%)	15 (23.4)
Pulmonary embolism (n) (%)	9 (14.1)
Pulmonary arterial aneurysm (n) (%)	6 (9.4)
Ascending aorta aneurysm (n) (%)	1 (1.6)
Cardiac involvement (n) (%)	5 (2.4)
- Pericarditis (n) (%)	1 (1.6)
-Myocarditis (n) (%)	1 (1.6)
- Intra cardiac thrombosis (n) (%)	2 (3.1)
- Myocardial infarction (n) (%)	1 (1.6)

Comparative study between patients with (group 1) and without cardiac or vascular involvement (group 2) revealed significant prevalence of males in group 1 (81.3% vs 62.4%) ($p = 0.007$), and increased frequency of patients with erythema nodosum (17.2% vs 6.7%) ($p = 0.019$) and with orchitis (10.9% vs 3.4%) ($p = 0.047$) (Exact Fisher test) (Table 3).

Multivariable analysis performed on this model showed that predictive factors for cardiac or vascular involvement were male gender (OR = 3.043, 95% CI = 1.436–6.447, $p = 0.004$), erythema nodosum (OR = 4.134, 95% CI = 1.541–11.091, $p = 0.005$) and neurologic involvement (OR = 2.46, 95% CI = 1.02–5.89, $p = 0.043$) (Table 4).

Discussion

Cardiac and vascular involvement in BD is rarely reported in African countries. To the best of our knowledge, this study is the first to focus on cardiac and vascular spectrum in BD patients in a Tunisian cohort.

Cardiac and vascular involvement is frequent in our cohort, diagnosed in 30% of our patients. It is estimated to range from 7 to 46%, [3] according to the published data, and to affect about 27% in the Tunisian multicenter study of 519 patients [4]. Predictive factors of cardiac and vascular involvement found in our cohort were male gender (OR = 3.043, 95% CI = 1.436–6.447, $p = 0.004$), erythema nodosum (OR = 4.134, 95% CI = 1.541–11.091, $p = 0.005$) and neurologic involvement (OR = 2.46, 95%

Table 3 Comparison of clinical features in Behçet Disease patients with and without vascular involvement

	Patients with cardiovascular involvement (group1) (n = 64)	Patients without cardiovascular involvement (group 2) (n = 149)	P value
Sex			
- Males (n) (%)	52(81.3)	93(62.4)	**0.007***
- Females (n) (%)	12(18.8)	56(37.6)	
Age (years)	31.5	30.21	0.43
Familiar history of BD (n) (%)	5 (8.9)	22(15.8)	0.2
Oral aphthosis (n) (%)	63(98.4)	147(98.7)	0.9
Genital ulcerations (n) (%)	53(82.8)	125(83.9)	0.84
Pseudofolliculitis (n) (%)	54(84.4)	115(77.2)	0.23
Erythema nodosum (n) (%)	11(17.2)	10(6.7)	**0.019***
Ophthalmic involvement (n) (%)	20(31.3)	47(31.5)	0.96
Neurological involvement (n) (%)	12(18.8)	14(9.4)	0.056
Orchitis (n) (%)	7(10.9)	5(3.4)	**0.047*** (exact Fisher test)

*$p < 0.05$

CI = 1.02–5.89, $p = 0.043$). All studies dealing with cardiac or vascular involvement in BD are unanimous on the fact that the frequency of these complications is higher in males [4–7]. Some authors found that eye involvement, genital ulcers and arthritis were less frequent in vasculo-BD patients [8], which was not the case in our study.

Cardiac or vascular complications revealed the disease in 12.5% of cases in our patients. In the study of Fei et al. [6], 27.5% of patients presented with vascular involvement as the initial manifestation.

There is a broad spectrum of cardiac and vascular involvement in BD patients and we found that vascular manifestations are more frequent than cardiac ones.

Table 4 Predictive factors independently associated with cardiovascular involvement in patients with BD in multivariate analysis

Variable	Odds ratio	95% CI	p value
Male gender	3.043	1.436–6.447	0.004*
Erythema nodosum	4.134	1.541–11.091	0.005*
Neurological involvement	2.462	1.028–5.893	0.043*

CI confidence interval; *$p < 0.05$

Cardiac involvement is accounting for 1 to 6% [5] and occurred in 2.4% of patients in our study. The main types of cardiac features are pericarditis, valvular insufficiency, intra cardiac thrombosis and myocardial infarction. Pericardial involvement has been reported as the most common manifestation in some series [3, 9]. Clinical presentation may be acute pericarditis, recurrent pericarditis, constrictive pericarditis, hemorrhagic pericarditis tamponade or even asymptomatic pericardial effusion [3, 5]. But unlike literature findings, pericarditis was not the first most frequent cardiac feature in our cohort (1.6%), it was intra cardiac thrombosis (3.1% of cases). This probably could be explained by the asymptomatic character of pericarditis which can be missed as echocardiography was not systematically done for all the patients. Intra cardiac thrombosis is generally considered one of the serious cardiac complications which may cause pulmonary embolism [3] like in one of our patients or cerebral emboli by passing through the patent foramen ovale. The right ventricle is usually involved, which was the case of all our patients [3]. But it has been demonstrated that the left ventricle can also be involved [10, 11].

Myocardial infarction diagnosed in one of our patients was caused by coronary aneurysm. Coronary lesions are usually proximal [5] and some of them may be asymptomatic [3]. Sinus Valsalva aneurysms may occur alone or with other sinus aneurysms and may lead to acute or chronic aortic failure [3].

We reported a rare case of myocarditis revealing BD which was diagnosed in a patient with fever and chest pain confirmed with MRI findings. Few data is found in this field, Geri et al. [5] reported only one case in a series of 52 European patients and two cases were reported in a Japanese autopsy series [12].

Vascular system involvement emerged in approximately 1.8 to 51.6% of BD patients affecting all sizes of arteries and veins and accounting for the major cause of mortality [6]. It was estimated at 34.27% in our study.

Vascular lesions mainly consist in venous and arterial thrombosis and various types of arterial aneurysms. Venous lesions were more common in our cohort reaching 85.9% in agreement of literature findings which demonstrated that venous lesions were more frequently affected than arterial lesions [6]. Venous involvement can affect lower extremities as well as upper limb. Others including inferior vena cava, Budd-Chiari syndrome (hepatic vein thrombosis) and mesenteric vein thrombosis are rarely seen [13].

Arterial involvement is less common than venous one [3]. It consists in thrombosis or aneurysms. Pulmonary embolism, although found in 14.1% in our study, is thought to be rare in the literature given that the thrombi in the inflamed veins of the lower extremities are strongly adherent. [6, 14]. Aneurysms are considered to be the most severe complications given the high risk of rupture [6]. They mainly affect pulmonary arteries (9.4% in our cohort) but can be located in systemic circulation. We described the first case of ascending aortic aneurysm associated with deep vein thrombosis revealing BD. Few articles reported cases of Hughes Stovin Syndrome revealing BD. It's a rare entity defined as thrombophlebitis associated with pulmonary aneurysms [15]. Few cases were reported with associated aneurysm of the systemic circulation such bronchial, external carotid, iliac artery aneurysm and left hepatic artery [16] but no association with ascending aorta aneurysm was reported.

Treatment of BD is still based on a low level of evidence [3, 17]. All of our patients were treated with colchicine associated to steroids and immunosuppressors in 46 and 26.6% of cases, respectively. Corticosteroids and immunosuppressive agents like Cyclophasphamide are usually used for the management of cardiac lesions or if there is evidence of severe vascular manifestations. Thrombotic complications too may require immunosuppressors given that vascular inflammation plays a major role in thrombus formation. However treatment of arterial aneurysms remains challenging. Anticoagulant treatment should be administered cautiously with a close control in association to steroids and immunosuppressors given the risk of bleeding.

Surgical treatment may be problematic leading to pseudo aneurysms. Therefore surgical treatment should not be applied in the active phase of the disease [6].

The major limitation of our work is that it is a retrospective study especially faced to the incompleteness in data collection. It would be interesting to prospectively monitor how BD patients with predictive risk factors will evolve and how many will develop cardiac or vascular features.

Conclusion

Cardiac and vascular involvement in BD is frequent in the Tunisian context having sometimes threatening complications. It can occur during follow up or reveal the disease as the initial manifestation. Vascular manifestations are the most frequent affecting both veins and arteries. Deep venous thromboses are most common. Cardiac involvement can affect all layers ranging from pericarditis to intra cardiac thrombosis and myocardial infarction. We found that male gender is more prone to developing such complications in addition to patients presenting with erythema nodosum or neurologic involvement, needing therefore close monitoring.

Management of cardiac and vascular involvement in Behçet disease is still lacking standardization as treatment is still based on a low level of evidence. Cardiologists should always be aware of such disease as they could be the first physicians to deal with the cardiac and vascular complications.

Authors' contributions

MK: wrote the manuscript and done the bibliography research. SS: corrected the statistics. R. Kahloun: corrected the language and the final form of the manuscript. R. Klii, SH, and IK: participates with data. All authors read and approved the final manuscript.

Author details

[1]Internal Medicine and Endocrinology Department, Fattouma Bourguiba University Hospital, 1st June Avenue, 5000 Monastir, Tunisia. [2]Physical Medicine and Rehabilitaion Department, Fattouma Bourguiba University Hospital, Monastir, Tunisia. [3]Ophtalmology Department, Fattouma Bourguiba University Hospital, Monastir, Tunisia.

References

1. Alpsoy E. Behcet's disease: a comprehensive review with a focus on epidemiology, etiology and clinical features, and management of mucocutaneous lesions. J Dermatol. 2016;43:620–32.
2. International Study Group for Behçet's disease. Criteria for diagnosis of Behçet's disease. Lancet. 1990;335:1078–80.
3. Demirelli S, Degirmenci H, Inci S, Arisoy A. Cardiac manifestations in Behcet's disease. Intractable Rare Dis Res. 2015;4(2):70–75.
4. B'chir Hamzaoui S, Harmel A, Bouslama K, Abdallah M, Ennafaa M, M'rad S, le groupe tunisien d'étude Sur la maladie de Behçet, et al. Behçet's disease in Tunisia. Clinical study of 519 cases. La Revue de médecine interne. 2006;27:742–50.
5. Geri G, Wechsler B, Thi Huong du L, Isnard R, Piette JC, Amoura Z, et al. Spectrum of cardiac lesions in Behçet disease. A series of 52 patients and review of the literature. Medicine. 2012;91:25–34.
6. Fei Y, Li X, Lin S, Song X, Wu Q, Zhu Y, et al. Major vascular involvement in Behçet's disease: a retrospective study of 796 patients. Clin Rheumatol. 2013;32:845–52.
7. Bang D, Lee JH, Lee ES, Lee S, Choi JS, Kim YK, et al. Epidemiologic and clinical survey of Behcet's disease in Korea: the first multicenter study. J Korean Med Sci. 2001;16(5):615–8.
8. Sakane T, Takeno M, Suzuki N, Inaba G. Behçet's disease. Engl J Med. 1999;341(17):1284–91.
9. Bono W, Filali-Ansary N, Mohattane A, Tazi-Mezalek Z, Adnaoui M, Aouni M, et al. Cardiac and pulmonary artery manifestations during Behçet's disease. Rev Med Interne. 2000;21:905–7.
10. Fekih M, Fennira S, Ghodbane L, Zaouali RM. Intracardiac thrombosis: unusual complication of Behcet's disease. Tunis Med. 2004;82:785–90.
11. Darie C, Knezinsky M, Demolombe-Rague S, Pinède L, Périnetti M, Ninet JF, et al. Cardiac pseudotumor revealing Behcet's disease. Rev Med Interne. 2005;26:420–4.
12. Lakhanpal S, Tani K, Lie JT, Katoh K, Ishigatsubo Y, Ohokubo T. Pathologic features of Behçet's syndrome: a review of Japanese autopsy registry data. Hum Pathol. 1985;16:790–5.
13. Ma WG, Zheng J, Zhu JM, Liu YM, Li M, Sun LZ. Aortic regurgitation caused by Behçet's disease: surgical experience during an 11-year period. J Card Surg. 2012;27:39–44.
14. Tohmé A, Aoun N, El-Rassi B, Ghayad E. Vascular manifestations of Behçet's disease. Eighteen cases among 140 patients. Joint Bone Spine. 2003;70:384–9.
15. Jambeih R, Salem G, Huard DR, Jones KR, Awab A. Hughes Stovin syndrome presenting with hematuria. Am J Med Sci. 2015;(5):425–6.
16. Balci NC, Semelka RC, Noone TC, Worawattanakul S. Multiple pulmonary aneurysms secondary to Hughes-Stovin syndrome: demonstration by MR angiography. J Magn Reson Imaging. 1998;(6):1323–5.
17. Hatemi G, Silman A, Bang D, Bodaghi B, Chamberlain AM, Gul A, et al. EULAR recommendations for the management of Behcet disease. Ann Rheum Dis. 2008;67:1656–62.

3

Guidelines of the Brazilian Society of Rheumatology for the treatment of systemic autoimmune myopathies

Fernando Henrique Carlos de Souza[1], Daniel Brito de Araújo[2], Verônica Silva Vilela[3], Mailze Campos Bezerra[4], Ricardo Santos Simões[1], Wanderley Marques Bernardo[1], Renata Miossi[1], Bernardo Matos da Cunha[5] and Samuel Katsuyuki Shinjo[6*]

Abstract

Background: Recommendations of the Myopathy Committee of the Brazilian Society of Rheumatology for the management and therapy of systemic autoimmune myopathies (SAM).

Main body: The review of the literature was done in the search for the Medline (PubMed), Embase and Cochrane databases including studies published until June 2018. The Prisma was used for the systematic review and the articles were evaluated according to the levels of Oxford evidence. Ten recommendations were developed addressing the management and therapy of systemic autoimmune myopathies.

Conclusions: Robust data to guide the therapeutic process are scarce. Although not proven effective in controlled clinical trials, glucocorticoid represents first-line drugs in the treatment of SAM. Intravenous immunoglobulin is considered in induction for refractory cases of SAM or when immunosuppressive drugs are contra-indicated. Consideration should be given to the early introduction of immunosuppressive drugs. There is no specific period determined for the suspension of glucocorticoid and immunosuppressive drugs when individually evaluating patients with SAM. A key component for treatment in an early rehabilitation program is the inclusion of strength-building and aerobic exercises, in addition to a rigorous evaluation of these activities for remission of disease and the education of the patient and his/her caregivers.

Keywords: Dermatomyositis, Guidelines, Polymyositis, Systemic autoimmune myopathies, Treatment

Background

Systemic autoimmune myopathies (SAM) are a heterogeneous group of autoimmune diseases associated with high morbidity and functional disability [1]. Considering its epidemiological, clinical, laboratory and histopathological features, SAM can be classified as dermatomyositis, juvenile dermatomyositis, clinically amyopathic dermatomyositis, polymyositis, inclusion body myositis, immune-mediated necrotizing myopathies and cancer-associated myopathies [1, 2].

Treatments of SAM include not only inflammatory process suppression, but also prevention against musculoskeletal tissue and extra-muscular organ damages. However, robust data are scarce and the therapeutic process is based mainly on observational studies, retrospective analysis and/or small samples of patients [3, 4].

Therefore, the purpose of these recommendations is to guide the treatment of adult patients with SAM, highlighting dermatomyositis and polymyositis, according to current evidence in the literature, facilitating access to available therapies and minimize irreversible disease damages.

Methods

A systematic literature review was performed with the following databases: Medline (Pubmed), Embase and Cochrane. The research strategy was performed

* Correspondence: samuel.shinjo@gmail.com
[6]Disciplina de Reumatologia, Faculdade de Medicina, Universidade de Sao Paulo, Av. Dr. Arnaldo, 455, 3° andar, sala 3150 - Cerqueira César, Sao Paulo CEP: 01246-903, Brazil
Full list of author information is available at the end of the article

according to each "PICO" question (Patient, Intervention, Control and Outcome) elaborated by rheumatologists with experience in the treatment of SAM.

The following English terms were used in the systematic review of the literature: (Muscular Disease OR Myopathies OR Muscle Disorders OR Muscle Disorders OR Myopathic Conditions OR Myopathic Conditions) AND (Autoimmune OR Autoimmune Disease OR Autoimmune Diseases OR Systemic OR Polymyositis OR Idiopathic Polymyositis OR Idiopathic OR Dermatomyositis OR Dermatopolymyositis OR Dermatopolymyositis OR Myositis OR Inflammatory Muscle Diseases OR Inflammatory Myopathy OR Inflammatory Myopathies OR Inclusion Body Myositis OR Inclusion Body Myopathy, Cyclosporine OR Cyclophosphamide OR Methotrexate OR Azathioprine OR Infliximab OR Tumor Necrosis Factor - alpha AND (Therapy / Broad [filter]).

With the application of the random filter, the terms related to each modality of induction treatment for patients with SAM were added.

Inclusion criteria for studies in this systematic review were: randomized and controlled trials (RCTs) addressing SAM treatment, extension studies made from RCTs with the criteria mentioned and systematic reviews with RCT meta-analyzes. In some cases, historical cohort studies and review articles were included and, in the absence of RCTs for specific modalities of therapy, open studies or low quality cohort studies were included.

The steps in this systematic review of the literature followed the Prisma guidelines [5]. The selected studies were evaluated and the degree of recommendation for each question was based on the level of evidence from the studies (Tables 1 and 2) [6–8]. Ten recommendations were developed to address different aspects of SAM therapy (Table 3).

Table 1 Categories of evidence in studies

Níveis	Evidências
1a	Systematic review and RCT meta-analysis
1b	At least one RCT with narrow confidence interval
2a	Systematic review and meta-analysis of cohort studies
2b	At least one cohort study or low quality RCT
3a	Systematic review and meta-analysis of case-control studies
3b	At least one case control study
4	At least one case series or cohort study and low quality case-control studies
5	Expert opinion without critical evaluation explicit or based on physiology, bench research or "fundamental principles"

RCT randomized clinical trial

Table 2 Degrees of recommendation for each evidence

Degree	Definition
A	Consistent level 1 studies
B	Consistent level 2 or 3 studies or extrapolations from level 1 studies
C	Level 4 studies or extrapolations of level 2 or 3 studies
D	Level 5 evidence or studies of any level with inconsistency or inconclusiveness

Recommendations

What are the general and educational recommendations for SAM?

Literature review and analysis. In general, the education of individuals with SAM, as well as their families and/or caregivers, is of great importance, since they are looking for environmental adaptations and implementation of rehabilitation programs aiming to maintain/improve the patient's quality of life.

Immunodeficient patients due to the use of medications should be advised about hygiene, maintenance of good nutritional status, avoidance of vaccines with live infectious agents and contact with infectious contagious diseases (B) [9].

When pulmonary dysfunction results from weakness of the diaphragmatic muscles and thoracic muscular wall, respiratory rehabilitation (kinesiotherapy) may be indicated to reduce dyspnea and increase exercise capacity (B) [10].

In case where muscle weakness at the level of the upper third of the esophagus leads to dysphagia, regurgitation or aspiration, dietary changes and swallowing training may be employed. In selected cases, cricopharyngeal myotomy and botulinum toxin application may be necessary (B) [9] (C) [11, 12]. In more severe patients a nasogastric tube or gastrostomy feeding may be recommended to reduce the risk of aspiration and pneumonia (C) [13] (D) [9].

What are some precautions before immunosuppression in patients with SAM?

Literature review and analysis. Glucocorticoids (GC) affect the adaptive and innate immunity processes and increase the risk of acute infections and reactivation of chronic infections caused by fungi, bacteria, viruses and parasites, which can lead to serious disseminated diseases (B) [14]. In addition to specific prophylactic and vaccine recommendations, the use of antibiotics at the first signs of bacterial infection is required (B) [14].

Pneumonia by *Pneumocystis jiroveci* is a complication in immunocompromised patients and is seen in individuals submitted to high doses GC or other immunosuppressive treatments (B) [15, 16] (C) [17, 18]. Despite the controversies and lack of available evidence, prophylaxis

Table 3 Recommendations for the treatment of systemic autoimmune myopathies

"PICO" questions	Recommendations
1. What are the general and educational recommendations for SAM?	The education of individuals with SAM, as well as their families and/or caregivers, is of great importance, since they are looking for environmental adaptations and implementation of rehabilitation programs aiming to maintain/improve the patient's quality of life. Physical therapy and occupational therapy play a prominent role in the rehabilitation and therapeutic process of patients with SAM (degree of recommendation B)
2. What are some precautions before immunosuppression in patients with SAM?	Immunosuppressive drugs are associated with an increased risk for infections. Therefore, obtaining a thorough medical history with extensive investigation of family history and by directing personnel to obtain information related to the patient's immunization schedule and infections or other diseases that occur with immunosuppression is of key importance. In general, the risk of these infections is related to the total dose and duration of immunosuppressive drug. The patient's vaccination status should be evaluated and documented at the first moment after diagnosis of the condition that guides the immunosuppressive drug and the recommended vaccines should be administered as soon as possible. If possible, the delayed vaccine should be given prior to the start of the immunosuppressive drug. Vaccines composed of live attenuated viruses should be administered at least four weeks before the start of the immunosuppressive drug (degree of recommendation B, C, D)
3. What treatment is recommended in the initial phase of SAM?	The administration of GC via oral route is the first-line treatment in cases of SAM (degree of recommendation C). Immunosuppressive drugs with methotrexate, azathioprine and cyclosporine may be associated with a reduction in GC doses (degree of recommendation B)
4. Which drug treatments are recommended for refractory SAM cases?	Evidence suggests that the treatment of refractory cases of SAM with intravenous immunoglobulin, tacrolimus, cyclosporine, cyclophosphamide, azathioprine, methotrexate, abatacept, tocilizumab and rituximab, as monotherapy or in combination, appear to improve muscle strength, CK levels and lung function. However, more controlled studies with greater numbers of patients for evaluation (degree of recommendation B) of efficacy and tolerability are needed. Anti-TNFα agents are not recommended (degree of recommendation C)
5. What initial dose of glucocorticoids should be used and for how long in patients with SAM?	Despite the lack of controlled studies, evidence indicates that first-line treatment should be the administration of GC, starting doses of prednisone or its equivalent potency range from 0.5 to 1.0 mg/kg/day given on a fractional basis, daily or on alternate days. In severe cases, MP pulse therapy should be considered (1 g/day for three consecutive days followed by a regimen with oral GC). Duration and need for association with other immunosuppressive agents are determined by the response of the disease to therapy (degree of recommendation B)
6. How long should SAM patients receive immunosuppressive / immunomodulatory drugs after discontinuation of GC?	There is no established timeframe that determines how long treatment with immunosuppressive/immunomodulatory drugs should be maintained after GC are discontinued. Follow-up evaluations of these individuals should be scheduled according to clinical evolution and changes observed during treatment monitoring (degree of recommendation B)
7. What is the evidence on the benefit of immunosuppressive / immunomodulatory drugs association (association versus exchange) in SAM?	Evidence points to the benefit of the association of immunosuppressive/immunomodulatory drugs in patients with SAM, especially in cases of adverse events with the use of GC in monotherapy, the "sparing" effect of GC, or precautions against the failure to obtain a complete clinical response. Agents such as intravenous immunoglobulin, mycophenolate mofetil, cyclosporine, azathioprine and methotrexate, used alone or in combination appear to contribute to improvement in muscle strength, CK levels and lung function, with no significant difference in efficacy between the treatment schemes (azathioprine with methotrexate, cyclosporine with methotrexate and intramuscular methotrexate with oral methotrexate and azathioprine) (degree of recommendation A)
8. What is the role of rehabilitation, physical exercise and physiotherapy in the treatment of SAM?	The implementation of a physical exercise program (resistance or aerobic physical training or the combination of these two) seems to be safe and beneficial in adult patients with SAM and should be used as a complement to pharmacological treatments in all stages of the disease to maximize muscle performance and aerobic capacity, as well as minimize the risk of side effects caused by GC treatment, for example. Individuals with active disease indication of physical exercises should preferably be instituted as early as possible and be supervised by a physiotherapist in close collaboration with an attending physician to strengthen the muscle groups involved with passive and active exercises (degree of recommendation B)

Table 3 Recommendations for the treatment of systemic autoimmune myopathies *(Continued)*

"PICO" questions	Recommendations
9. How to monitor disease activity (biomarkers) in patients with SAM?	Evidence has pointed to the possibility of using objective measures, in the form of identification and dosage of molecules that present the potential to discriminate the activity of the disease and predict its damage. (degree of recommendation B)
10 How to define activity versus remission of SAM in clinical practice?	Despite limitations in the study of myopathies, assessment of disease activity or remission is based mainly on clinical presentation and complementary examinations. International groups such as the IMACS have defined instruments that have not yet been fully validated and are largely based on a subjective assessment conducted by both patient and physician on the disease status. It is important to recognize that there is no single gold standard measure to assess disease activity. (degree of recommendation D)

CK creatine phosphokinase, *GC* glucocorticoid, *IMACS* International Myositis Assessment and Clinical Studies Group, *SAM* systemic autoimmune myopathies, *SAM* systemic autoimmune myopathies, *TNF* tumor necrosis factor

for pneumocystosis should be considered, particularly in the presence of risk factors (e.g., interstitial lung diseases - ILD, other immunosuppressive drugs, patients with anti-MDA-5), for patients who use ≥20 mg/day of prednisone or its equivalent for a period of more than four weeks (B) [19, 20] (D) [21] (C) [22–24].

Due to the risk of reactivation of latent tuberculosis, patients undergoing immunosuppressive therapy who present a positive tuberculin test (≥ 5 mm), even with a chest X-ray without evidence of a cicatricial lesion are candidates for prophylaxis (C) [25]. Doses equal to or higher than 15 mg/day of prednisone for a period of more than one month or another immunosuppressive therapy are considered as a risk for the progression of tuberculosis from its latent form to the active form (B) [26–28]. Screening for exposure to tuberculosis, as well as obtaining the patient's medical history, can identify risk factors such as contact with an infected person, residence in an endemic area or abuse of illicit substances. In these individuals, prophylaxis with isoniazid should be considered at a dose of 5 to 10 mg/kg per body weight (maximum dose of 300 mg/day) for 9 months [29].

In immunosuppressed patients, an infestation caused by *Strongyloides stercoralis* is associated with a high mortality rate even years after exposure (B) [30]. Screenings should be considered in patients with risk factors (e.g., travels to or inhabitants of endemic or high incidence areas of the disease) and who are initiating therapy with immunosuppressive drugs such as GC. Although there is no evidence guiding the prophylaxis of strongylodiasis, ivermectin with immunosuppressive drugs and pulse therapy with methylprednisolone prior to the start of treatment is considered in endemic areas (A) [31] (D) [32].

Immunosuppressive drugs may lead to a lack of vaccinal immune response or the development of active infections when exposed to vaccines consisting of live attenuated viruses. At the moment, there is no solid evidence on the recommendation of the vaccine process of immunocompromised individuals, but for those

requiring high doses of GC (≥ 20 mg/day of prednisone or its equivalent for more than two weeks), vaccination is recommended for *Haemophilus influenzae* type B and the hepatitis A and B, human papillomavirus, influenza, *Neisseria meningitidis*, measles, mumps and rubella, *Streptococcus pneumoniae* and tetanus (B) [33, 34]. Individuals who have not received the updated vaccines should receive the vaccine prior to taking immunosuppressive drugs, especially those composed of live viruses due to its contraindication during immunosuppression (D) [35, 36].

Due to the lack of data, specific recommendations guiding the start of treatment with immunosuppressive drugs after immunization with live-attenuated virus vaccines vary. A minimum waiting period of two to four weeks, an estimated time to allow the establishment of an immune response and elimination of live viruses, is advocated (A) [37].

Vigorous hydration to increase urine output and intravenous 2-mercaptethane sulfonate (MESNA) were recommended for prophylaxis of cyclophosphamide-induced hemorrhagic cystitis (C) [38].

Patients should be assessed for fracture risk and bone preserving agents and be prescribed calcium and vitamin D supplementation (B) [39]. Bisphosphonates remain the first choice of treatment in GC-treated patients with high fracture risk (A) [40].

What drug treatment is indicated in the initial treatment of SAM?

Literature review and analysis. Although they have not been tested in controlled clinical trials, GC represent first-line drugs in the treatment of SAM with recommended initial doses of 0.5 to 1.0 mg/kg/day of prednisone for at least 4 weeks (C) [41–43]. (Fig. 1). However, depending on the severity of the disease, lower doses, which are associated with fewer adverse events, can be used. In severe cases, such as patients with marked muscle weakness, ulcerated skin lesions, ILD and severe dysphagia, the use of intravenous methylprednisolone

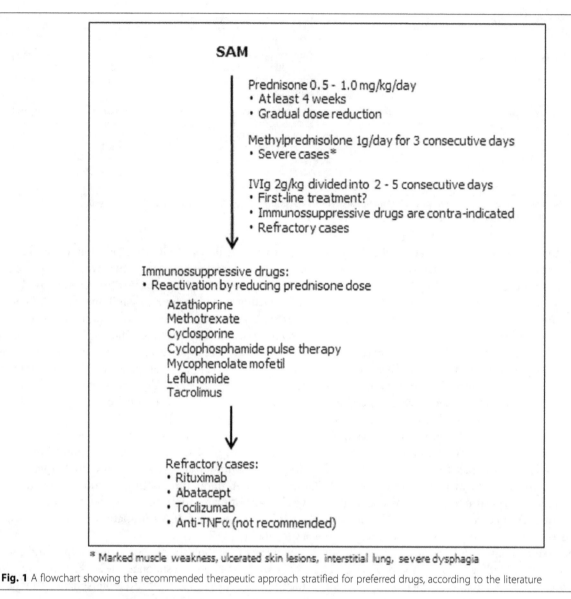

* Marked muscle weakness, ulcerated skin lesions, interstitial lung, severe dysphagia

Fig. 1 A flowchart showing the recommended therapeutic approach stratified for preferred drugs, according to the literature

(MP) pulse therapy (1 g/day for three consecutive days) followed by a high dose of GC via oral route should be considered (C) [44] (B) [41].

There have no sufficient studies showing the appropriate timing for initiating GC. However, it is possible that an early drug intervention allows a rapid remission of the disease, a lower frequency of relapses and/or a good prognosis of MAS (C) [45, 46]. Moreover, the GC treatment should not be postponed in order to perform an appropriate investigation (e.g., muscle biopsy) (C) [47, 48]. Of note, GC use does not influence the presence or the degree of inflammatory cell infiltration found in muscle biopsies in dermatomyositis / polymyositis with clinical and laboratory disease activity (C) [47, 48].

GC typically results in the normalization of serum levels of muscle enzymes and clinical improvement in muscle strength. However, more than half of patients (B) [49] do not present a complete response to the use of

these drugs, and several factors may contribute to response to treatment including disease subtype, onset of therapy, antibody profile or the presence of cancer [41].

Patients with a long period between the muscle symptoms onset and the institution of drug treatment are less likely to present a complete response to GC (B) [49].

Among those who do not present clinical improvement with GC, the reassessment of the diagnosis, the development of myopathy induced by the use of GC or the appearance of malignancy should be verified (D) [50]. For those who present reactivation of the disease by reducing GC doses, methotrexate, azathioprine and/or cyclosporine are the most frequently used in clinical practice, despite the absence of controlled trials evaluating their efficacy (B) [44, 51–55].

The use of intravenous immunoglobulin (dose of 2 g/kg divided into 2 to 5 days) is considered for refractory cases of SAM or when immunosuppressive drugs are contra-indicated, such as during of an infectious process (B) [54]. Evidence, however, on the efficacy of intravenous immunoglobulin as first-line treatment of SAM is controversial (B) [56, 57] (A) [58].

What are the recommended drug treatments for refractory SAM cases?

Literature review and analysis. Patients with SAM who failed conventional therapy were treated with oral tacrolimus (0.075 mg/kg/day) and showed an improvement in muscle strength, a reduction in levels of CK and a mean dose of GC (C) [59].

Case reports have demonstrated favorable results for cyclosporine use (mean dose of 3.5 mg/kg/day) in refractory SAM patients which an improvement in serum levels of CK and muscle strength (C) [60–63].

Intravenous cyclophosphamide pulses in patients with refractory SAM result in improved muscle strength (C) [64, 65]. In addition, it is possible that its association with methotrexate normalizes the serum levels of CK (C) [65].

Mycophenolate mofetil (1.0 g to 1.5 g twice a day) may be an effective GC-sparing therapy for the treatment of some patients with SAM [66]. This response was based on an improvement in skin disease as judged clinically, an increase in strength and/or an ability to decrease or discontinue concomitant therapies (C) [66].

Leflunomide appears to be effective and safe as an adjuvant drug in refractory dermatomyositis with primarily cutaneous activities (C) [67].

Intravenous immunoglobulin, alone or in combination with immunosuppressive drugs, has a good therapeutic response, mainly in refractory cases (C) [68] (B) [69, 70].

Clinical trials analyzed patients with refractory SAM treated with anti TNFs [71–73]. Among the patients who completed the study, there was no improvement in muscle strength [72]. In fact, some patients presented an exacerbation of their disease, elevation of muscle enzyme levels, unchanged rashes [69] and no significant treatment effect on functional outcome [74]. Thus, the use of anti-TNFs are not recommended.

A phase IIb clinical trial evaluating the efficacy of abatacept in patients with refractory SAM demonstrated few serious adverse effects in approximately half of the patients' responses based on the criteria established by the International Myositis Assessment and Clinical Studies Group (IMACS) (B) [75].

Tocilizumab demonstrated efficacy in reports of patients with refractory polymyositis, with a normalization of CK levels, resolution of muscle inflammation in magnetic resonance imaging and reduction of GC doses (C) [76].

Although numerous reports and case series have demonstrated the beneficial effects of rituximab, experience in refractory SAM is still limited (C) [77–81] (B) [82–84].

A multicenter clinical trial known as the "Rituximab In Myositis" trial did not reach its primary endpoint (response in the 8th week in the group treated early in relation to the late intervention group), but in the 44th week of follow-up, the majority of patients (83%) reached the definition of response to treatment based on the criteria established by the IMACS [85]. In this study, serious adverse events attributed to rituximab were observed, most of which were represented by infections (B) [82]. Reanalysis of the data obtained in this study was conducted, and individuals who were positive for the anti-synthase and anti-Mi-2 autoantibodies presented better clinical responses (B) [86].

A multicenter phase II study evaluated the efficacy of rituximab in individuals with SAM with anti-synthetase autoantibodies refractory to conventional treatment (GC and at least two immunosuppressive drugs) demonstrated that the majority of these patients had an increase in the Manual Muscle Testing (MMT)-8 followed by a reduction of CK levels and a reduction in the dose of GC (B) [87].

What initial dose of GC should be used and for how long in patients with SAM?

Literature review and analysis. With different regimens of use and routes of administration, the generally recommended starting doses of prednisone, or its equivalent, range from 0.5 to 1.0 mg/kg/day given in divided doses, daily or every other day (C) [88] (B) [89–91]. Although there are no controlled clinical trials evaluating the optimal rate of GC reduction, dose reduction should be based on the activity of the disease and the presence of extra-muscular involvement (B) [89–91].

Studies have indicated the maintenance of the initial dose over a period of 4 to 8 weeks with monitoring of serum CK levels and muscle strength in addition to other disease manifestations [41, 92, 93]. After this period of time, as long as the disease has been controlled, GC dose can be reduced by 20 to 25% every four weeks until the daily dose of 5 to 10 mg is reached, at which point a stable dose of GC is maintained for another year, depending on the clinical course (C) [41, 92, 93].

In severe cases, MP pulse therapy should be considered (1 g/day for three consecutive days followed by a regimen with oral GC) (C) [41, 42, 92, 93] (B) [41–44, 49, 93, 94].

Although it is considered a first-line drug, studies have shown that more than half of the patients fail to obtain a complete clinical response to CG in monotherapy and adding other immunosuppressive drugs in often necessary (B) [95, 96].

How long should SAM patients receive immunosuppressive / immunomodulatory drugs after GC discontinuation?

Literature review and analysis. There is no conclusive evidence to establish how long patients with SAM should receive treatment with immunosuppressive and/ or immunomodulatory drugs following the discontinuation of GC therapy [97, 98]. Overall, studies show that after disease remission, drug doses can be reduced gradually. Initially, GC dose reduction is suggested and, subsequently, in the maintenance of clinical and laboratory parameters, a reduction in the doses of immunosuppressive/immunomodulatory drugs can be attempted. There is no predetermined treatment duration (B) [97, 98].

What is the evidence on the benefit of association vs. exchange immunosuppressive/immunomodulatory drugs in SAM?

Literature review and analysis. Few comparative studies between immunosuppressive/immunomodulatory drugs support the prescription superiority of one medication over another, between monotherapies or combination treatments [3, 52–54, 66, 68–70, 99–105].

In a long-term follow-up, individuals who received MTX and combination of methotrexate and azathioprine showed an improvement in functional status beyond the need for lower doses of maintenance GC (B) [52, 53].

A randomized clinical trial did not verify the difference in muscle function tests in patients who had failed to obtain a clinical response with GC alone and who were randomized to treatment with cyclosporine, methotrexate or cyclosporine/methotrexate combination therapy (B) [100].

Despite weak evidence, studies including a small number of patients have shown improvement in the evolution of extra-muscular disease, muscle strength and inflammatory markers in individuals who did not respond to conventional therapy and who used mycophenolate mofetil in monotherapy or in association (C) [70, 101]. Evidence points mainly to associated therapy for improvements in lung function tests in patients with SAM and ILD (C) [104, 105].

What is the role of rehabilitation, physical exercise and physiotherapy in the treatment of SAM?

Literature review and analysis. Physical rehabilitation through physical exercises and physical therapy for muscle strengthening are beneficial and safe for patients with SAM when indicated two to three weeks after exacerbation of the disease, however this has not always been the guidance since, historically, these patients were discouraged from exercising because of the possibility of disease relapse or damage (B, D) [106–110].

There was evidence of improvement in aerobic capacity and isometric muscle strength without signs of increased inflammation among individuals randomized to exercise assessed by serum levels of CK (B) [111] (C) [112, 113]. Numerous studies have demonstrated the safety and positive results of supervised physical exercise in muscular function indicated for patients with SAM (B) [110] (A) [111]. Moreover, physical exercise can prevent the process of muscle atrophy caused by inflammation, physical inactivity and treatment with GC (D) [114].

In addition to improving muscle strength and increasing maximal oxygen uptake through resistance training, patient experienced the reduced expression of pro-inflammatory and pro-fibrotic genes, with significant positive impact on molecular profile and improvement in functional capacity (B) [115–119].

Evidence indicates that physical exercise has the potential to reduce disease activity in established cases of SAM and aerobic exercises may be more effective in reducing disease activity than strength and resistance exercises (B) [119–121].

How to monitor disease activity (biomarkers) in patients with SAM?

Literature review and analysis. Levels of interleukin (IL)-6, IL-8, TNF and interferon gamma induced protein 10 (IP-10) can be used as biomarkers to monitor disease activity and pulmonary involvement (B) [122–125].

Several cytokines have been identified as a possible prognosis biomarker in SAM: TNF-related apoptosis-inducing ligand, IL-8, macrophage migration inhibitory factor, monocyte chemoattractant protein-1, leukemia inhibitory factor, IP-10 and interferon-α2 showed significant changes after treatment with methotrexate (B) [126, 127].

It was also verified that the loss of muscle strength was associated with changes in the serum levels of IL-8, IL-12 and stromal cell-derived factor 1 (B) [125].

Additional results showed that changes in serum levels of cytokines (IL-6, IL-8 and TNFα) were positively correlated with changes in the evaluation of muscular strength and visual analogue scale regardless of treatment (B) [125].

Levels of some biomarkers, such as TNF-α-activating factor B, were elevated in some subgroups of patients with SAM, especially those with active or positive anti-Jo-1 disease (B) [128].

Elevated serum levels of the Krebs von den Lungen-6 are directly associated with pulmonary involvement with a manifestation of ILD, and these levels are inversely correlated to the variables studied through the pulmonary function test, which presents findings corresponding to a restrictive respiratory pattern (B) [129–131].

Other proposed biomarkers that are elevated in patients with active SAM, are represented by adipokines such as MRP8/14, galectin-9, TNF-type II receptor, CXCL10, and myositis-specific antibodies (B) [132–136].

Autoantibody titers demonstrated association with disease activity. A decrease in serum levels of anti-Mi-2, anti-Jo-1 and TIF-1 after treatment of SAM was detected in many cases (B) [137]. High levels of serum ferritin was also found in patients with SAM and ILD, and evidence suggests that this may be used as a prognostic marker (B) [137].

Of note, high serum levels of CK are the hallmark of muscle involvement [138]. CK is released in the serum in case of muscle damage and is the most sensitive muscle enzyme in the acute phase of the disease. Moreover, elevation in serum aldolase, myoglobin, lactate dehydrogenase, aspartate aminotransferase and alanine aminotransferase also occur [138].

Some patients have selectively increased serum levels of aldolase, which could be associated with syndromes including myopathies with discomfort and weakness, systemic disorders and pathology in perimysial muscle connective tissue (C) [139].

How to define activity versus remission of SAM in clinical practice?

Literature review and analysis. The IMACS has developed an assessment tool that provides appropriate clinical measures of disease status and which, together, assesses 6 items related to its activity. These items include overall evaluation of disease activity perceived by the patient and physician, accessed by an Likert scale or analogue visual scale; muscle strength assessed by MMT; muscle function measured by the Health Assessment Questionnaire Disability Index (HAQ-DI); and muscle enzyme sera and extra-muscular manifestations of the disease assessed by the Myositis Disease Activity Assessment Tool (MDAAT) (D) [140]. In addition to the MDAAT, the IMACS defined the Myositis Damage Index (MDI) to included irreversible damage from the disease [140].

To evaluate the cutaneous lesions of dermatomyositis, the IMACS developed the CDASI (Cutaneous Disease Activity Score), which assigns scores to active and chronic skin lesions [141]. It is important to note that the IMACS used a consensus methodology to define the clinical response criteria, establishing as a complete clinical response a period of 6 months or more with no evidence of disease activity during treatment and definition for clinical remission as a period equal to or greater than 6 months of inactive disease in the absence of any therapy (D) [141]. According to the IMACS, response to treatment is defined as an improvement of more than 30% in 3 IMACS items, excluding the MMT-8 [141]. The IMACS's assessment of response to treatment is therefore dichotomous, allowing us to state only whether or not there was improvement [141].

Considering the need for sensitive response criteria at different levels of improvement, the recent ACR/EULAR initiative validated a tool. According to the score, improvement is defined as minimal, moderate or greater. This new assessment tool should be used in upcoming clinical studies evaluating new therapies for SAM [142].

In addition to serum dosage of muscle enzymes, imaging techniques can identify changes in the muscle structure of SAM patients. Magnetic resonance imaging (MRI) has been used to evaluate disease activity, guide therapeutic decisions and select the biopsy site when necessary (B) [143]. Patients with active disease may present areas of edema and muscular necrosis in T2-weighted images [143]. In this same examination, areas of muscular atrophy, fatty degeneration, fibrosis and calcification can be evidenced in T1-weighted sequences (B) [144] (D) [145]. It is important to emphasize that there is not yet a universally accepted standardization of the MRI protocol to be used.

Conclusions

Robust data to guide the therapeutic process are scarce. Decision-making is based mainly on observational studies, many of which are retrospective in nature and include a small number of patients.

Although not proven effective in controlled clinical trials, GC represents first-line drugs in the treatment of SAM. Intravenous immunoglobulin is considered in induction for refractory cases of SAM or when immunosuppressive drugs are contra-indicated.

Consideration should be given to the early introduction of immunosuppressive drugs, especially azathioprine, methotrexate and cyclosporine, considering the association of these drugs and, in refractory cases, the use of rituximab. There is no specific period determined for the suspension of GC and immunosuppressive drugs when individually evaluating patients with SAM.

A key component for treatment in an early rehabilitation program is the inclusion of strength-building and aerobic exercises, in addition to a rigorous evaluation of these activities for remission of disease and the education of the patient and his/her caregivers.

Abbreviations

CK: Creatine phosphokinase; GC: Glucocorticoid; IL: Interleukin; ILD: Interstitial lung disease; IMACS: International Myositis Assessment and Clinical Studies Group; MDAAT: Myositis Disease Activity Assessment Tool; MMT: Manual Muscle Testing; MP: Methylprednisolone; PICO: Patient, Intervention, Control and Outcome; RCT: Randomized controlled trials; SAM: Systemic autoimmune myopathies; TNF: Tumor necrosis factor

Acknowledgements

Not applicable.

Authors' contributions
All authors contributed equally to write and review the manuscript. All authors read and approved the final manuscript.

Author details
[1]Hospital das Clinicas HCFMUSP, Faculdade de Medicina, Universidade de Sao Paulo, São Paulo, SP, Brazil. [2]Universidade Federal de Pelotas (UFP), Pelotas, RS, Brazil. [3]Universidade do Estado do Rio de Janeiro (UERJ), Rio de Janeiro, RJ, Brazil. [4]Hospital Geral de Fortaleza (HGF), Fortaleza, CE, Brazil. [5]Rede Sarah de Hospitais de Reabilitação, Brasília, Brazil. [6]Disciplina de Reumatologia, Faculdade de Medicina, Universidade de Sao Paulo, Av. Dr. Arnaldo, 455, 3° andar, sala 3150 - Cerqueira César, Sao Paulo CEP: 01246-903, Brazil.

References
1. Feldman BM, Rider LG, Reed AM, Pachman LM. Juvenile dermatomyositis and other idiopathic inflammatory myopathies of childhood. Lancet. 2008; 371:201–12.
2. Lundberg IE, Tjamlund A, Bottai M, Pikington C, de Visser M, Alfredson L, et al. 2017 European league against rheumatism/ American College of Rheumatology classification criteria for adult and juvenile idiopathic inflammatory myopathies and their major subgroups. Arthritis Rheum. 2017; 69:2271–82.
3. Gordon PA, Winer JB, Hoogendijk JE, Choy EH. Immunosuppressant and immunomodulatory treatment for dermatomyositis and polymyositis. Cochrane Database Syst Rev. 2012:CD003643.
4. Leclair V, Lundberg IE. Recent clinical trials in idiopathic inflammatory myopathies. Curr Opin Rheumatol. 2017;29:652–65.
5. Iberati A, Altman DG, Tetzlaff J, Mulrow C, Gøtzsche PC, Ioannidis JP, et al. The PRISMA statement for reporting systematic reviews and meta-analyses of studies that evaluate healthcare interventions: explanation and elaboration. BMJ. 2009;339:b2700.
6. Oxford centre for evidence-based medicine - Levels of evidence (March 2009) - CEBM. 2009.
7. Guyatt GH, Oxman AD, Kunz R, Falck-Ytter Y, Vist GE, Liberati A, GRADE Working Group, et al. Going from evidence to recommendations. BMJ. 2008; 336:1049–51.
8. Guyatt GH, Oxman AD, Vist GE, Kunz R, Falck-Ytter Y, Alonso-Coello P, GRADE Working Group, et al. GRADE: an emerging consensus on rating quality of evidence and strength of recommendations. BMJ. 2008;336:924–6.
9. Kuhn MA, Belafsky PC. Management of cricopharyngeus muscle dysfunction. Otolaryngol Clin N Am. 2013;46:1087–99.
10. Oh TH, Brumfield KA, Hoskin TL, Stolp KA, Murray JA, Brassford JR. Dysphagia in inflammatory myopathy: clinical characteristics, treatment strategies, and outcome in 62 patients. Mayo Clin Proc. 2007;82:441–7.
11. Schrey A, Airas L, Jokela M, Pulkkinen J. Botulinum toxin alleviates dysphagia of patients with inclusion body myositis. J Neurol Sci. 2017;380:142–7.
12. Moerman M, Callier Y, Dick C, Vermeersch H. Botulinum toxin for dysphagia due to cricopharyngeal dysfunction. Eur Arch Otorhinolaryngol. 2002;259:1–3.
13. Sanei-Moghaddam A, Kumar S, Jani P, Brierley C. Cricopharyngeal myotomy for cricopharyngeus stricture in an inclusion body myositis patient with hiatus hernia: a learning experience. BMJ Case Rep. 2013;2013.
14. Marie I, Mcnard JF, Hachulla E, Chérin P, Benveniste O, Tiev K, et al. Infectious complications in polymyositis and dermatomyositis: a series of 279 patients. Semin Arthritis Rheum. 2011;41:48–60.
15. Gerhart JL, Kalaaji AN. Development of *Pneumocystis carinii* pneumonia in patients with immunobullous and connective tissue disease receiving immunosuppressive medications. J Am Acad Dermatol. 2010;62:957–61.
16. Li J, Huang XM, Fang WG, Zeng XJ. *Pneumocystis carinii* pneumonia in patients with connective tissue disease. J Clin Rheumatol. 2006;12:114–7.
17. Ward MM, Donald F. *Pneumocystis carinii* pneumonia in patients with connective tissue diseases: the role of hospital experience in diagnosis and mortality. Arthritis Rheum. 1999;42:780–9.
18. Bachelez H, Schremmer B, Cadranel J, Mouly F, Sarfati C, Agbalika F, et al. Fulminant *Pneumocystis carinii* pneumonia in 4 patients with dermatomyositis. Arch Intern Med. 1997;157:1501–3.
19. Yale SH, Limper AH. *Pneumocystis carinii* pneumonia in patients without acquired immunodeficiency syndrome: associated illness and prior corticosteroid therapy. Mayo Clin Proc. 1996;71:5–13.
20. Kadoya A, Okada J, Iikuni Y, Kondo H. Risk factors for *Pneumocystis carinii* pneumonia in patients with polymyositis/dermatomyositis or systemic lupus erythematosus. J Rheumatol. 1996;23:1186–8.
21. Wolfe RM, Peacock JE Jr. *Pneumocystis pneumonia* (PCP) and the rheumatologist: which patients are at risk and how can PCP be prevented? Curr Rheumatol Rep. 2017;19:35.
22. Aymonier M, Abed S, Boy T, Barazzutti H, Fournier B, Morand JJ. Dermatomyositis associated with anti-MDA5 antibodies and *Pneumocystis pneumonia*: two lethal cases. Ann Dermatol Venereol. 2017;144:279–83.
23. Stern A, Green H, Paul M, Vidal L, Leibovici L. Prophylaxis for *Pneumocystis pneumonia* (PCP) in non-HIV immunocompromised patients. Cochrane Database Syst Rev. 2014:CD005590.
24. Utsunomiya M, Dobashi H, Odani T, Saito K, Yokogawa N, Nagasaka K, et al. Optimal regimens of sulfamethoxazole-trimethoprim for chemoprophylaxis of *Pneumocystis pneumonia* in patients with systemic rheumatic diseases: results from a non-blinded, randomized controlled trial. Arthritis Res Ther. 2017;19:7.
25. Ravn P, Munk ME, Andersen AB, Lundgren B, Nielsen LN, Lillebaek T, et al. Reactivation of tuberculosis during immunosuppressive treatment in a patient with a positive QuantiFERON-RD1 test. Scand J Infect Dis. 2004;36:499–501.
26. Jick SS, Lieberman ES, Rahman MU, Choi HK. Glucocorticoid use, other associated factors, and the risk of tuberculosis. Arthritis Rheum. 2006;55:19–26.
27. Chan MJ, Wen YH, Huang YB, Chuang HY, Tain YL, Lily Wang YC, et al. Risk of tuberculosis comparison in new users of anti-tumour necrosis factor and with existing disease-modifying antirheumatic drug therapy. J Clin Pharm Ther. 2018;43:256–64.
28. Kim HA, Yoo CD, Baek HJ, Lee EB, Ahn C, Han JS, et al. *Mycobacterium tuberculosis* infection in a corticosteroid-treated rheumatic disease patient population. Clin Exp Rheumatol. 1998;16:9–13.
29. Health Surveillance Guide, 2017, Ministry of Health.
30. Lam CS, Tong MK, Chan KM, Siu YP. Disseminated strongyloidiasis: a retrospective study of clinical course and outcome. Eur J Clin Microbiol Infect Dis. 2006;25:14–8.
31. Santiago M, Leito B. Prevention of strongyloides hyperinfection syndrome: a rheumatological point of view. Eur J Intern Med. 2009;20:744–8.
32. Davis JS, Currie BJ, Fisher DA, Huffam SE, Anstey NM, Price RN, et al. Prevention of opportunistic infections in immunosuppressed patients in the tropical top end of the Northern Territory. Commun Dis Intell Q Rep. 2003; 27:526–32.
33. Shinjo SK, de Moraes JC, Levy-Neto M, Aikawa NE, de Medeiros Ribeiro AC, Schahin Saad CG, et al. Pandemic unadjuvanted influenza a (H1N1) vaccine in dermatomyositis and polymyositis: immunogenicity independent of therapy and no harmful effect in disease. Vaccine. 2012;31:202–6.
34. Guissa VR, Pereira RM, Sallum AM, Aikawa NE, Campos LM, Silva CA, et al. Influenza a H1N1/2009 vaccine in juvenile dermatomyositis: reduced immunogenicity in patients under immunosuppressive therapy. Clin Exp Rheumatol. 2012;30:583–8.
35. Bruhler S, Eperon G, Ribi C, Kyburz D, van Gompel F, Visser LG, et al. Vaccination recommendations for adult patients with autoimmune inflammatory rheumatic diseases. Swiss Med Wkly. 2015;145:w14159.
36. Papadopoulou D, Sipsas NV. Comparison of national clinical practice guidelines and recommendations on vaccination of adult patients with autoimmune rheumatic diseases. Rheumatol Int. 2014;34:151–63.
37. van Assen S, Elkayam O, Agmon-Levin N, Cervera R, Doran MF, Dougados M, et al. Vaccination in adult patients with auto-immune inflammatory rheumatic diseases: a systematic literature review for the European league against rheumatism evidence-based recommendations for vaccination in adult patients with auto-immune inflammatory rheumatic diseases. Autoimmun Rev. 2011;10:341–52.
38. Matz EL, Hsieh MH. Review of advances in uroprotective agents for cyclophosphamide and ifosfamide-induced hemorrhagic cystitis. Urology. 2017;100:16–9.
39. Cooper C, Bardin T, Brandi ML, Cacoub P, Caminis J, Civitelli R, et al. Balancing benefits and risks of glucocorticoids in rheumatic diseases and other inflammatory joint disorders: new insights from emerging data. An expert consensus paper from the European Society for Clinical and Economic Aspects of Osteoporosis and Osteoarthritis (ESCEO). Aging Clin Exp Res. 2016;28:1–16.
40. Lems WF, Saag K. Bisphosphonates and glucocorticoid-induced osteoporosis: cons. Endocrine. 2015;49:628–34.
41. Bolosiu HD, Man L, Rednic S. The effect of methylprednisolone pulse therapy in polymyositis/dermatomyositis. Adv Exp Med Biol. 1999;455:349–57.
42. Winkelmann RK, Mulder DW, Lambert EH, Howard FM Jr, Diessner GR. Course of dermatomyositis-polymyositis: comparison of untreated and cortisone-treated patients. Mayo Clin Proc. 1968;43:545 56.

43. Hoffman GS, Franck WA, Raddatz DA, Stallones L. Presentation, treatment, and prognosis of idiopathic inflammatory muscle disease in a rural hospital. Am J Med. 1983;75:433–8.

44. Matsubara S, Hirai S, Sawa Y. Pulsed intravenous methylprednisolone therapy for inflammatory myopathies: evaluation of the effect by comparing two consecutive biopsies from the same muscle. J Neuroimmunol. 1997;76:75–80.

45. Naji P, Shahram F, Nadji A, Davatchi F. Effect of early treatment in polymyositis and dermatomyositis. Neurol India. 2010;58:58–61.

46. De Souza FHC, Miossi R, Shinjo SK. Necrotising myopathy associated with anti-signal recognition particle (anti-SRP) antibody. Clin Exp Rheumatol. 2017;35:766–71.

47. Pinhata MM. Nascimento, Marie SK, Shinjo SK. Does previous corticosteroid treatment affect the inflammatory infiltrate found in polymyositis muscle biopsies? Clin Exp Rheumatol. 2015;33:310–4.

48. Shinjo SK, Nascimento JJ, Marie SK. The effect of prior corticosteroid use in muscle biopsies from patients with dermatomyositis. Clin Exp Rheumatol. 2015;33:336–40.

49. Joffe MM, Love LA, Leff RL, Fraser DD, Targoff IN, Hicks JE, et al. Drug therapy of the idiopathic inflammatory myopathies: predictors of response to prednisone, azathioprine, and methotrexate and a comparison of their efficacy. Am J Med. 1993;94:379–87.

50. Fry CS, Nayeem SZ, Dillon EL, Sarkar PS, Tumurbaatar B, Urban RJ, et al. Glucocorticoids increase skeletal muscle NF-κB inducing kinase (NIK): links to muscle atrophy. Physiol Rep. 2016;4.

51. Newman ED, Scott DW. The use of low-dose oral methotrexate in the treatment of polymyositis and dermatomyositis. J Clin Rheumatol. 1995;1:99–102.

52. Bunch TW, Worthington JW, Combs JJ, Ilstrup DM, Engel AG. Azathioprine with prednisone for polymyositis. A controlled, clinical trial. Ann Intern Med. 1980;92:365–9.

53. Bunch TW. Prednisone and azathioprine for polymyositis: long-term follow-up. Arthritis Rheum. 1981;24:45–8.

54. Schiopu E, Phillips K, MacDonald PM, Crofford LJ, Somers EC. Predictors of survival in a cohort of patients with polymyositis and dermatomyositis: effect of corticosteroids, methotrexate and azathioprine. Arthritis Res Ther. 2012;14:R22.

55. Yu KH, Wu YJ, Kuo CF, See LC, Shen YM, Chang HC, et al. Survival analysis of patients with dermatomyositis and polymyositis: analysis of 192 Chinese cases. Clin Rheumatol. 2011;30:1595–601.

56. Cherin P, Piette JC, Wechsler B, Bletry O, Ziza JM, Laraki R, et al. Intravenous gamma globulin as first line therapy in polymyositis and dermatomyositis: an open study in 11 adult patients. J Rheumatol. 1994;21:1092–7.

57. Göttfried I, Seeber A, Anegg B, Rieger A, Stingl G, Volc-Platzer B. High dose intravenous immunoglobulin (IVIG) in dermatomyositis: clinical responses and effect on sIL-2R levels. Eur J Dermatol. 2000;10:29–35.

58. Anh-Tu Hoa S, Hudson M. Critical review of the role of intravenous immunoglobulins in idiopathic inflammatory myopathies. Semin Arthritis Rheum. 2017;46:488–508.

59. Oddis CV, Sciurba FC, Elmagd KA, Starzl TE. Tacrolimus in refractory polymyositis with interstitial lung disease. Lancet. 1999;353:1762–3.

60. Chang HK, Lee DH. Successful combination therapy of cyclosporine and methotrexate for refractory polymyositis with anti-Jo-1 antibody: a case report. J Korean Med Sci. 2003;18:131–4.

61. Mitsunaka H, Tokuda M, Hiraishi T, Dobashi H, Takahara J. Combined use of cyclosporine a and methotrexate in refractory polymyositis. Scand J Rheumatol. 2000;29:192–4.

62. Qushmaq KA, Chalmers A, Esdaile JM. Cyclosporin a in the treatment of refractory adult polymyositis/dermatomyositis: population based experience in 6 patients and literature review. J Rheumatol. 2000;27:2855–9.

63. Villalba L, Hicks JE, Adams EM, Sherman JB, Gourley MF, Leff RL, et al. Treatment of refractory myositis: a randomized crossover study of two new cytotoxic regimens. Arthritis Rheum. 1998;41:392–9.

64. Nakashima S, Mori M, Miyamae T, Ito S, Ibe M, Aihara Y, et al. Intravenous cyclophosphamide pulse therapy for refractory juvenile dermatomyositis. Ryumachi. 2002;42:895–902.

65. Hirano F, Tanaka H, Nomura Y, Matsui T, Makino Y, Fukawa E, et al. Successful treatment of refractory polymyositis with pulse intravenous cyclophosphamide and low-dose weekly oral methotrexate therapy. Intern Med. 1993;32:749–52.

66. Edge JC, Outland JD, Dempsey JR, Callen JP. Mycophenolate mofetil as an effective corticosteroid sparing therapy for recalcitrant dermatomyositis. Arch Dermatol. 2006;142:65–9.

67. De Souza RC, De Souza FHC, Miossi R, Shinjo SK. Efficacty and safety of leflunomide as na adjuvante drug in refractory dermatomyositis with primarily cutaneous activity. Clin Exp Rheumatol. 2017;35:1011–3.

68. Saito E, Koike T, Hashimoto H, Miyasaka N, Ikeda Y, Hara M, et al. Efficacy of high-dose intravenous immunoglobulin therapy in Japanese patients with steroid-resistant polymyositis and dermatomyositis. Mod Rheumatol. 2008;18:34–44.

69. Dalakas MC, Illa I, Dambrosia JM, Soueidan SA, Stein DP, Otero C, et al. A controlled trial of high-dose intravenous immune globulin infusions as treatment for dermatomyositis. N Engl J Med. 1993;329:1993–2000.

70. Cherin P, Pelletier S, Teixeira A, Laforet P, Genereau T, Simon A, et al. Results and long-term followup of intravenous immunoglobulin infusions in chronic, refractory polymyositis: an open study with thirty-five adult patients. Arthritis Rheum. 2002;46:467–74.

71. Wendling D, Prati C, Ornetti P, Toussirot E, Streit G. Anti TNF-alpha treatment of a refractory polymyositis. Rev Med Interne. 2007;28:194–5.

72. Dastmalchi M, Grundtman C, Alexanderson H, Mavragani CP, Einarsdottir H, Helmers SB, et al. A high incidence of disease flares in an open pilot study of infliximab in patients with refractory inflammatory myopathies. Ann Rheum Dis. 2008;67:1670–7.

73. Iannone F, Scioscia C, Falappone PC, Covelli M, Lapadula G. Use of etanercept in the treatment of dermatomyositis: a case series. J Rheumatol. 2006;33:1802–4.

74. Amato AA, Tawil R, Kissel J, Barohn R, McDermott MP, Pandya S, et al. A randomized, pilot trial of etanercept in dermatomyositis. Ann Neurol. 2011;70:427–36.

75. Tjärnlund A, Tang Q, Wick C, Dastmalchi M, Mann H, Tomasová Studýnková J, et al. Abatacept in the treatment of adult dermatomyositis and polymyositis: a randomised, phase IIb treatment delayed-start trial. Ann Rheum Dis. 2018;77:55–62.

76. Narazaki M, Hagihara K, Shima Y, Ogata A, Kishimoto T, Tanaka T. Therapeutic effect of tocilizumab on two patients with polymyositis. Rheumatology (Oxford). 2011;50:1344–6.

77. Mahler EA, Blom M, Voermans NC, van Engelen BG, van Riel PL, Vonk MC, et al. Rituximab treatment in patients with refractory inflammatory myopathies. Rheumatology (Oxford). 2011;50:2206–13.

78. Mok CC, Ho LY, To CH. Rituximab for refractory polymyositis: an open-label prospective study. J Rheumatol. 2007;34:1864–8.

79. Noss EH, Hausner-Sypek DL, Weinblatt ME. Rituximab as therapy for refractory polymyositis and dermatomyositis. J Rheumatol. 2006;33:1021–6.

80. Sánchez-Fernández SÁ, Carrasco Fernández JA, Rojas Vargas LM. Efficacy of rituximab in dermatomyositis and polymyositis refractory to conventional therapy. Reumatol Clin. 2013;9:117–9.

81. Frikha F, Rigolet A, Behin A, Fautrel B, Herson S, Benveniste O. Efficacy of rituximab in refractory and relapsing myositis with anti-Jo-1 antibodies: a report of two cases. Rheumatology (Oxford). 2009;48:1166–8.

82. Unger L, Kampf S, Lüthke K, Aringer M. Rituximab therapy in patients with refractory dermatomyositis or polymyositis: differential effects in a real-life population. Rheumatology (Oxford). 2014;53:1630–8.

83. Levine TD. Rituximab in the treatment of dermatomyositis: an open-label pilot study. Arthritis Rheum. 2005;52:601–7.

84. Lambotte O, Kotb R, Maigne G, Blanc FX, Goujard C, Delfraissy JF. Efficacy of rituximab in refractory polymyositis. J Rheumatol. 2005;32:1369–70.

85. Oddis CV, Reed AM, Aggarwal R, Rider LG, Ascherman DP, Levesque MC, RIM Study Group, et al. Rituximab in the treatment of refractory adult and juvenile dermatomyositis and adult polymyositis: a randomized, placebo-phase trial. Arthritis Rheum. 2013;65:314–24.

86. Reed AM, Crowson CS, Hein M, de Padilla CL, Olazagasti JM, Aggarwal R, RIM Study Group, et al. Biologic predictors of clinical improvement in rituximab-treated refractory myositis. BMC Musculoskelet Disord. 2015;16:257.

87. Allenbach Y, Guiguet M, Rigolet A, Marie I, Hachulla E, Drouot L, et al. Efficacy of rituximab in refractory inflammatory myopathies associated with anti-synthetase auto-antibodies: an open-label, phase II trial. PLoS One. 2015;10:e0133702.

88. van der Kooi AJ, de Visser M. Idiopathic inflammatory myopathies. Handb Clin Neurol. 2014;119:495–512.

89. Dalakas MC. Inflammatory muscle diseases. N Engl J Med. 2015;372:1734–47.

90. Nzeusseu A, Brion F, Lefèbvre C, Knoops P, Devogelaer JP, et al. Functional outcome of myositis patients: can a low-dose glucocorticoid regimen achieve good functional results? Clin Exp Rheumatol. 1999;17:441–6.

91. van de Vlekkert J, Hoogendijk JE, de Haan RJ, Algra A, van der Tweel I, van der Pol WL, et al. Dexa myositis trial. Oral dexamethasone pulse therapy

versus daily prednisolone in sub-acute onset myositis, a randomized clinical trial. Neuromuscul Disord. 2010;20:382 9.

92. Uchino M, Yamashita S, Uchino K, Hara A, Koide T, Suga T, et al. Long-term outcome of polymyositis treated with high single-dose alternate-day prednisolone therapy. Eur Neurol. 2012;68:117–21.

93. Seshadri R, Feldman BM, Ilowite N, Cawkwell G, Pachman LM. The role of aggressive corticosteroid therapy in patients with juvenile dermatomyositis: a propensity score analysis. Arthritis Rheum. 2008;59:989–95.

94. Raghu P, Manadan AM, Schmukler J, Mathur T, Block JA. Pulse dose methylprednisolone therapy for adult idiopathic inflammatory myopathy. Am J Ther. 2015;22:244–7.

95. Mathur T, Manadan AM, Thiagarajan S, Hota B, Block JA. Corticosteroid monotherapy is usually insufficient treatment for idiopathic inflammatory myopathy. Am J Ther. 2015;22:350–4.

96. Mosca M, Neri R, Pasero G, Bombardieri S. Treatment of the idiopathic inflammatory myopathies: a retrospective analysis of 63 Caucasian patients longitudinally followed at a single center. Clin Exp Rheumatol. 2000;18:451–6.

97. Bronner IM, van der Meulen MF, de Visser M, Kalmijn S, van Venrooij WJ, Voskuyl AE, et al. Long-term outcome in polymyositis and dermatomyositis. Ann Rheum Dis. 2006;65:1456–61.

98. Marie I, Hachulla E, Hatron PY, Hellot MF, Levesque H, Devulder B, et al. Polymyositis and dermatomyositis: short term and longterm outcome, and predictive factors of prognosis. J Rheumatol. 2001;28:2230–7.

99. Vencovsk J, Jarosov K, Machcek S, Studnkov J, Kafkov J, Bartunková J, et al. Cyclosporine a versus methotrexate in the treatment of polymyositis and dermatomyositis. Scand J Rheumatol. 2000;29:95–102.

100. Ibrahim F, Choy E, Gordon P, Dor CJ, Hakim A, Kitas G, et al. Second-line agents in myositis: 1-year factorial trial of additional immunosuppression in patients who have partially responded to steroids. Rheumatology (Oxford). 2015;54:1050–5.

101. Pisoni CN, Cuadrado MJ, Khamashta MA, Hughes GR, D'Cruz DP. Mycophenolate mofetil treatment in resistant myositis. Rheumatology (Oxford). 2007;46:516–8.

102. Majithia V, Harisdangkul V. Mycophenolate mofetil (CellCept): an alternative therapy for autoimmune inflammatory myopathy. Rheumatology (Oxford). 2005;44:386–9.

103. Dagher R, Desjonqures M, Duquesne A, Quartier P, Bader-Meunier B, Fischbach M, et al. Mycophenolate mofetil in juvenile dermatomyositis: a case series. Rheumatol Int. 2012;32:711–6.

104. Mira-Avendano IC, Parambil JG, Yadav R, Arrossi V, Xu M, Chapman JT, et al. A retrospective review of clinical features and treatment outcomes in steroid resistant interstitial lung disease from polymyositis / dermatomyositis. Respir Med. 2013;107:890–6.

105. Morganroth PA, Kreider ME, Werth VP. Mycophenolate mofetil for interstitial lung disease in dermatomyositis. Arthritis Care Res (Hoboken). 2010;62:1496–501.

106. Cea G, Bendahan D, Manners D, Hilton-Jones D, Lodi R, Styles P, et al. Reduced oxidative phosphorylation and proton efflux suggest reduced capillary blood supply in skeletal muscle of patients with dermatomyositis and polymyositis: a quantitative 31P - magnetic resonance spectroscopy and MRI study. Brain. 2002;125:1635–45.

107. Englund P, Nennesmo I, Klareskog L, Lundberg IE. Interleukin-1 alpha expression in capillaries and major histocompatibility complex class I expression in type II muscle fibers from polymyositis and dermatomyositis patients: important pathogenic features independent of inflammatory cell clusters in muscle tissue. Arthritis Rheum. 2002;46:1044–55.

108. Loell I, Lundberg IE. Can muscle regeneration fail in chronic inflammation: a weakness in inflammatory myopathies? J Intern Med. 2011;269:243–57.

109. Varjú C, Pethö E, Kutas R, Czirják L. The effect of physical exercise following acute disease exacerbation in patients with dermato/polymyositis. Clin Rehabil. 2003;17:83–7.

110. Bertolucci F, Neri R, Dalise S, Venturi M, Rossi B, Crisari C. Abnormal lactate levels in patients with polymyositis and dermatomyositis: the benefits of a specific rehabilitative program. Eur J Phys Rehabil Med. 2014;50:161–9.

111. Wiesinger GF, Quittan M, Aringer M, Seeber A, Volc-Platzer B, Smolen J, et al. Improvement of physical fitness and muscle strength in polymyositis/dermatomyositis patients by a training programme. Br J Rheumatol. 1998;37:196–200.

112. Hicks JE, Miller F, Plotz P, Chen TH, Gerber L. Isometric exercise increases strength and does not produce sustained creatinine phosphokinase increases in a patient with polymyositis. J Rheumatol. 1993;20:1399–401.

113. Escalante A, Miller L, Beardmore TD. Resistive exercise in the rehabilitation of polymyositis/dermatomyositis. J Rheumatol. 1993;20:1340–4.

114. Nader GA, Lundberg IE. Exercise as an anti-inflammatory intervention to combat inflammatory diseases of muscle. Curr Opin Rheumatol. 2009;21:599–603.

115. Nader GA, Dastmalchi M, Alexanderson H, Grundtman C, Gernapudi R, Esbjörnsson M, et al. A longitudinal, integrated, clinical, histological and mRNA profiling study of resistance exercise in myositis. Mol Med. 2010;16:455–64.

116. Munters LA, Loell I, Ossipova E, Raouf J, Dastmalchi M, Lindroos E, et al. Endurance exercise improves molecular pathways of aerobic metabolism in patients with myositis. Arthritis Rheumatol. 2016;68:1738–50.

117. Boehler JF, Hogarth MW, Barberio MD, Novak JS, Ghimbovschi S, Brown KJ, et al. Effect of endurance exercise on microRNAs in myositis skeletal muscle - a randomized controlled study. PLoS One. 2017;12:e0183292.

118. Alexanderson H, Munters LA, Dastmalchi M, Loell I, Heimbürger M, Opava CH, et al. Resistive home exercise in patients with recent-onset polymyositis and dermatomyositis - a randomized controlled single-blinded study with a 2-year followup. J Rheumatol. 2014;41:1124–32.

119. Alemo Munters L, Dastmalchi M, Katz A, Esbjörnsson M, Loell I, Hanna B, et al. Improved exercise performance and increased aerobic capacity after endurance training of patients with stable polymyositis and dermatomyositis. Arthritis Res Ther. 2013;15:R83.

120. Alemo Munters L, Dastmalchi M, Andren V, Emilson C, Bergegård J, Regardt M, et al. Improvement in health and possible reduction in disease activity using endurance exercise in patients with established polymyositis and dermatomyositis: a multicenter randomized controlled trial with a 1-year open extension follow-up. Arthritis Care Res (Hoboken). 2013;65:1959–68.

121. Tiffreau V, Rannou F, Kopciuch F, Hachulla E, Mouthon L, Thoumie P, et al. Post rehabilitation functional improvements in patients with inflammatory myopathies: the results of a randomized controlle trial. Arch Phys Med Rehabil. 2017;98:227–34.

122. López De Padilla CM, Crowson CS, Hein MS, Strausbauch MA, Aggarwal R, Levesque MC, et al. Interferon-regulated chemokine score associated with improvement in disease activity in refractory myositis patients treated with rituximab. Clin Exp Rheumatol. 2015;33:655–63.

123. Gono T, Kaneko H, Kawaguchi Y, Hanaoka M, Kataoka S, Kuwana M, et al. Cytokine profiles in polymyositis and dermatomyositis complicated by rapidly progressive or chronic interstitial lung disease. Rheumatology (Oxford). 2014;53:2196–203.

124. Olazagasti JM, Niewold TB, Reed AM. Immunological biomarkers in dermatomyositis. Curr Rheumatol Rep. 2015;17:68.

125. Badrising UA, Tsonaka R, Hiller M, Niks EH, Evangelista T, Lochmüller H, et al. Cytokine profiling of serum allows monitoring of disease progression in inclusion body myositis. J Neuromuscul Dis. 2017;4:327–35.

126. Krystufková O, Vallerskog T, Helmers SB, Mann H, Putová I, Belácek J, et al. Increased serum levels of B cell activating factor (BAFF) in subsets of patients with idiopathic inflammatory myopathies. Ann Rheum Dis. 2009;68:836–43.

127. Reed AM, Peterson E, Bilgic H, Ytterberg SR, Amin S, Hein MS, et al. Changes in novel biomarkers of disease activity in juvenile and adult dermatomyositis are sensitive biomarkers of disease course. Arthritis Rheum. 2012;64:4078–86.

128. Kobayashi N, Kobayashi I, Mori M, Sato S, Iwata N, Shiguemura T, et al. Increased serum B cell activating factor and a proliferation-inducing ligand are associated with interstitial lung disease in patients with juvenile dermatomyositis. J Rheumatol. 2015;42:2412–8.

129. Kubo M, Ihn H, Yamane K, Kikuchi K, Yazawa N, Soma Y, et al. Serum KL-6 in adult patients with polymyositis and dermatomyositis. Rheumatology (Oxford). 2000;39:632–6.

130. Fathi M, Barbasso Helmers S, Lundberg IE. KL-6: a serological biomarker for interstitial lung disease in patients with polymyositis and dermatomyositis. J Intern Med. 2012;271:589–97.

131. Chen F, Lu X, Shu X, Peng Q, Tian X, Wang G. Predictive value of serum markers for the development of interstitial lung disease in patients with polymyositis and dermatomyositis: a comparative and prospective study. Intern Med J. 2015;45:641–7.

132. Nistala K, Varsani H, Wittkowski H, Vogl T, Krol P, Shah V, et al. Myeloid related protein induces muscle derived inflammatory mediators in juvenile dermatomyositis. Arthritis Res Ther. 2013;15:R131.

133. Olazagasti JM, Hein M, Crowson CS, de Padilla CL, Peterson E, Baechler EC, et al. Adipokine gene expression in peripheral blood of adult and juvenile dermatomyositis patients and their relation to clinical parameters and disease activity measures. J Inflamm (Lond). 2015;12:29.

134. Bellutti Enders F, van Wijk F, Scholman R, Hofer M, Prakken BJ, van Royen-Kerkhof A, de Jager W. Correlation of CXCL10, tumor necrosis factor receptor type II, and galectin 9 with disease activity in juvenile dermatomyositis. Arthritis Rheumatol. 2014;66:2281–9.

135. McHugh NJ, Tansley SL. Autoantibodies in myositis. Nat Rev Rheumatol. 2018;14:290–302.

136. Aggarwal R, Oddis CV, Goudeau D, Koontz D, Qi Z, Reed AM, et al. Autoantibody levels in myositis patients correlate with clinical response during B cell depletion with rituximab. Rheumatology (Oxford). 2016;55:991–9.

137. Ishizuka M, Watanabe R, Ishii T, Machiyama T, Akita K, Fujita Y, et al. Long-term follow-up of 124 patients with polymyositis and dermatomyositis: statistical analysis of prognostic factors. Mod Rheumatol. 2016;26:115–20.

138. Dalakas MC. Polymyositis and dermatomyositis. Lancet. 2003;362:971–82.

139. Nozaki K, Pestronk A. High aldolase with normal creatine kinase in serum predicts a myopathy with perimysial pathology. J Neurol Neurosurg Psychiatry. 2009;80:904–8.

140. Rider LG, Giannini EH, Harris-Love M, Joe G, Isenberg D, Pilkington C, International Myositis Assessment and Clinical Studies Group, et al. Defining clinical improvement in adult and juvenile myositis. J Rheumatol. 2003;30:603–17.

141. Oddis CV, Rider LG, Reed AM, Ruperto N, Brunner HI, Koneru B, International Myositis Assessment and Clinical Studies Group, et al. International consensus guidelines for trials of therapies in the idiopathic inflammatory myopathies. Arthritis Rheum. 2005;52:2607–15.

142. Aggarwal R, Rider L, Ruperto N, Bayat N, Erman B, Feldman BM, et al. 2016 American College of Rheumatology (ACR)- European league against rheumatism (EULAR) criteria for minimal, moderate and major clinical response for adult dermatomyositis and polymyositis: an international myositis assessment and clinical studies group/ pediatric rheumatology international trials organization collaborative initiative. Ann Rheum Dis. 2017;76:792–801.

143. Abdul-Aziz R, Yu CY, Adler B, Bout-Tabaku S, Lintner KE, Moore-Clingenpeel M, et al. Muscle MRI at the time of questionable disease flares in juvenile dermatomyositis (JDM). Pediatr Rheumatol Online J. 2017;15:25.

144. Yao L, Yip AL, Shrader JA, Mesdaghinia S, Volochayev R, Jansen AV, et al. Magnetic resonance measurement of muscle T2, fat-corrected T2 and fat fraction in the assessment of idiopathic inflammatory myopathies. Rheumatology (Oxford). 2016;55:441–9.

145. Day J, Patel S, Limaye V. The role of magnetic resonance imaging techniques in evaluation and management of the idiopathic inflammatory myopathies. Semin Arthritis Rheum. 2017;46:642–9.

4

Brazilian recommendations on the safety and effectiveness of the yellow fever vaccination in patients with chronic immune-mediated inflammatory diseases

Gecilmara Salviato Pileggi[1,34*] (iD), Licia Maria Henrique Da Mota[2], Adriana Maria Kakehasi[3], Alexandre Wagner De Souza[4], Aline Rocha[5], Ana Karla Guedes de Melo[6], Caroline Araujo M. da Fonte[7], Cecilia Bortoletto[8], Claiton Viegas Brenol[9], Claudia Diniz Lopes Marques[10], Cyrla Zaltman[11], Eduardo Ferreira Borba[12], Enio Ribeiro Reis[13], Eutilia Andrade Medeiros Freire[14], Evandro Mendes Klumb[14], Georges Basile Christopoulos[15], Ieda Maria M. Laurindo[16], Isabella Ballalai[17], Izaias Pereira Da Costa[18], Lessandra Michelin[19], Lilian David de Azevêdo Valadares[20], Liliana Andrade Chebli[21], Marcus Lacerda[22], Maria Amazile Ferreira Toscano[23], Michel Alexandre Yazbek[24], Rejane Maria R. De Abreu Vieira[25], Renata Magalhães[26], Renato Kfouri[27], Rosana Richtmann[28], Selma Da Costa Silva Merenlender[29], Valeria Valim[30], Marcos Renato De Assis[31], Sergio Candido Kowalski[32] and Virginia Fernandes Moça Trevisani[33]

Abstract

Background: In Brazil, we are facing an alarming epidemic scenario of Yellow fever (YF), which is reaching the most populous areas of the country in unvaccinated people. Vaccination is the only effective tool to prevent YF. In special situations, such as patients with chronic immune-mediated inflammatory diseases (CIMID), undergoing immunosuppressive therapy, as a higher risk of severe adverse events may occur, assessment of the risk-benefit ratio of the yellow fever vaccine (YFV) should be performed on an individual level.

Main body of the abstract: Faced with the scarcity of specific orientation on YFV for this special group of patients, the Brazilian Rheumatology Society (BRS) endorsed a project aiming the development of individualized YFV recommendations for patients with CIMID, guided by questions addressed by both medical professionals and patients, followed an internationally validated methodology (GIN-McMaster Guideline Development). Firstly, a systematic review was carried out and an expert panel formed to take part of the decision process, comprising BRS clinical practitioners, as well as individuals from the Brazilian Dermatology Society (BDS), Brazilian Inflammatory Bowel Diseases Study Group (GEDIIB), and specialists on infectious diseases and vaccination (from Tropical Medicine, Infectious Diseases and Immunizations National Societies); in addition, two representatives of patient groups were included as members of the panel. When the quality of the evidence was low or there was a lack of evidence to determine the recommendations, the decisions were based on the expert opinion panel and a Delphi approach was performed. A recommendation was accepted upon achieving ≥80% agreement among the panel, including the patient representatives. As a result, eight recommendations were developed regarding the

(Continued on next page)

* Correspondence: gecilmara@gmail.com
[1]SBR. Faculdade de Ciências da Saúde de Barretos – FACISB, Barretos, São Paulo, Brazil
[34]School of Medical Science Barretos- FACISB, Avenue Masonic Lodge Renovadora 68, No. 100 - Airport Neighborhood, Barretos/SP 14785-002, Brazil
Full list of author information is available at the end of the article

(Continued from previous page)

safety of YFV in patients with CIMID, considering the immunosuppression degree conferred by the treatment used. It was not possible to establish recommendations on the effectiveness of YFV in these patients as there is no consistent evidence to support these recommendations.

Conclusion: This paper approaches a real need, assessed by clinicians and patient care groups, to address specific questions on the management of YFV in patients with CIMID living or traveling to YF endemic areas, involving specialists from many areas together with patients, and might have global applicability, contributing to and supporting vaccination practices. We recommended a shared decision-making approach on taking or not the YFV.

Background

Yellow fever: Disease and vaccine

Yellow fever (YF) is an infectious zoonotic disease caused by an RNA arbovirus, belonging to the *family Flaviviridae*, transmitted by hematophagous insects, especially of the genera *Aedes* and *Haemagogus*. In Brazil, the main sylvatic cycle of transmission involves mostly *Haemagogus* mosquitos. The disease is both, endemic and epidemic, in tropical regions of South America and Africa, and its clinical spectrum is highly variable, ranging from asymptomatic to severe disease, with a 50% mortality risk [1, 2].

In Brazil, although YF is endemic in the North and Central West regions, it has become epidemic outside the Legal Amazon in the last five years. The YF transmission cycle occasionally re-emerges and, in the last decade, an increase in viral circulation has been observed throughout the country [3, 4]. From July 2016 to March 2017, 691 cases and 220 deaths were confirmed; an increase was noticed during the same period of the following year, when the records increased to 1127 cases and 328 deaths (http://portalms.saude.gov.br/boletim-epidemiologico, access December, 2018).

Vaccination is the only effective measure to prevent YF. The rapid recognition of disease outbreaks in high-risk areas, followed by the vaccination of 60 to 80% of the population is crucial to prevent epidemics [5].

The YFV is composed of an attenuated live virus, specific pathogen free (SPF) strain 17D or equivalent, cultivated in chicken embryo eggs, and has been used for the prevention of the disease since 1937. It is considered highly immunogenic, capable of immunizing 95 to 99% of adults and approximately 90% of infants (< 2 years) one week after application [3, 6, 7]. However, on the other hand, the YFV is related to a potential risk of inducing an adverse event following vaccination (AEFV) [8].

According to the World Health Organization (WHO), an AEFV is defined as any harmful medical occurrence after vaccination, classified as local or systemic, even without a clear causal relationship traced back to the vaccine. In general, AEFVs are mild and transitory. They generally occur three to seven days after vaccination and usually last no longer than three to seven days. Local manifestations (pain, erythema, and induration at the injection site) or systemic manifestations, such as malaise, tiredness, low fever, mild headache or myalgia may occur [3, 6, 7].

The major concern regarding an AEFV is when it is reported as a severe adverse event (SAE), characterized by hospitalization required for at least 24 h, significant dysfunction, and/or persistent secondary or congenital abnormality and even death or risk of death [9]. Although rare, SAEs can occur, particularly post-primary vaccination, mainly during immunization campaigns in areas with no prior vaccine recommendation [10, 11]. SAEs related to the YFV are extremely rare and the risk of dying from YF is considered higher than vaccination-associated risks [5].

In Brazil, there are two vaccines available, derived from the same strain, with very similar and comparable response profiles and reactogenicity – YFV 17DD (Biomanguinhos©) and 17D-204 (Sanofi Pasteur©) [3, 6, 7, 12]. The current Brazilian immunization schedule recommends a single subcutaneous 0.5 ml dose at nine months of age [6] and is contraindicated in some groups, as follows [3, 5, 13]:

- infants younger than nine months for routine immunization or younger than six months during an epidemic;
- pregnant women or breastfeeding children under six months of age, except during YF outbreaks, when the risk of infection is high;
- severe allergies to egg protein;
- history of severe adverse reactions to previous doses;
- organ transplantation;
- previous history of thymus disease (myasthenia gravis, thymoma, thymus absence or surgical removal);
- severe immunodeficiency of any nature.

The most serious SAE related to YFV is associated with viscerotropic disease (YEL-AVD), an acute post-vaccination dysfunction that usually appears one to four weeks after vaccination, with clinical manifestations ranging from a mild multisystem disease to multiple organ failure and death. Virological and pathological findings during necropsies of vaccinated patients showed the replication and uncontrolled dissemination of the 17D or 17DD virus. The initial symptoms are nonspecific, similar to YF manifestations. The most serious condition associated with YEL-AVD is characterized by hypotension, hemorrhage, and acute renal and respiratory failure, with an overall case–fatality rate of approximately 50% [14, 15].

According to Staples et al. (2017), at least 100 cases of YEL-AVD had been reported worldwide and none were reported after revaccination until February 2017. In the United States, the incidence of YEL-AVD is 0.25–0.4/ 100,000 doses and in Brazil, 21 cases were reported from 2007 to 2012, at a rate of 0.04 cases per 100,000 administered doses. In 2009, during the vaccination campaign in the State of São Paulo, 0.31 cases per 100,000 doses applied were observed, and in Rio Grande do Sul, the frequency observed was 0.11 per 100,000 doses applied [16].

Another SAE is the yellow fever vaccine-associated neurotropic disease (YEL-AND), which although not related to death, can cause hypersensitive reactions, neurological manifestations (encephalitis, meningitis, Guillain-Barré syndrome, etc.), and autoimmune diseases, involving the central and peripheral nervous system [9, 17].

A single-dose vaccination has been implemented since April 2017, however due to conflicting results on immunity in long-term YFV studies it is still under debate among vaccination experts [6, 18–21].

According to the WHO, the use of fractional-dose YFV is a good strategy to avoid disease outbreaks as this strategy rapidly increases vaccination coverage in areas of risk [22]. Recently in Brazil, the Ministry of Health started a campaign using YFV fractionated-dose due to the current epidemic quickly spreading over the most populous states.

Due to the current epidemiological setting, the vaccination against the YF virus will be extended and recommended across the country. It is intended to be gradually incorporated as part of the basic vaccination schedule in all Brazilian States from July 2018 [4].

Yellow fever vaccine: Assessment of the immunogenicity

YFV is one of the most immunogenic vaccines. The highly effective and long-lasting immunity caused by 17D makes it an important research target for the development of vaccines against related viruses and for understanding the attenuation and immunological induction processes for highly effective vaccines in general [23]. Studies have demonstrated that humoral immunity is a primary protective element in previously exposed individuals, and a single vaccine may provide protection against global strains of the YF virus [18, 23]. Approximately 90% of 17D-

immunized individuals are shown to be producing neutralizing antibodies on the tenth day after vaccination, and almost 100% are doing so by day 30 [21].

The post-immunization humoral responses to YFV can be measured by the plaque reduction neutralization test (PRNT). This is the gold standard correlation of protection method, which is considered when more than 80% of virus neutralization at 1:10 dilution is detected in the serum. The micro-PRTN90 has a sensitivity of 100% and specificity of 94.7% for the yellow fever virus [24].

Other methods, such as the Indirect Immunofluorescence Test (IFA), used to evaluate IgG antibodies, present false positives with various viruses of the *Flaviviridae* family, and although highly sensitive, it does not reach the specificity of the PRNT. The specificity of these tests is impaired in patients with Dengue fever history [25]. Thus, the neutralizing antibodies remain accepted as a correlate of protection against the YF virus.

To date, there is no other adequate method to evaluate the response to YFV in humans besides neutralizing antibodies. Nevertheless, new alternatives based on the complex modulation of innate immune cytokines induced by YFV are being studied [26]. In addition, CD4+ and CD8+ T cells strongly respond to 17D, with CD4+ T reaching their highest level between seven and 14 days and CD8+ T between 14 and 30 days after vaccination. These cells slowly decline over time, but remain detectable for more than 25 years, while another group of self-renewing and highly responsive 17D-specific memory cells remains stable during the same 25-year period. Complementary studies in humans are required regarding cytokine and CD4+ and CD8+ T cell counts in order to assess their real benefit as a vaccine response marker [27].

Studies published to date (WHO, ACIP, and CDC) have shown that approximately 88% of healthy individuals remain seropositive for more than ten years after the YFV [20]. On the other hand, Brazilian studies have demonstrated a fall in protection after 5–10 years in some groups [6, 24]. It is crucial to obtain further understanding about the YFV immunogenicity in patients with CIMID, particularly in Brazil, since it is an endemic area with frequent outbreaks of the disease.

Yellow fever vaccine in specific situations of immunosuppression

In some situations, there is a higher risk of AEFV, and it is important to evaluate the risk-benefit ratio on an individual basis. In cases of moderate to severe acute febrile illnesses, postponement of the vaccine is recommended until resolution of the condition. Blood or organ donors should wait for four weeks after vaccination before donating; the immunosuppression degree of patients with CIMID, undergoing immunosuppressive therapy, should be established in order to evaluate the safety of receiving the YFV [3].

The CIMID concept is used to collectively describe a group of heterogeneous diseases that share common inflammatory pathways and deregulation in the immune system. These are responsible for chronic inflammation, such as rheumatoid arthritis (RA), ankylosing spondylitis (AS), psoriasis, psoriatic arthritis (PsoA), multiple sclerosis (MS), systemic lupus erythematosus (SLE), and inflammatory bowel diseases (IBD), such as Crohn's disease and ulcerative colitis [28]. These diseases affect approximately 5–8% of the population and cause significant morbidity, mortality, and a high risk of infection [29].

The treatment of these diseases is based mainly on immunosuppressive or immunomodulatory agents to control chronic inflammation. The use of these medications, with different mechanisms of action, besides changes in the immune system inherent in the underlying disease, lead to variable degrees of immunosuppression and, consequently, increase susceptibility to infections, which is considered the major cause of morbidity and mortality in this population [30]. As a result, the immunogenicity of vaccines may be reduced. Furthermore, the administration of live attenuated vaccines (LAV) bears the potential risk of invasive infection with the attenuated vaccine strain and should generally be avoided in patients under immunosuppressive therapy; this being the reason why these vaccines are generally contraindicated in this population [31, 32].

According to the Brazilian Ministry of Health, the recommendation for YF vaccination is based on the routine immunization of the population exposed to the virus, residents or subjects travelling to endemic regions, in the absence of contraindications. There are still some controversial issues regarding contraindication, and they require caution, as well as the elderly population (over sixty years old), and patients with different immunosuppression degrees [3].

For patients with CIMID, it is essential to take into account the risk of (rare) post-vaccination adverse events and the protection provided by a highly effective vaccine against a potentially lethal illness without specific treatment. When evaluating the risk of severe AEFVs, we should consider the underlying disease, its severity, level of activity, and immunosuppression degree. At the same time, we should consider the risk of contracting the YF virus in areas of vaccine recommendation [15, 33, 34].

It is important to emphasize that none of the review articles or consensus formed by the panels of experts have established specific recommendations or absolute contraindications against the indication of LAV in patients with CIMID, considering the particular differences between the diseases and their treatment. Based on the knowledge that the only effective measure to prevent YF is vaccination, and

that many immunocompromised patients have been inadvertently vaccinated without presenting an SAE [35], these panels of specialists agree that there is no absolute contraindication for YFV in this setting and the risk and benefits should be considered individually.

In this context, management should be individualized, according to the underlying disease, medications used and their doses, replication capacity of the attenuated vaccine virus, and risk of infection. Risks related to LAV potentially involve viral replication capability (elevated with the YFV agent), availability of an antiviral agent (such as acyclovir for varicella), immunoglobulins (passive immunity), or an antimicrobial agent.

We conducted a systematic literature review on the safety and effectiveness of the YFV in patients with CIMID, guided by the most frequent questions addressed by healthcare professionals and patients on this issue. Thus, the objective of this study was to develop individualized YFV recommendations for this special group of patients.

Methods

This was an initiative of the Brazilian Rheumatology Society (BRS); to develop YFV-specific recommendations for this special group of patients, considering the national epidemiological scenario, based on scientific evidence.

Study method

To develop the recommendations, the BRS followed an internationally validated methodology, according to the GIN-McMaster Guideline Development Checklist (https:// cebgrade.mcmaster.ca/guidelinechecklistonline.html). The Society counted on a work group comprised of clinical practitioners with expertise in different CIMID types, such as the Brazilian Dermatology Society (BDS) and the Brazilian Inflammatory Bowel Diseases Study Group (GEDIIB). In addition, the BRS invited experts on infectious diseases and vaccination (from Tropical Medicine, Infectious Diseases and Immunization National Societies) to take part in the process.

The chair of the group (GSP) was chosen and endorsed by the BRS, who defined groups to run the process of developing recommendations: the oversight committee, composed of five rheumatologists (LM, AMK, SK, MRA, VMFT), specialists in systematic reviews and the Grading of Recommendations Assessment, Development and Evaluation Working Group (GRADE), and a postgraduate student from the Evidence Based Medicine postgraduate program (APR).

The oversight committee was responsible for defining the questions that guided the recommendations via weekly Skype meetings, keeping the guideline development on track, the goals and objectives, timeline, task assignments, documenting the decisions, and proposing the methodology for all steps. The committee was also in charge of including and developing search strategies, running searches and selection of evidence, and critically appraising the existing evidence and establishing methods for identifying additional evidence.

The other workgroup, the panel members, was composed of experts representing the above-mentioned societies and two representatives of National groups of patients (PT, ET). These representatives are both very engaged in continuous education and advocacy and have sufficient knowledge on CIMID diseases, regularly giving on-line and presential support to patients around Latin America. They did not receive any incentive to participate in the panel and did not receive any tool to help their decisions during the recommendation development process. They participated in all steps of the process, which were transparent to all members, and their votes had the same weight as all others.

Search strategy
The systematic literature review was performed in electronic and manual databases, using terms derived from the main question of the study, formulated using PICO format (terms described in Table 1).

Analysis of the methodological quality of the studies
For this evaluation, the Cochrane Collaboration risk of bias table was used for the intervention studies [36]. For observational studies, we used the Newcastle-Ottawa Quality Assessment Scale [37]. Studies that received scores equal to or greater than six were considered to have good methodological quality.

Quality of evidence
The quality of the evidence (QoE) reported in this systematic literature review was analyzed based on the GRADE approach [38]. As studies with different levels of evidence were included in the recommendation development, the oversight committee chose to split them into two categories: in comma-separated sequences or in intervals, separated by hyphens [39].

Delphi methodology
When the quality of the evidence was low or there was a lack of evidence, the opinion of the expert panel was used to support the decisions to determining the recommendations.

To achieve consensus among panel members, Delphi methodology was employed [40]. A face-to-face meeting was arranged and held on November 30, 2017 to present the literature reviewed to the panel and train them on Delphi methodology voting, where all participants should anonymously assign a score from 0 to 100 on a continuous scale to each recommendation, with 0 indicating total disagreement and 100 absolute agreement.

Recommendations were refined and voted on by all work groups (oversight and panel) through a series of three online Delphi rounds supervised by the chair (GSP). From these grades, a final level of agreement (LoA) score was allocated to each recommendation. It was a consensus for all work groups that a recommendation was accepted when it achieved ≥80% agreement among the panel, including the patient representatives.

Sample
We included all the studies found by the search strategy specified above, with no language restrictions.

Eligibility criteria
Studies included: clinical trials, observational studies, and case studies on the effectiveness and/or safety of YFV that included CIMID patients with or without treatment.

Intervention
The YFV was considered as the intervention when compared to placebo.

Outcomes
For assessing YFV safety, the following aspects were considered:

- AEFV, most severe adverse events (SAE), including YEL-AVD and YEL-AND,

Table 1 Terms used for the literature review search using the PICO Format

Population with or without treatment	Patients with rheumatoid arthritis OR juvenile idiopathic arthritis OR systemic lupus erythematosus OR systemic sclerosis OR psoriatic arthritis OR spondyloarthritis OR Sjögren's syndrome OR vasculitis OR inflammatory myopathy OR dermatomyositis OR psoriasis OR Crohn's disease OR ulcerative colitis
Intervention	yellow fever vaccine
Comparison	Placebo OR no intervention
Outcomes	immunization, safety, severe adverse events, viscerotropic disease associated with yellow fever vaccine, immunogenicity, response, effectiveness, efficacy, seroconversion, disease activity: DAS28, ACR 30/50/70. BASDAI, SLEDAI, HAQ / CHAQ, VASDAI, CMAS, MMT

Terms used for the search related to treatment: abatacept, acitretin, adalimumab, anti-CD20, anti-IL-1, anti-IL-6, anti-IL17, anti-IL23, anti-JAK, anti-TNF, azathioprine, belimumab, canakinumab, certolizumab, cyclophosphamide, CTLA4 IgG, etanercept, golimumab, hydroxychloroquine, infliximab, leflunomide, methotrexate, methylprednisolone, mycophenolate mofetil, prednisolone, prednisone, rituximab, secukinumab, sulfasalazine, tacrolimus, tocilizumab, tofacitinib, ustequikinumab

- risk of infection with attenuated vaccine strain,
- relapse or worsening of underlying disease activity.

The response to YFV was evaluated considering the following terms as surrogates for efficacy: immunogenicity, seroconversion, and effectiveness.

Questions defined using PICO format

Initial questions regarding YFV safety in patients with CIMID, receiving or not immunosuppressive medications, were divided according to vaccine exposure to primary vaccination and revaccination (re-exposure) (see Table 2).

Study selection and data extraction

Two reviewers independently assessed the titles and abstracts of all studies selected by the search strategy group. The full texts of the eligible studies were then retrieved. Two reviewers selected the studies to be included, and disagreements were resolved either by consensus or by the opinion of a third reviewer. A standard data extraction sheet was developed for this review. For the eligible studies, two reviewers extracted the data independently. The discrepancies were resolved by discussion or, where necessary, by consulting a third reviewer.

Results

Studies selected and data extracted

From the entire database search, 175 articles were identified, and nine additional studies were selected from other sources (congress abstracts). Among the 184, only 36 were eligible and 148 were excluded, either for not meeting the inclusion criteria (113) or for being duplicates (35). After evaluating the 36 selected studies, a further 19 were excluded for methodological reasons; they were not observational studies or randomized clinical trials. Finally, 17 studies were selected for qualitative analysis and none for quantitative analysis. The flow chart in Fig. 1 depicts the selection process for Systematic Reviews.

Eleven of the 17 selected studies were observational (cohort, case control, or cross-sectional studies) and 6 were case series. Based on these 11 observational studies, a total of 692 patients were included for the safety analyses. The participants were subjects who had received the YFV despite a diagnosis of CIMID and no SAE was reported. There was no difference in AEFV occurrence between patients and healthy individuals [35, 41–48].

Recently, Valim et al. (2017) carried out an observational study evaluating the safety of selected patients with rheumatic diseases after a primary YF vaccination. The authors enrolled 241 patients with rheumatic diseases for whom no SAE was reported and 40 healthy controls [46]. This is an ongoing study and we had access to only partial results from a conference abstract.

Table 2 Questions used to formulate the recommendations

1. Are there specific restrictions on the indication of YFV in patients with CIMID baseline disease, activity, or medication use facing a yellow fever outbreak?

2. Is the risk of SAE following primary or booster YFV vaccination higher in patients with CIMID? Is this related to disease type or activity?

3. Is the risk of SAE following primary and booster YFV vaccination higher in patients using corticosteroid or CsDMARD, TsDMARD or JAK inhibitors?

4. Is the risk of SAE after primary or booster YFV vaccination higher in patients with CIMID using immunosuppressive drugs (azathioprine, cyclophosphamide, cyclosporine, mycophenolate mofetil/acid) or bDMARD?

5. Should an interval be recommended between YFV application (primary or booster) and initiation or restart of medications for CIMID treatment?

6. Should a minimum interval be recommended between discontinuation of medications for CIMID treatment and YFV application (primary or booster)?

7. Does the concomitant application of other vaccines interfere in the YFV response in patients receiving or not CIMID treatment?

8. Is there any contraindication of YFV in close contacts or people living with CIMID patients?

9. Does the use of immunomodulatory and/or immunosuppressive agents in patients with CIMID interfere in the YFV response or long-term efficacy?

YFV: yellow fever vaccine; CIMID: chronic immune-mediated inflammatory diseases; DMARD: disease modifying anti-rheumatic drugs; csDMARD conventional synthetic DMARD – methotrexate, leflunomide, sulfasalazine and antimalarials (hydroxychloroquine and chloroquine); tsDMARD: synthetic target-specific DMARD – tofacitinib; bDMARD: biological DMARD – tumor necrosis factor inhibitors/TNFi (adalimumab, certolizumab, etanercept, golimumab, infliximab), T-lymphocyte costimulation modulator (abatacept), anti-CD20 (rituximab), and IL-6 receptor blocker (tocilizumab)

All included studies had methodological limitations regarding the design or development and did not describe adequate statistical analysis data to evaluate the magnitude of effect. In addition, we only had access to the partial results of three included studies at the time of our review, as they were conference abstracts from ongoing studies [43, 46, 47]. For this reason, we could not estimate the effect or quality of evidence.

Three studies [21, 42, 48] did not include randomly selected controls and the vaccinated group was not homogeneous, with very different sample sizes in the control group and intervention group. Only one study (Scheinberg 2010) included randomly selected controls and included a homogeneous sample [44].

Scheinberg et al. (2010) carried out a study with 17 patients with RA who received a YFV booster during treatment with methotrexate and infliximab. In 15 patients, serology was analyzed by immunofluorescence before and after vaccination. The results were compared with a control group. The YFV was administered 30 days after the last infusion of anti-TNF. Of 17 patients, only one did not seroconvert. Although there was a trend towards lower antibody titers in the

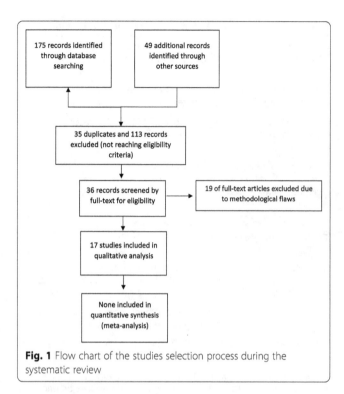

Fig. 1 Flow chart of the studies selection process during the systematic review

RA group, unfortunately, the authors did not apply any statistical tests [44].

Five observational studies [41, 42, 44, 45, 48] evaluated the neutralizing antibodies to YFV in 180 patients with CIMID using immunosuppressant drugs, including corticosteroids, synthetic or biological. The authors concluded that all immunocompromised patients were able to develop a protective response to the yellow fever booster. The quality of evidence was very poor.

Oliveira et al. (2015) analyzed the presence of neutralizing antibodies in 31 patients diagnosed with rheumatic diseases who had been inadvertently vaccinated with a booster of YFV (without the physician's knowledge) [45] during a YF outbreak (2007–2008). Twenty-three subjects with RA, five with SLE, two with ES, and one with ankylosing spondylitis were included in the study. The patients were taking various immunomodulatory drugs, such as MTX, leflunomide, infliximab, or rituximab. A plaque reduction neutralization test (PRNT) was performed to evaluate the immunogenicity to the YFV, with values ≥794 mIU/ml considered protective. In total, 27 out of 31 (87%) presented protective titers of neutralizing antibodies. The lowest PRNT value was in a patient who had used rituximab prior to the booster [45].

Another observational study collected data from patients using corticosteroids who were planning to travel to endemic regions for YF. The control group consisted of healthy individuals matched for age and history of YFV. The safety and immunogenicity of the 17D vaccine was

evaluated. Forty participants in the study group and 77 in the control group were enrolled. The main diseases of the study group were RA and other CIMIDs. The dose of prednisone or equivalent ranged from 5 to 20 mg/day, and 71% had been using the drug for more than 15 days before the YFV, with an average of ten months of use [48]. There were no serious adverse events; however, the patient group presented a higher frequency of mild reactions, with relative risk (RR) = 8.0 and a 95% confidence interval (CI): 1.4–45.9. In this study, the neutralizing antibodies were also measured by PRNT. All participants had titers ≥1:10. There were no differences between the groups that received primary or booster YFV [48]. It is important to mention they specifically evaluated patients vaccinated while using corticosteroids. However, the dosage was low, not reaching immunosuppressive doses. Furthermore, as the study was not blind, bias may have occurred [48].

Recently, Wieten et al. (2016) studied 15 immunocompromised patients who were vaccinated inadvertently or after a risk-benefit analysis had been performed by the attending physician. Neutralizing antibodies were measured by PRNT, and an analysis of PBMC (peripheral blood mononuclear cells) and T cells as well as analysis of the cytokine profile produced by CD8+ lymphocytes specific for the yellow fever virus were performed. The results were compared to a control group composed of 41 healthy individuals who were matched for age, sex, and time of vaccination [41, 42].

The neutralizing antibody dosage was similar between groups, with 100% of the immunocompromised individuals and 96.7% of the control group presenting protective levels. Specific CD8+ cells, were also comparable in relation to the frequency, with a gradual decline over the years after vaccination. Other results showed that there were no significant differences in the phenotypic and cytotoxic profile of specific T cells. The production of cytokines was also equivalent between the groups [41, 42].

This was the first study to analyze the profile of the immunological alterations post the YFV in immunocompromised individuals, although the sample was small and became even smaller when the authors performed the analysis of subgroups.

In another study, Wieten et al. (2016) analyzed blood samples from 15 immunocompromised patients and 12 healthy controls in order to compare PRNT and serology values by immunofluorescence. Of the patients evaluated, 11 were on methotrexate, two on etanercept, one on prednisone, and one on leflunomide. The medication was withdrawn around two to six weeks in three patients. Using the PRNT method, 100% of the study group demonstrated protective levels of neutralizing antibodies compared to 83.3% of the control group. Regarding immunofluorescence serology, only 47% of the study group was seropositive, and no sample was positive in the control group. There was no correlation between PRNT and immunofluorescence [21, 41, 42].

A recent Brazilian study by Ferreira et al. (2017), performed a long-term follow-up including 144 RA patients treated with immunomodulatory and immunosuppressive specific drugs who were inadvertently vaccinated. The authors evaluated the humoral and cellular immunity profile to YFV and demonstrated a reduced frequency of memory lymphocytes among previously vaccinated patients when compared to healthy controls. Based on this data, the authors concluded that patients taking synthetic or biological drugs were unprotected by the 17DD YFV after a five-year follow-up [43]. This is an ongoing study and we had access to only partial results from a conference abstract.

There are some case reports in the literature to support these results, such as a 63-year-old woman diagnosed with Crohn's disease who received the 17D vaccine during the use of adalimumab. The vaccine was given four days before the next dose, which is usually administered every 14 days. Blood samples were collected on days 12, 18, and 26 post-immunization for viral RNA analysis and detection of neutralizing antibodies. There were no adverse effects. No viremia was detected on day 12, and from day 18 onward, protective levels of neutralizing antibodies were recorded. In this case, it is important to point out that it was the primary dose [49].

All the studies were judged as very low quality of evidence due to methodological limitations, including small sample sizes and lack of statistical data to evaluate the magnitude of the effect. Another limitation identified was a wide range of follow-up and analyses applied in the studies, varying from six days to eight years.

Additionally, given the lack of consensus on defining immunosuppression degrees among national and international Societies and evidence to support this strategy, the Brazilian societies involved in the treatment of patients with CIMID assembled to discuss and vote on it, aiming to standardize these definitions and enable establishment of recommendations. A panel of 22 specialists, representing several committees of the BRS, in addition to two representatives of the Brazilian Society of Dermatology (BDS), the Brazilian Infectious Diseases Society (BIDS), and the study group on Inflammatory Bowel Diseases (GEDIIB), conducted a careful literature review. This step was followed by anonymous voting to categorize the immunosuppression degree of patients with CIMID. For this classification, more than 80% agreement was required among the members for each item, applied to develop the recommendations for vaccine indication or contraindication.

Complete information on this part of the guidelines process will be published in a separate paper by the same work group (Manuscript in preparation).

Table 3 summarizes the position of the BRS and the immunosuppression degree conferred by the drugs used to treat patients with CIMID, considering the class of medication and mechanism of action.

As a result, eight recommendations were developed regarding the safety of YFV in patients with CIMID and the immunosuppression degree conferred by the treatment used.

Since there was no consistent evidence to support any kind of conclusion or position for the last question formulated as part of the primary objective, on the immunogenicity to YFV in patients with CIMID, the unanimous decision of the panel of members was that it was not possible to establish recommendations on the effectiveness, in the short and long-term, of YFV in these patients; therefore, the results on this issue will only be described.

Recommendations

1. *YFV should not be administered to patients with CIMID under high immunosuppression. For patients with a low degree or no immunosuppression, it is recommended that the risk of the vaccine be assessed individually. This evaluation should be performed by a physician, preferably the specialist assisting the patient (QoE: very low, LoA: > 90% of agreement).*

2. *YFV should not be administered to patients with CIMID with high activity of the underlying disease. However, in clinically stable patients or those with no activity of the underlying disease there is no contraindication to vaccination. The risk to vaccinate in these situations should be assessed individually by a physician, preferably the specialist assisting the patient (QoE: very low, LoA: > 90% of agreement)*

3. *YFV should not be administered to patients with CIMID using a high dose of corticosteroid. The risk of vaccinating patients receiving low doses should be assessed individually by a physician, preferably the specialist assisting the patient (QoE: very low, LoA: > 90% of agreement).*

We emphasize an individual-based evaluation, ideally shared decision making (SDM) [50], considering the risks and benefits of vaccination, especially in a high-risk epidemiological setting, because of the severity and mortality rate related to YF infection, as

Table 3 Immunosuppression degree conferred by drugs used to treat patients with chronic immune-mediated inflammatory diseases: Positioning of the Brazilian Societies of Rheumatology, Dermatology and Study Groups on Inflammatory Bowel Diseases

Non-immunosuppressed

Those clinically stable under the following conditions:
No drug treatment
Only using sulfasalazine or hydroxychloroquine or mesalazine or acitretin
Using topical, inhaled, peri or intra-articular corticosteroids

Low immunosuppression degree

Using:
Methotrexate at a dose of ≤0.4 mg/kg/week or ≤ 20 mg/week
Leflunomide at a dose of ≤20 mg/day[a]
Corticosteroid at a dose of ≤20 mg/day (or 2 mg/kg/day for patients weighing < 10 kg) prednisone or equivalent

High immunosuppression degree

Using:
Corticosteroid at a dose of ≥20 mg/day (or > 2 mg/kg/day for patients weighing < 10 kg) prednisone or equivalent, for a period ≥14 days
Pulsotherapy with methylprednisolone
Immunosuppressants as mycophenolate mofetil or sodic, cyclosporine, cyclophosphamide, tacrolimus, azathioprine
JAK inhibitors, such as tofacitinib[b]
b-DMARD

bDMARD: biologic disease modifying anti-rheumatic drugs; As the dosage of serum level of leflunomide is difficult and the studies on the risk of vaccinating individuals taking leflunomide at the usual doses are lacked, in cases requiring vaccination, a drug elimination regimen of 8 g of cholestyramine 3 times/day for 11 days or 50 g of activated charcoal 4 times/day for 11 days must be prescribed (similar to Sanofi Pasteur Laboratory recommendation when a woman taking leflunomide become pregnant). If the leflunomide plasma level determination is available it is recommended to reach nondetectable levels (i.e., below 0.02 mg/l) before vaccination

well as the possible adverse events of the YFV in an immunosuppression context [8, 13].

The Center for Diseases Control and Prevention (CDC) used the GRADE system to evaluate the evidence of SAE following YFV and 1255 cases with a report of SAE following YFV were identified. For the majority (84%) of subjects, it was unknown if the SAE occurred following a primary or booster dose of the vaccine. Furthermore, it was not known how many of the 437 million doses of YFV were administered as a primary or booster dose. Of the 201 subjects for whom SAE was reported, the dose type was known, whereas 14 (7%) occurred following a booster dose of vaccine [13, 19, 51–55].

In this systematic review, YEL-AVD was reported for 72 subjects; in 41 (57%) it was unknown if the event occurred following a primary or booster dose of the vaccine. Of the 31 subjects for whom the dose type was known, one (3%) subject had YEL-AVD after receiving a booster dose of the vaccine; no laboratory testing was performed for that case [10, 11, 14, 15, 34, 52, 56–60]. In the same review, YFV-AND was reported for 218

subjects. For 108 (50%) subjects it was not known whether YEL-AVD occurred following a primary or booster dose of the vaccine. Of the 110 subjects for whom the dose type was known, three (3%) subjects reported YFV-AND after receiving a booster dose of the vaccine. All three cases were reported as an autoimmune-mediated event rather than direct vaccine viral invasion of the central nervous system and no specific laboratory testing was available to assess vaccine causality [10, 17, 52, 56–59, 61, 62].

SAE in altered immune status patients
It is well established that YFV is contraindicated in people with a thymus disorder associated with abnormal immune cell function, such as thymoma or myasthenia gravis. YFV is contraindicated in people with AIDS or other clinical HIV manifestations, including patients with CD4+ T lymphocyte values $< 200/mm^3$ or < 15% of total lymphocytes for children aged < 6 years. This recommendation is based on the potential increased risk of encephalitis in this population. It is also contraindicated in patients with primary immunodeficiencies, as well as those with malignant neoplasms or transplants.

There are no data regarding possible increased adverse events or decreased vaccine effectiveness after YFV administration to patients with other chronic medical conditions (such as renal disease, hepatitis C virus infection, diabetes mellitus, and CIMID). Factors to be considered when assessing a patient's general level of immune competence include disease severity and activity, complications, comorbidities, and current treatment programs, mainly immunosuppressants. As there are no specific data on the use of YFV in these populations to date, the use of LAV is contraindicated according to the majority of package inserts in these therapies.

According to CDC, there are no data available on disease activity and medication used in nine patients diagnosed or potentially diagnosed with autoimmune diseases who developed YEL-AVD by the year 2016 and could potentially be under treatment with immunosuppressive agents. Four out of nine patients were older than 60 years, and two had a previous history of thymectomy – both situations are considered a risk factor for YEL-AVD [11]. According to the CDC and Advisory Committee on Immunization Practices (ACIP) recommendations, there are no contraindications or precautions for this special group of patients regarding underlying diseases. However, the contraindications should be carefully observed, and consideration given to the precautions for vaccination when patients are receiving immunosuppressive therapy, following the recommendations for immunosuppressed individuals [12, 13, 19].

Nevertheless, there are some studies performed in Brazil that have shown no SAE related to YFV. The first, published by Mota et al. (2009), reported retrospective data from 70 patients with various rheumatic diseases such as RA, SLE, Spo, and systemic sclerosis (SyS) who were inadvertently vaccinated with YFV. All participants were receiving immunosuppressive therapy. Among them, 22.8% reported mild adverse events such as rash, headache, and myalgia. There were no serious adverse events, hospitalizations, or deaths due to immunization [35].

Recently, Valim et al. (2017), enrolled 241 patients with rheumatic diseases for whom no SAE was reported, s described above [46]. Additionally, case reports of patients with CIMID using synthetic or biological DMARDs were described without any reported of SAE [33, 35, 41, 42, 44, 45, 49, 63–67].

Since there are scarce data on LAV, such as YFV, in patients with CIMID, guidelines on vaccination for this group are less evidence-based than other immunosuppressive conditions. In addition, it is almost impossible to establish a real causal correlation between an AEFV related to YFV and a CIMID, as this group of diseases encompasses a range of clinical presentation conditions and multivariate manifestations, as well as they have particular differences considering the type of treatment, in general inducing immunosuppressive drugs. These all variables together inducing a wide variation in the immunosuppression degree, which could be further related to susceptibility to infections and can be considered a cause of SAE per se.

Therefore, this section provides recommendations based on the best data available and the practices of experienced clinicians. A special comment about the fractional YFV dose campaign should be highlighted, as, besides the balance between risk/benefits, it is also necessary to consider the shortage of the vaccine. In this situation, if there is an endorsement by national health authorities, our advice is to follow the same recommendations regarding the vaccination safety in patients with CIMID.

4. *Revaccination with YFV should not be administered to patients with CIMID under high immunosuppression. In specific situations in which a booster is necessary, the risk of vaccinating patients with a low or no immunosuppression degree should be assessed individually by a physician, preferably the specialist assisting the patient (QoE: Very low, LOA: > 90% of agreement)*

Although booster doses of YFV are not recommended in current epidemiological settings in Brazil, this is a matter of debate. For ACIP and CDC, a booster is recommended for special groups, such as those with HIV, post-transplant patients, and may be considered for travelers who received their previous dose of YFV ≥10 years ago and plan to remain for a prolonged period in endemic or ongoing outbreak areas [13, 19].

5. *In situations of risk, when YFV is indicated, a minimum interval of four weeks is recommended between application of the vaccine and the initiation or resumption of treatment with immunomodulatory and immunosuppressive drugs (QoE: very low, LOA: > 90% of agreement).*

6. *In situations of risk, when YFV is indicated, a minimum period after the suspension of medications prior to the application of the vaccine is recommended, varying according to the immunosuppression degree. Advice on treatment discontinuation should be individualized and given by a specialist (QoE: very low, LOA: > 90% of agreement).*

There is no strong and consistent evidence to be used as the foundation for establishing recommendations about whether patients with CIMID should be undergoing therapy or not when receiving LAV. The majority of healthcare work in this field follows guidelines based on the experience of other specialists, who manage immunosuppressive therapy in their clinical practice more frequently (e.g. oncologists).

Papadopoulou and Sipsas (2014) performed a search for all the guidelines available on the vaccination of adult patients with CIMID. The authors identified specific protocols in 21 national rheumatology societies, all of them built on an expert opinion panel. Points of agreement include avoiding the use of LAV in immunosuppressed patients. However, the most important differences were based on the immunosuppression degree of patients under different treatments, such as the steroid dose that induces immunosuppression, the time interval between LAV, and the initiation of immunosuppressive treatment. The authors concluded that these significant differences among national recommendations on immunizations in patients with CIMID reflected the lack of evidence-based data [32].

A defined safety period between the onset or withdrawal from immunosuppressive therapy and a vaccination with LAV in patients with CIMID has not been studied; subsequently, the majority of the guidelines are based on expert opinion. There is consensus between the guidelines among the international societies regarding the period recommended between LAV and therapy onset, which is at least one month [30, 31, 33, 68]. However, there is no consensus among these experts on how long the temporary discontinuation of immunosuppressive medication should be before vaccination with LAV.

Thus, considering the epidemiological scenario in Brazil and the need for a specific recommendation on YFV for this population, we were motivated to defend our position that the immunosuppression degree induced by the treatment should be the basis for an individualized and safer approach to the vaccination of patients with CIMID. Complete information regarding this study can be found in another publication from this group (Manuscript in preparation). The recommended period that clinicians should wait, after discontinuation of therapy, to administer a live vaccine, is shown in Table 4.

> 7. *When YFV is indicated to patients with CIMID, it is recommended that it not be applied concurrently with another live attenuated virus vaccine, primarily with MMR (measles, mumps, and rubella). When indicated, a 28-day interval between the application of these vaccines is recommended (QoE: Very low, LOA: > 90% agreement)*

There is no evidence that inactivated vaccines interfere in the immune response to the yellow fever vaccine. Therefore, inactivated vaccines can be administered either simultaneously or at any time before or after the yellow fever vaccination. The ACIP recommends that the YFV should be administered either simultaneously or 30 days apart from other live viral vaccines as the immune response to one live virus vaccine might be impaired if administered within 30 days of another LAV [2, 69]. One study involving the simultaneous administration of YFV and MMR vaccines in children found a decrease in the immune response to yellow fever, mumps, and rubella when the vaccines were given on the same day versus 30 days apart. Additional studies are needed to confirm these findings, but they suggest that, if possible, the yellow fever and MMR vaccines should be administered 30 days apart.

> 8. *There is no contraindication of YFV in those in close contact with immunocompromised patients, since the transmission of the vaccine virus without vector participation is documented only through breast milk, blood donation, and, possibly, by accidental contact with biological materials (QoE: Very low, LOA: > 90% of agreement)*

Healthy and immunocompetent subjects living with immunocompromised patients can and should receive LAV as well as inactivated vaccines, such as MMR, the rotavirus vaccine, varicella, and shingles. In addition, these subjects can safely receive vaccines recommended for travelers, such as typhoid fever and yellow fever [70].

According to the CDC, there is no evidence that people receiving YFV can eliminate the vaccine virus through any specimens [19]. Although detected in the urine of vaccinated individuals, the presence of the yellow fever vaccine virus has never been related to this route of transmission [71].

There is a theoretical risk of YFV being transmitted through blood products, but patients should be allowed to donate two to four weeks after vaccination [72, 73]. In April 2009, the transmission of the yellow fever vaccine virus through breast milk was documented in Brazil for the first time [73, 74].

Discussion

The development of tailored recommendations for indicating YFV to patients with CIMID, receiving immunosuppressive therapy or not, was a pragmatic project in the field of rheumatology and related specialties. Given the paucity of scientific literature on vaccination for this particular group of patients, the most suitable approach to be adopted was to gather specialists from different areas, together with patients, in an attempt to define the recommendations in a setting with a high YF burden, in light of the knowledge that recommendations in the literature in different settings may not be the most appropriate for this specific group.

Table 4 Minimal period recommended between therapy withdrawal and yellow fever vaccination in patients with CIMID

Drug	Interval between withdrawal and YFV
Prednisone > 20 mg/day or pulse methylprednisolone	At least one month
Hydroxychloroquine, sulfasalazine, acitretin, methotrexate ≤20 mg/week, or leflunomide 20 mg/day[a]	Consider vaccination without interval
Methotrexate > 20 mg/week	At least 1 month
Azathioprine, mycophenolate mofetil or sodic, cyclosporine, tacrolimus, or cyclophosphamide	At least 3 months
Tofacitinib	At least 2 weeks
Anti-cytokines and co-stimulation inhibitor	4–5 half-lives[b]
B-lymphocyte depletors	6–12 months

the medical criterion to carry out the drug elimination protocol before indicating the vaccine [b]based on pharmacological half-life, except for B-lymphocyte depletors

Strengths

To our knowledge, this is the first paper to address specific questions, using a Guidelines Grade approach, involving specialists from many areas and patients, on the management of YFV in patients with CIMID living or traveling to YF endemic areas. This paper approaches a real need, assessed by clinicians and patient care groups and might have global applicability, contributing to and supporting vaccination practices.

Additionally, the participation of patients is inedited in the decision process as a motivation to shared decision-making (SDM). It has been argued that SDM represents the pinnacle of patient-centered care; well-informed preference-based patient decisions might lead to safer, more cost-effective healthcare, which in turn might result in improved health outcomes. In practice, these SDMs are seen to occur to a limited extent. In this process, although a patient may not want to make any final decision, they should still be involved in the development of important but difficult recommendations, such as eliciting their concerns and views. Knowledge and awareness among both professionals and patients, as well as tools and skills training, are needed for SDM to become widely implemented [75].

Limitations

Due to the lack of evidence in the literature to help the development of these recommendations, they were mainly based on expert opinion and panel making decisions. Further research and advances will lead to future revisions and updates.

Thus, in particular here, we consider essential a SDM approach on taking the YFV or not, since these recommendations were based on few evidences and mostly in expert opinion.

Conclusions

The number of patients with CIMID is increasing as well as those exposed to therapy with a varied range of immunosuppressive degrees. In Brazil, we are facing an alarming epidemic scenario of YF, which is reaching the most populous areas in the country in unvaccinated people.

The majority of vaccination guidelines for this special population do not define recommendations or measures to plan the YFV for this particular group. Thus, given the urgent need for specific recommendations on YFV for this population and the lack of available evidence in the literature, the Brazilian Society of Rheumatology gathered a panel of experts, including representatives from five other related Societies, together with patients, to build these recommendations, prioritizing the vaccination safety and motivation for SDM. These are summarized in Table 5.

Last but not least, our work group would like to address a particular concern of great importance that should be given to the vaccine effectiveness. Due to the lack of evidence regarding short or long-term responses to the primary vaccination, we were not able to draw any recommendations or even advice in this field. However, we consider it fundamental to inform patients with CIMID, who have been inadvertently vaccinated under immunosuppression, that they may not have developed a proper response to the vaccine, so they are advised to take care when exposed to YF high-risk areas, until protection is confirmed by a post vaccination test (PRNT).

Finally, we hope this document will encourage all health professionals involved in the care of this special group of patients, to incorporate vaccination planning into their clinical practice, considering both safety and satisfactory immunogenicity.

Table 5 List of recommendations for yellow fever vaccine (YFV) administration in patients with CIMID

1. YFV should not be administered to patients with CIMID under high immunosuppression. For patients with a low degree or no immunosuppression, it is recommended to assess individually the risk of the vaccine. This evaluation should be performed by a physician, preferably the specialist assisting the patient

2. YFV should not be administered to patients with CIMID with high activity of the underlying disease. However, in clinically stable patients or those with no activity of the underlying disease there is no contraindication to vaccination. The risk to vaccinate in these situations should be assessed individually by a physician, preferably the specialist assisting the patient

3. YFV should not be administered to patients with CIMID using a high dose of corticosteroid. The risk of vaccinating patients receiving low doses should be assessed individually by a physician, preferably the specialist assisting the patient

4. Revaccination with YFV is not recommended for patients with CIMID under high immunosuppression. In specific situations in which a booster is necessary, the risk of vaccinating patients with a low or no immunosuppression degree should be assessed individually by a physician, preferably the specialist assisting the patient

5. In situations of risk, when YFV is indicated, a minimum interval of four weeks is recommended between application of the vaccine and the initiation or resumption of treatment with immunomodulatory and immunosuppressive drugs

6. In situations of risk, when YFV is indicated, a minimum period after the suspension of medications prior to the application of the vaccine is recommended, varying according to the immunosuppression degree. Advice on treatment discontinuation should be individualized and given by a specialist

7. When YFV is indicated in patients with CIMID, it is recommended that it not be applied concurrently with another live attenuated virus vaccine, primarily with the MMR (measles, mumps, and rubella). When indicated, a 28-day interval between the application of these vaccines is recommended

8. There is no contraindication of YFV in those in close contact with immunocompromised patients, since the transmission of the vaccine virus without vector participation is documented only through breast milk, blood donation, and, possibly, by accidental contact with biological materials

Abbreviations

ACIP: Advisory Committee on Immunization Practices; ACR: American College of Rheumatology; AEFV: Adverse Event Following Vaccination; AIDS: Acquired Immunodeficiency Syndrome; AS: Ankylosing Spondylitis; BDM: Brazilian Dermatology Society; bDMARD: Biological Disease-Modifying Drugs; BIDS: Brazilian Infectious Diseases Society; BRS: Brazilian Rheumatology Society; CDC: Centers for Diseases Control and Prevention; CIMID: Chronic Immune-Mediated Inflammatory Diseases; csDMARD: Conventional Synthetic Disease-Modifying Drugs; DMARD: Disease Modifying Anti-Rheumatic Drugs; EULAR: European League Against Rheumatism; GEDIIB: Inflammatory Bowel Diseases Study Group; GRADE: Grading of Recommendations Assessment, Development and Evaluation Working Group; HIV: Human Immunodeficiency Virus; IBD: Inflammatory Bowel Diseases; IFA: Indirect Immunofluorescence Test; IFIT: Tetracyclic Peptide Repeats; IL: Interleukin; IRF: Interferon Regulator Factor; LAV: Live Attenuated Vaccines; LoA: Level of Agreement; MMR: Measles-Mumps-Rubella; MS: Multiple Sclerosis; PBMC: Peripheral Blood Mononuclear Cells; PCR: C-reactive protein; PRNT: Plaque Reduction Neutralization Test; PsoA: Psoriatic Arthritis; QoE: Quality of the Evidence; RA : Rheumatoid Arthritis; RNA : Ribonucleic Acid; RR: Relative Risk; SAE: Serious Adverse Event; SDM: Shared decision-making; SLE: Systemic Lupus Erythematosus; SPF : Specific Pathogen Free; Spo: Spondyloarthropathies; STAT: Transcription Activator; SyS: Systemic Sclerosis; TLR: Toll-like receptor; TNF: Tumor Necrosis Factor; TNFi: Tumor Necrosis Factor Inhibitors; tsDMARD: Synthetic Target-Specific Disease-Modifying Drugs; WHO: World Health Organization; YEL-AND: Yellow Fever Vaccine-Associated Neurotropic Disease; YEL-AVD: Yellow Fever Vaccine-Associated Viscerotropic Disease; YF: Yellow Fever; YFV: Yellow Fever Vaccine

Acknowledgements

The authors would like to thank Priscila Torres and Eduardo Tenorio, both patients from the supporting groups *Encontrar/Grupar* and *Superando o Lupus* for participating in the panel and attending the meeting. Furthermore, we would like to give special thanks to Dr. Jose Tupinanbá Sousa Vasconcelos, scientific director of SBR, for the fundamental support to this work.

Authors' contributions

The oversight committee was involved in searching the literature and selecting studies. All the authors contributed to analyzing the studies, and drafting or critically revising the manuscript for important intellectual content. All of them gave their final approval of the version to be published and have sufficiently participated in the study to take public responsibility for the content; and agree to be accountable for all aspects of the study in ensuring that questions related to the accuracy or integrity of any part of the study are appropriately investigated and resolved.

Competing interests

Adriana Maria Kakehasi Research funds: CNPq, SBR, FAPEMIG Support for Scientific Events: Abbvie, BMS, Janssen Lecture Fees: UCB, Janssen, Pfizer, Roche, BMS Clinical research: Roche, Pfizer Advisory board: Janssen, Roche, BMS, Pfizer.

Alexandre Wagner S de Souza has received financial support as an advisory board member for Roche. Financial competing interest: none.

Caroline Araújo Magnata da Fonte: none.

Clayton Brenol Has received personal or institutional support from Abbvie, Bristol, Janssen, Pfizer and Roche; has delivered speeches at events related to this work and sponsored by Abbvie, Pfizer and Roche. Financial competing interest: none.

Claudia Marques: Non-financial and financial competing interests related to this publication

Cyrla Zaltman: Non-financial and financial competing interests related to this publication

Eduardo Ferreira Borba was supported by grants from Conselho Nacional de Desenvolvimento Científico e Tecnológico (CNPq #307226/2014-0). Financial competing interest: none.

Gecilmara Salviato Pileggi has received fees for lectures and talks at events related to this study sponsored by Abbvie, Janssen, and UCB. The authors declare no financial competing interest.

Georges Basile Christopoulos: none

Ieda M M Laurindo – has no competing interests related to this work. Financial competing interests: none.

Isabella Ballalai: has received funding for meetings related to this work sponsored by the Brazilian Ministry of Health (CTAI-PNI), fees for lectures and advisory board sponsored by Sanofi Pasteur, Pfizer and MSD.

Izaias Pereira da Costa Non-financial competing interests

Lessandra Michelin has received funding for meetings related to this work sponsored by the Brazilian Ministry of Health (CTAI-PNI). Financial competing interest: none.

Licia Maria Henrique da Mota Has received personal or institutional support from Abbvie, Janssen, Pfizer and Roche; has delivered speeches at events related to this work and sponsored by Abbvie, Janssen, Pfizer, Roche and UCB. Financial competing interest: none.

Lilian David de Azevêdo Valadares has received for lectures fees and speeches at events related to this work sponsored by Janssen and Novartis. Financial competing interest: none.

Liliana Andrade Chebli has received for lecture fees and speeches at events not related to this work sponsored by Takeda. Financial competing interest: none.

Marcos Renato de Assis has received personal or institutional support from Apsen and Lilly; has given lectures and/or consultancy to Novartis, UCB and Janssen not related to this work. Financial competing interest: none.

Marcus Vinícius Guimarães de Lacerda has no conflict of interest.

Michel Alexandre Yazbek has no competing interests related to this work. Financial competing interests: none.

Rejane Maria Rodrigues de Abreu Vieira has no conflicts of interest.

Renato Kfouri has received fees for lectures and advisory board sponsored by Sanofi Pasteur.

Rosana Richtmann has received for lectures fees sponsored by Abbvie, Pfizer and MSD. Financial competing interest: none.

Selma Merenlender is presently supported by SRRJ.

Valéria Valim has no competing interest.

Author details

[1]SBR. Faculdade de Ciências da Saúde de Barretos – FACISB, Barretos, São Paulo, Brazil. [2]SBR. Serviço de Reumatologia do Hospital Universitário de Brasília, Universidade de Brasília, Brasília, Brazil. [3]SBR. Faculdade de Medicina, Universidade Federal de Minas Gerais, Belo Horizonte, Brazil. [4]SBR. Escola Paulista de Medicina, Universidade Federal de São Paulo, São Paulo, Brazil. [5]Pós graduanda do programa de Medicina Baseada em Evidências, Universidade Federal do Estado de São Paulo (UNIFESP), São Paulo, Brazil. [6]SBR. Hospital Universitário Lauro Wanderley, Universidade Federal da Paraíba (UFPB), João Pessoa, Brazil. [7]SBR. Hospital Getulio Vargas, Recife, Brazil. [8]SBD. Faculdade de Medicina do ABC, Santo Andre, Brazil. [9]SBR. Hospital de Clínicas de Porto Alegre, Universidade Federal do Rio Grande do Sul, Porto Alegre, Brazil. [10]SBR. Hospital das Clínicas, Universidade Federal de Pernambuco, Recife, Brazil. [11]GEDIIB. Presidente do GEDIIB 2017-2019, Universidade Federal do Rio de Janeiro, Rio de Janeiro, Brazil. [12]SBR. Hospital das Clinicas, Faculdade de Medicina, Universidade de Sao Paulo, Sao Paulo, Brazil. [13]SBR. Diretor médico do Centro de infusão do Hospital Humanitas, Varginha, Brazil. [14]SBR. Unidade Docente Assistencial de Reumatologia, Universidade do Estado do Rio de Janeiro, Rio de Janeiro, Brazil. [15]SBR. Presidente da Sociedade Brasileira de Reumatologia, Maceió-AL, Brazil. [16]SBR. Escola de Medicina da Universidade Nove de Julho, São Paulo, Brazil. [17]SBIm. Vice-Presidente da Sociedade Brasileira de Imunizações (SBIm), SBiM, Rio de Janeiro, Brazil. [18]SBR. Professor da Faculdade de Medicina da Universidade Federal do Mato Grosso do Sul, Cuiabá, Brazil. [19]SBI. Professora na faculdade de Medicina, Universidade de Caxias do Sul, Caxias do Sul, Brazil. [20]SBR. Reumatologista. Hospital Getulio Vargas, Recife, Brazil. [21]GEDIIB, Faculdade de Medicina da Universidade Federal de Juiz de Fora, Juiz de Fora, Brazil. [22]SMBT. Instituto Leônidas e Maria Deane (Fiocruz - Amazônia), Fundação de Medicina Tropical Dr. Heitor Vieira Dourado (FMT-HVD), Maceio-AL, Brazil. [23]SBR. Medica reguladora da Secretaria Estadual da Saúde de Santa Catarina, Florianópolis, Brazil. [24]SBR. Escola de Medicina, Universidade Estadual de

Campinas, Campinas, Brazil. [25]SBR. Hospital Geral de Fortaleza e Universidade de Fortaleza, Fortaleza, Brazil. [26]SBD. Faculdade de Medicina da Universidade Estadual de Campinas, Campinas, Brazil. [27]SBIm. Presidente do Departamento de Imunizações da Sociedade Brasileira de Pediatria (SBP), Maceio-AL, Brazil. [28]SBI. Instituto de Infectologia Emilio Ribas, Maceio-AL, Brazil. [29]SBR. Presidente da SRRJ. Chefe do Serviço de Reumatologia do Hospital Estadual Eduardo Rabelo RJ, Rio de Janeiro, Brazil. [30]SBR. Faculdade de Medicina, Universidade Federal do Espírito Santo, Vitória, Brazil. [31]SBR. Escola Médica de Marilia, Marilia, Brazil. [32]SBR. Universidade federal do Paraná, Curitiba, Brazil. [33]SBR. Universidade Federal de São Paulo (UNIFESP), São Paulo; Universidade Santo Amaro (UNISA), Sao Paulo, Brazil. [34]School of Medical Science Barretos-FACISB, Avenue Masonic Lodge Renovadora 68, No. 100 - Airport Neighborhood, Barretos/SP 14785-002, Brazil.

References

1. Monath TP. Yellow fever: an update. Lancet Infect Dis. 2001;1:11–20.
2. Staples JE, Gershman M, Fischer M, Centers for Disease C, Prevention. Yellow fever vaccine: recommendations of the advisory committee on immunization practices (ACIP). MMWR Recomm Rep. 2010;59(RR-7):1–27.
3. Brasil: Febre amarela - Guia para Profissionais de Saúde. Ministério da Saúde do Brasil.Brasília; 2018.
4. Febre amarela: Ministério da Saúde atualiza casos no país. In:[http://portalms.saude.boletim-epidemiologico/noticias/agencia-saude/42940-febre-amarela-ministerio-da-saude-atualiza-casos-no-pais-6]. Acess in 24/nov/2018.
5. Verma R, Khanna P, Chawla S. Yellow fever vaccine: an effective vaccine for travelers. Hum Vaccin Immunother. 2014;10(1):126–8.
6. Campi-Azevedo AC, Costa-Pereira C, Antonelli LR, Fonseca CT, Teixeira-Carvalho A, et al. Booster dose after 10 years is recommended following 17DD-YF primary vaccination. Hum Vaccin Immunother. 2016; 12(2):491–502.
7. Cavalcante KR, Tauil PL. Epidemiological characteristics of yellow fever in Brazil, 2000-2012. Epidemiol Serv Saude. 2016;25(1):11–20.
8. Lindsey NP, Schroeder BA, Miller ER, Braun MM, Hinckley AF, Marano N, et al. Adverse event reports following yellow fever vaccination. Vaccine. 2008; 26(48):6077–82.
9. WHO. Immunization Safety Surveillance: Guidelines for Immunization Programme Managers on Surveillance of Adverse Events Following Immunization Regional Office for the Western Pacific Region. World Health Organization. Manila: WHO Press; 2013.
10. Breugelmans JG, Lewis RF, Agbenu E, Veit O, Jackson D, Domingo C, et al. Adverse events following yellow fever preventive vaccination campaigns in eight African countries from 2007 to 2010. Vaccine. 2013;31(14):1819–29.
11. Whittembury A, Ramirez G, Hernandez H, Ropero AM, Waterman S, Ticona M, et al. Viscerotropic disease following yellow fever vaccination in Peru. Vaccine. 2009;27(43):5974–81.
12. Ferreira CC, Campi-Azevedo AC, Peruhype-Magalhaes V, Costa-Pereira C, Albuquerque CP, Muniz LF, Yokoy de Souza T, et al. The 17D-204 and 17DD yellow fever vaccines: an overview of major similarities and subtle differences. Expert Rev Vaccines. 2018;17(1):79–90.
13. Chiodini J. The CDC yellow book app 2018. Travel Med Infect Dis. 2017.
14. Gershman MD, Staples JE, Bentsi-Enchill AD, Breugelmans JG, Brito GS, Camacho LA, et al. Viscerotropic disease: case definition and guidelines for collection, analysis, and presentation of immunization safety data. Vaccine. 2012;30(33):5038–58.
15. Thomas RE. Yellow fever vaccine-associated viscerotropic disease: current perspectives. Drug Des Devel Ther. 2016;10:3345–53.
16. Staples JE, Gershman MD. Yellow fever vaccines. In: Plotkin SAOW, Offit PA, Edwards KM, editors. Vaccine. 7th ed. Philadelhia: Elsevier; 2017.
17. Martins R, Pavao AL, de Oliveira PM, dos Santos PR, Carvalho SM, Mohrdieck RF, et al. Adverse events following yellow fever immunization: report and analysis of 67 neurological cases in Brazil. Vaccine. 2014;32(49):6676–82.
18. Gotuzzo E, Yactayo S, Cordova E. Efficacy and duration of immunity after yellow fever vaccination: systematic review on the need for a booster every 10 years. Am J Trop Med Hyg. 2013;89(3):434–44.
19. Staples JE, Bocchini JA, Rubin L Jr, Fischer M. Yellow fever vaccine booster doses: recommendations of the advisory committee on immunization practices, 2015. MMWR Morb Mortal Wkly Rep. 2015; 64(23):647–50.
20. Amanna IJ, Slifka MK. Questions regarding the safety and duration of immunity following live yellow fever vaccination. Expert Rev Vaccines. 2016; 15(12):1519–33.
21. Wieten RW, Jonker EF, van Leeuwen EM, Remmerswaal EB, Ten Berge IJ, de Visser AW, et al. A single 17D yellow fever vaccination provides lifelong immunity; characterization of yellow-fever-specific neutralizing antibody and T-cell responses after vaccination. PLoS One. 2016;11(3):e0149871.
22. Ahuka-Mundeke S, Casey RM, Harris JB, Dixon MG, Nsele PM, Kizito GM, et al. Immunogenicity of fractional-dose vaccine during a yellow fever outbreak - preliminary report. N Engl J Med. 2018.
23. Watson AM, Klimstra WB. T cell-mediated immunity towards yellow fever virus and useful animal models. Viruses. 2017;9(4).
24. Simoes M, Camacho LA, Yamamura AM, Miranda EH, Cajaraville AC, da Silva Freire M. Evaluation of accuracy and reliability of the plaque reduction neutralization test (micro-PRNT) in detection of yellow fever virus antibodies. Biologicals. 2012;40(6):399–404.
25. Mercier-Delarue S, Durier C, Colin de Verdiere N, Poveda JD, Meiffredy V, Fernandez Garcia MD, et al. Screening test for neutralizing antibodies against yellow fever virus, based on a flavivirus pseudotype. PLoS One. 2017;12(5):e0177882.
26. Silva ML, Martins MA, Espirito-Santo LR, Campi-Azevedo AC, Silveira-Lemos D, Ribeiro JG, et al. Characterization of main cytokine sources from the innate and adaptive immune responses following primary 17DD yellow fever vaccination in adults. Vaccine. 2011;29(3):583–92.
27. Fuertes Marraco SA, Soneson C, Cagnon L, Gannon PO, Allard M, Abed Maillard S, et al. Long-lasting stem cell-like memory CD8+ T cells with a naive-like profile upon yellow fever vaccination. Sci Transl Med. 2015;7(282):282ra248.
28. Bayry J, Radstake TR. Immune-mediated inflammatory diseases: progress in molecular pathogenesis and therapeutic strategies. Expert Rev Clin Immunol. 2013;9(4):297–9.
29. Youinou P, Pers JO, Gershwin ME, Shoenfeld Y. Geo-epidemiology and autoimmunity. J Autoimmun. 2010;34(3):J163–7.
30. Buhler S, Eperon G, Ribi C, Kyburz D, van Gompel F, Visser LG, et al. Vaccination recommendations for adult patients with autoimmune inflammatory rheumatic diseases. Swiss Med Wkly. 2015;145:w14159.
31. van Assen S, Agmon-Levin N, Elkayam O, Cervera R, Doran MF, Dougados M, et al. EULAR recommendations for vaccination in adult patients with autoimmune inflammatory rheumatic diseases. Ann Rheum Dis. 2011;70(3):414–22.
32. Papadopoulou D, Sipsas NV. Comparison of national clinical practice guidelines and recommendations on vaccination of adult patients with autoimmune rheumatic diseases. Rheumatol Int. 2014;34(2):151–63.
33. Croce E, Hatz C, Jonker EF, Visser LG, Jaeger VK, Buhler S. Safety of live vaccinations on immunosuppressive therapy in patients with immune-mediated inflammatory diseases, solid organ transplantation or after bone-marrow transplantation - a systematic review of randomized trials, observational studies and case reports. Vaccine. 2017;35(9):1216–26.
34. Monath TP. Review of the risks and benefits of yellow fever vaccination including some new analyses. Expert Rev Vaccines. 2012;11(4):427–48.
35. Mota LM, Oliveira AC, Lima RA, Santos-Neto LL, Tauil PL. Vaccination against yellow fever among patients on immunosuppressors with diagnoses of rheumatic diseases. Rev Soc Bras Med Trop. 2009;42(1):23–7.
36. Higgins JPTGS. Cochrane handbook for systematic reviews of interventions, vol. Version 5.1.0: Cochrane Colaborations; 2011.
37. The Newcastle-Ottawa Scale (NOS) for assessing the quality of nonrandomised studies in meta-analyses [http://www.ohri.ca/programs/clinical_epidemiology/oxford.asp]. Accessed Dec 2018.
38. Guyatt GH, Oxman AD, Vist GE, Kunz R, Falck-Ytter Y, Alonso-Coello P, et al. GRADE: an emerging consensus on rating quality of evidence and strength of recommendations. BMJ. 2008;336(7650):924–6.
39. Howick J. CI, Glasziou P, Greenhalgh T, Heneghan C, Liberati A, Moschetti I, OCEBM Levels of Evidence Working Group et al. "The Oxford Levels of Evidence 2". . In.: Oxford Centre for Evidence-Based Medicine; 2011.
40. McMillan SS, King M, Tully MP. How to use the nominal group and Delphi techniques. Int J Clin Pharm. 2016;38(3):655–62.
41. Wieten RW, Goorhuis A, Jonker EFF, de Bree GJ, de Visser AW, van Genderen PJJ, et al. 17D yellow fever vaccine elicits comparable long-term immune responses in healthy individuals and immune-compromised patients. J Inf Secur. 2016;72(6):713–22.

42. Wieten RW, Jonker EF, Pieren DK, Hodiamont CJ, van Thiel PP, van Gorp EC, et al. Comparison of the PRNT and an immune fluorescence assay in yellow fever vaccinees receiving immunosuppressive medication. Vaccine. 2016;34(10):1247–51.

43. Ferreira CC, Campi-Azevedo ACV, Peruhype-Magalhães V, Freire LC, Albuquerque CP, Muniza LF, et al. Imunidade vacinal antiamarílica em pacientes com artrite reumatoide. Rev BrasReum. 57:381.

44. Scheinberg M, Guedes-Barbosa LS, Mangueira C, Rosseto EA, Mota L. Yellow fever revaccination during infliximab therapy. Arthritis Care Res (Hoboken). 2010;62(6):896–8.

45. Oliveira AC, Mota LM, Santos-Neto LL, Simoes M, Martins-Filho OA, Tauil PL. Seroconversion in patients with rheumatic diseases treated with immunomodulators or immunosuppressants, who were inadvertently revaccinated against yellow fever. Arthritis Rheumatol. 2015;67(2):582–3.

46. Valim V, Gouveia SA, de Lima SMB, Azevedo ACC, Carvalho AT, Pascoal VPM, et al. Eficácia e segurança da vacinação anti-amarílica a curto e longo prazo em pacientes com doenças reumáticas imunomediadas em tratamento. Rev Bras Reumatol. 2017;57:S 52–3.

47. Lira KLL, Balarini L, de Lima SMB, Azevedo ACC, de Carvalho AT, Paschoal VPM, et al. Vacinação anti-amarílica em pacientes com doenças reumáticas imunomediadas: análise retrospectiva. Rev Bras Reumat. 2017;57:S69.

48. Kerneis S, Launay O, Ancelle T, Iordache L, Naneix-Laroche V, Mechai F, et al. Safety and immunogenicity of yellow fever 17D vaccine in adults receiving systemic corticosteroid therapy: an observational cohort study. Arthritis Care Res (Hoboken). 2013;65(9):1522–8.

49. Nash ER, Brand M, Chalkias S. Yellow fever vaccination of a primary Vaccinee during adalimumab therapy. J Travel Med. 2015;22(4):279–81.

50. Charles C, Gafni A, Whelan T. Shared decision-making in the medical encounter: what does it mean? (or it takes at least two to tango). Soc Sci Med. 1997;44(5):681–92.

51. de Menezes Martins R, Fernandes Leal Mda L, Homma A. Serious adverse events associated with yellow fever vaccine. Hum Vaccin Immunother. 2015;11(9):2183–7.

52. Lindsey NP, Rabe IB, Miller ER, Fischer M, Staples JE. Adverse event reports following yellow fever vaccination, 2007-13. J Travel Med. 2016;23(5).

53. McNeil MM, Li R, Pickering S, Real TM, Smith PJ, Pemberton MR. Who is unlikely to report adverse events after vaccinations to the vaccine adverse event reporting system (VAERS)? Vaccine. 2013;31(24):2673–9.

54. Tafuri S, Gallone MS, Calabrese G, Germinario C. Adverse events following immunization: is this time for the use of WHO causality assessment? Expert Rev Vaccines. 2015;14(5):625–7.

55. Tozzi AE, Asturias EJ, Balakrishnan MR, Halsey NA, Law B, Zuber PL. Assessment of causality of individual adverse events following immunization (AEFI): a WHO tool for global use. Vaccine. 2013;31(44):5041–6.

56. Biscayart C, Carrega ME, Sagradini S, Gentile A, Stecher D, Orduna T, et al. Yellow fever vaccine-associated adverse events following extensive immunization in Argentina. Vaccine. 2014;32(11):1266–72.

57. Cottin P, Niedrig M, Domingo C. Safety profile of the yellow fever vaccine Stamaril(R): a 17-year review. Expert Rev Vaccines. 2013;12(11):1351–68.

58. Khromava AY, Eidex RB, Weld LH, Kohl KS, Bradshaw RD, Chen RT, et al. Yellow fever vaccine: an updated assessment of advanced age as a risk factor for serious adverse events. Vaccine. 2005;23(25):3256–63.

59. Kitchener S. Viscerotropic and neurotropic disease following vaccination with the 17D yellow fever vaccine, ARILVAX. Vaccine. 2004;22(17–18):2103–5.

60. Rafferty E, Duclos P, Yactayo S, Schuster M. Risk of yellow fever vaccine-associated viscerotropic disease among the elderly: a systematic review. Vaccine. 2013;31(49):5798–805.

61. Thomas RE, Lorenzetti DL, Spragins W, Jackson D, Williamson T. The safety of yellow fever vaccine 17D or 17DD in children, pregnant women, HIV+ individuals, and older persons: systematic review. Am J Trop Med Hyg. 2012;86(2):359–72.

62. Thomas RE, Lorenzetti DL, Spragins W, Jackson D, Williamson T. Active and passive surveillance of yellow fever vaccine 17D or 17DD-associated serious adverse events: systematic review. Vaccine. 2011;29(28):4544–55.

63. Caplan A, Fett N, Rosenbach M, Werth VP, Micheletti RG. Prevention and management of glucocorticoid-induced side effects: a comprehensive review: Infectious complications and vaccination recommendations. J Am Acad Dermatol. 2017;76(2):191–8.

64. Ekenberg C, Friis-Moller N, Ulstrup T, Aalykke C. Inadvertent yellow fever vaccination of a patient with Crohn's disease treated with infliximab and methotrexate. BMJ Case Rep. 2016;2016. https://doi.org/10.1136/bcr-2016-215403.

65. Lopez A, Mariette X, Bachelez H, Belot A, Bonnotte B, Hachulla E, et al. Vaccination recommendations for the adult immunosuppressed patient: a systematic review and comprehensive field synopsis. J Autoimmun. 2017;80:10–27.

66. Ruddel J, Schleenvoigt BT, Schuler E, Schmidt C, Pletz MW, Stallmach A. Yellow fever vaccination during treatment with infliximab in a patient with ulcerative colitis: a case report. Z Gastroenterol. 2016;54(9):1081–4.

67. Tarazona B, Diaz-Menendez M, Mato Chain G. International travelers receiving pharmacological immunosuppression: challenges and opportunities. Med Clin (Barc). 2017.

68. Brenol CV, da Mota LM, Cruz BA, Pileggi GS, Pereira IA, Rezende LS, et al. 2012 Brazilian Society of Rheumatology Consensus on vaccination of patients with rheumatoid arthritis. Rev Bras Reumatol. 2013;53(1):4–23.

69. Cetron MS, Marfin AA, Julian KG, Gubler DJ, Sharp DJ, Barwick RS, et al. Yellow fever vaccine. Recommendations of the advisory committee on immunization practices (ACIP), 2002. MMWR Recomm Rep. 2002;51(RR-17):1–11 quiz CE11-14.

70. Rubin LG, Levin MJ, Ljungman P, Davies EG, Avery R, Tomblyn M, et al. 2013 IDSA clinical practice guideline for vaccination of the immunocompromised host. Clin Infect Dis. 2014;58(3):309–18.

71. Domingo C, Yactayo S, Agbenu E, Demanou M, Schulz AR, Daskalow K, Niedrig M. Detection of yellow fever 17D genome in urine. J Clin Microbiol. 2011;49(2):760–2.

72. CDC. Transfusion-related transmission of yellow fever vaccine virus--California. MMWR Morb Mortal Wkly Rep 2010. 2009;59(2):34–7.

73. CDC. Transmission of yellow fever vaccine virus through breast-feeding - Brazil. MMWR Morb Mortal Wkly Rep 2010. 2009;59(5):130–2.

74. Kuhn S, Twele-Montecinos L, MacDonald J, Webster P, Law B. Case report: probable transmission of vaccine strain of yellow fever virus to an infant via breast milk. CMAJ. 2011;183(4):E243–5.

75. Stiggelbout AM, Pieterse AH, De Haes JC. Shared decision making: concepts, evidence, and practice. Patient Educ Couns. 2015;98(10):1172–9.

5

Evaluation of the safety and satisfaction of rheumatic patients with accelerated infliximab infusion

Jozélio Freire de Carvalho[1,2*], Maria Natividade Pereira dos Santos[1], Joyce Meyre Vieira de Oliveira[1], Andrea Nogueira S. Lanty Silva[1], Roberto Paulo Correia de Araujo[1,2] and Juliana Bahia Cardozo[1]

Abstract

Introduction: Infliximab infusion generally occurs in 2–4 h. Recent studies have suggested the possibility of accelerated infusion (1 h) of this drug.

Objective: To evaluate the safety of accelerated infliximab infusion in patients with rheumatic diseases. In addition, patient satisfaction was also assessed.

Methods: A prospective, single-center, non-randomized study with 34 patients with rheumatic diseases was conducted from July to November 2016. Patients with the following were excluded: history of allergic reaction to biologics, asthma or severe atopy. All patients previously received a 2- to 3-h infliximab infusion. The infusion rate was accelerated to 1 h, and premedication was excluded. The infusion was monitored in all patients.

Results: A total of 34 patients were included in the study [rheumatoid arthritis ($n = 16$), ankylosing spondylitis ($n = 15$), psoriatic arthritis ($n = 2$) and enteropathic arthropathy ($n = 1$)], with an average age of 48.7 ± 18.6 years; 55.5% of the patients were female, and 29.4% were white. The duration of disease was 9.5 ± 9.2 years, and the duration of infliximab use was 38.9 ± 27.6 months, with a mean dose per infusion of 414.2 ± 158.1 (range, 200–800) mg. The mean infliximab infusion time prior to the study was 2.2 ± 0.4 h. A total of 6 (17.6%) patients received premedication. The premedication was suspended. There were no adverse effects during or after infusion. Ninety-seven percent of the patients and 100% of the health workers were satisfied with the accelerated infusion.

Conclusion: Our data support the safe use of accelerated infliximab infusion in rheumatic patients, with high satisfaction among patients and health workers.

Keywords: Infliximab, Infusion, Immunobiologics, Rheumatoid arthritis, Ankylosing spondylitis, Psoriatic arthritis, Spondyloarthritis

Background

Immunobiological drugs have become increasingly used in the treatment of rheumatic diseases. An example is the use of inhibitors of tumor necrosis factor (anti-TNF) in the treatment of rheumatoid arthritis and spondyloarthritis [1]. However, the infusion of anti-TNF may lead to infusion-related complications, requiring its supervision and monitoring.

Infliximab, a chimeric anti-TNF monoclonal antibody, is an intravenous medication for which infusion of at least 2 h and a 1-h clinical observation period are recommended due to the risk of infusion-related complications [2]. In the modern world, where processes need to be faster both to reduce costs and to minimize the time spent by the patient using the hospital structure, there is a need to attempt to accelerate the infliximab infusion process. Many experiments, including meta-analyses, mainly regarding the treatment of inflammatory bowel diseases, have been performed that have demonstrated the safety of an accelerated infusion of this biologic [3].

* Correspondence: jotafc@gmail.com
[1]SOS Vida, Rheumatology Unit, Salvador, Bahia, Brazil
[2]Institute of Health Sciences, Universidade Federal da Bahia (Federal University of Bahia), Salvador, Bahia, Brazil

Regarding the treatment of rheumatic diseases, articles have already been published that have evaluated the safety of accelerated infliximab infusion rates of 30 min to 1 h [4–8]. However, we did not find any Brazilian studies that employed this infusion technique.

The aim of the present study was to evaluate the safety of accelerated infliximab infusion in patients with rheumatic diseases. Secondarily, the authors evaluated whether patients and health workers involved in this treatment were satisfied.

Methods

This prospective, single-center, non-randomized, open-label study included adult patients (> 18 years of age) with a confirmed diagnosis of rheumatic diseases using infliximab. The patients were included in the study if they presented with rheumatoid arthritis (RA) (American College of Rheumatology– ACR criteria) [9], ankylosing spondylitis (AS) [10], psoriatic arthritis (PsA) [11] and Crohn's disease [12] and were regularly monitored in our infusion clinic. Exclusion criteria were history of infusion reaction prior to immunobiological therapy, refusal to participate in the study and history of asthma or severe atopy. Clinical and laboratory data were obtained after consulting the medical records and performing the clinical examination. Ethical local committee approved this study.

Infusion protocol

Patients with RA received a dose of 3 or 5 mg/kg (if refractory to the previous dose), and patients with AS, PsA and Crohn's disease received 5 mg/kg, all receiving a stable dose, every 8 weeks. The accelerated infusion consisted of starting at half the rate in the first 15 min to check for infusion reaction; the remainder of the volume was infused in the remaining 45 min. Subsequently, the patients underwent post-infusion monitoring lasting 30 min. A nurse trained in infliximab infusion recorded all infusion data and monitored vital data during and after the infusion. In case of any adverse effects, the infusion was stopped immediately. Depending on the severity of the infusion reaction, the emergency response protocol consisted of decreasing the infusion rate, stopping the infusion and intravenously injecting diphenhydramine (50 mg), followed by methylprednisolone (125 mg) and, if necessary, adrenaline [13].

Satisfaction of patients and health workers

At the end of the last infusion, patient satisfaction was measured by answering the following question: "Did the change in infusion time improve your quality of life?" Responses ranged from 1 to 10 on a Likert scale. For health workers (nursing and nursing technicians) who dealt directly with the infusion, the following question

was asked: "Did the change in infusion time improve the quality of care?" Responses ranged from 1 to 10 on a Likert scale.

Statistical analysis

Descriptive statistics were used. Values are expressed as the means and standard deviations or medians or percentages. The data were entered into Microsoft Excel software for analysis.

Results

A total of 34 patients were included, with a mean age of 48.7 ± 18.6 years (19–79 years); 55.5% of the patients were female, and 29.4% were white. The patients had the following conditions: rheumatoid arthritis ($n = 16$), ankylosing spondylitis ($n = 15$), psoriatic arthritis ($n = 2$) and Crohn's disease (n = 1). The mean disease duration was 9.5 ± 9.2 years.

The mean duration of infliximab use was 38.9 ± 27.6 months. The mean dose per infliximab infusion was 414.2 ± 158.1 mg, ranging from 200 to 800 mg. Regarding other medications, 10 (29.4%) patients received methotrexate (5 RA, 4 AS and 1 PsA), 3 (8.8%) patients received leflunomide, and only 2 patients were taking prednisone 5 mg/day. Positive results for rheumatoid factor and anti-cyclic citrullinated peptide antibody (anti-CCP) were observed in 69 and 63% of the patients with RA, respectively. A total of 6 (17.6%) patients used premedication with corticoid and antihistamine.

The mean infusion time prior to the infliximab study was 2.2 ± 0.4 h, ranging from 2 to 3 h. A total of 6 (17.6%) patients received premedication: 3 patients with RA and 3 patients with AS.

After the accelerated infusion protocol was started, all patients stopped receiving premedication. There were no adverse effects during or after infusion in any of the patients included in this study. A mean of 2.7 ± 0.7 infusions per patient was performed during the study.

Regarding satisfaction, 97% answered the question: "Did the change in infusion time improve your quality of life?" with scores between 8 and 10. All (100%) health workers gave a score of 10 to the following question: "Did the change in infusion time improve the quality of care?"

It is assumed that there was a reduction of approximately 1 h 30 min in each patient's time in the hospital. This inference was based on the 1-h reduction in infusion time plus the 30 min saved by eliminating the need for premedication preparation and application.

Discussion

The present study demonstrates the safety of accelerated infliximab infusion in adult patients with rheumatic diseases, all without previous history of infusion reactions.

The relevance of the present study is supported by the rigorous patient selection criteria, with all the participants meeting the classification/diagnostic criteria for their diseases, along with the exclusion of people with prior allergic reactions or severe atopy. These criteria may justify the absence of adverse effects during the present study. In fact, if these conditions were not excluded, the risk of anaphylaxis could be increased.

A meta-analysis that included 10 studies comparing 1-h (8497 infusions) and 2-h (13,147 infusions) infliximab infusions showed a reduction in the rate of infusion reactions when the drug was administered for 1 h [1]. The present study did not result in any adverse infusion reactions during the study period.

Reactions to infliximab infusion occur in approximately 2–3% of infusions [14]. Interestingly, our study showed no adverse effects. In addition, accelerated infusion may increase adherence to treatment. Indeed, in patients with enteropathic arthropathy, poor adherence has been reported, ranging from 25 to 35%, which increases medical costs and hospitalization risk [15].

There are some limitations in the present study, the first being the relatively small number of patients included. To address this issue, new studies with large numbers of participants should be conducted. Another factor was the exclusion of patients with a previous history of severe atopy or infusion reaction, which may have contributed to the absence of adverse events. New studies that include individuals with a history of atopy could also be performed, obviously with careful monitoring and adequate preparation for an emergency intervention. The infliximab dose used here (3–5 mg/kg) may also preclude the capacity to extend its conclusions to larger doses, which are often used in refractory cases.

It should be noted that all patients included in this study were already undergoing treatment with infliximab. For new patients, the literature recommends that the first infusion or the induction phase be performed within the usual 2-h period.

In summary, the present study demonstrates the excellent tolerability of the accelerated infliximab infusion in adult patients with rheumatic diseases, without previous history of infusion reaction. In addition, the results of this study precluded the need for premedication. In addition, great satisfaction was expressed among both patients and health workers.

Authors' contributions

JF de C Idea about the manuscript, writting, data analysis, review; MNP dos S data collection, data analysis; JMV de O data collection, data analysisi, AN S. LS data collection, data analysis; RPC de A writting, data analysis, review; JBC writting, data analysis, review.

References

1. Titton DC, Silveira IG, Louzada-Junior P, Hayata AL, Carvalho HM, et al. Brazilian biologic registry: BiobadaBrasil implementation process and preliminary results. Rev Bras Reumatol. 2011;51:152–60.
2. de Moraes JC, Aikawa NE, Ribeiro AC, Saad CG, Carvalho JF, Pereira RM, Silva CA, Bonfá E. Immediate complications of 3,555 injections of anti-TNFα. Rev Bras Reumatol. 2010;50:165–75.
3. Neef HC, Riebschleger MP, Adler J. Meta-analysis: rapid IFX infusions are safe. Alimentary Pharmacology and Therapeuticc. 2013;38:365–76.
4. Bañuelos-Ramírez D, Ramirez-Palma MM, Balcazar-Sanchez ME, Sanchez-Alonso S. Rapid application of infliximab. Efficacy complications. Reumatol Clin. 2007;3:171–5.
5. Buch MH, Bryer D, Lindsay S, Rees-Evans B, Fairclough A, Emery P. Shortening infusion times for infliximab administration. Rheumatology (Oxford). 2006;45:485–6.
6. El Miedany Y, Palmer D. Infliximab infusion therapy in inflammatory arthritis: assessment of the accelerated infusion protocol in comparison to the standard infusion approach. Rheumatology (Oxford). 2011;50:97–97.
7. hergy WJ, Isern RA, Cooley DA, et al. Open label study to assess infliximab safety and timing of onset of clinical benefit among patients with rheumatoid arthritis. J Rheumatol. 2002;29:667–77.
8. Lee TW, Singh R, Fedorak RN. A one-hour infusion of infliximab during maintenance therapy is safe and well tolerated: a prospective cohort study. Aliment Pharmacol Ther. 2011;34:181.
9. Arnett FC, Edworthy SM, Bloch DA, Mcshane DJ, Fries JF, Coope NS, et al. The American rheumatism association 1987 revised criteria for the classification of rheumatoid arthritis. Arthritis Rheum. 1988;31:315–24.
10. Bennett PH, Wood PHN. Population studies of the rheumatic diseases. New York: Excerpta Medica; 1968. p. 456.
11. Moll JM, Wright V. Psoriatic arthritis. Semin Arthritis Rheum. 1973;3:55–78.
12. Dougados M, vander Linden S, Juhlin R, Huitfeldt B, Amor B, Calin A, et al. The European Spondylarthropathy study group preliminary criteria for the classification of spondylarthropathy. Arthritis Rheum. 1991;34:1218–27.
13. Protocolo de actuação em caso de reacção à infusão de infliximab. Grupo de Estudos de Artrite Reumatoide da Sociedade Portuguesa de Reumatologia. Acta Reum Port. 2005;30:355–9.
14. Van Assche G, Lewis JD, Lichtenstein GR, et al. The London position statement of the world congress of gastroenterology on biological therapy for IBD with the European Crohn's and colitis organisation: safety. Am J Gastroenterol. 2011;106:1594–602.
15. Kane SV, Chao J, Mulani PM. Adherence to infliximab maintenance therapy and health care utilization and costs by Crohn's disease patients. Adv Ther. 2009;26:936–46.

6

Home storage of biological medications administered to patients with rheumatic diseases

Glaucia Santin[1,2*] [iD], Mariana Moreira Magnabosco da Silva[2], Vinicius Augusto Villarreal[2], Leane Dhara Dalle Laste[2], Eduardo de Freitas Montin[2], Luis Eduardo Ribeiro Betiol[2] and Valderilio Feijó Azevedo[1,2]

Abstract

Background: The inadequate storage of biopharmaceuticals may result in an ineffective therapeutic response since poor conservation can lead to the emergence of protein aggregates and cause immunogenicity in patients, which can increase the risk of adverse events by inducing the production of anti-drug antibodies. This can also lead to significant economic losses for public health, given the high cost of these medicines. The aim of this study was to verify whether the home storage of biopharmaceuticals dispensed by the Unified Public System was in accordance with the manufacturers' specified standards and whether external variables interfered with the correct home storage.

Methods: This was a prospective observational study. Patients with a confirmed diagnosis of rheumatoid arthritis, ankylosing spondylitis or psoriatic arthritis who were using a biologic exclusively dispensed by Unified Public System were included. Storage temperature was measured by digital thermometer inserted into the refrigerator of the participant's home. Fisher's exact test was performed to cross-reference the temperature data and the qualitative variables obtained using an epidemiologic questionnaire. Mean, minimum, maximum values and standard deviation were described in the quantitative data. Mann-Whitney non-parametric test was performed to the association between temperature excursion and the number of people in the house.

Results: A total of 81 participants were included and 67 (82.71%) did not maintain home storage correctly. The maximum temperature observed among all patients was 15.5 °C, the minimum was − 4.4 °C and the average was 5.6 °C (standard deviation 2.8); 10 (12.3%) had at least one negative temperature measured. The average time for participants who had an inadequate temperature record was 8 h and 31 min. Nine participants (90%) who stored the medication into the shelf/drawer below the freezer had a temperature excursion ($p = 0.011$). Most of the participants (88.5%) who stored their biopharmaceutical near the back side, close to the wall of the refrigerator had a negative temperature record ($p < 0.001$).

Conclusion: Most of the study participants (82.71%) did not maintain adequate home storage conditions for their biopharmaceutical. Intrinsic factors of household refrigerators may be involved in temperature deviations.

Keywords: Biological drugs, Home storage, Rheumatic diseases

* Correspondence: glaucia_farma@hotmail.com
[1]Edumed Educação em Saúde, Rua Bispo Dom José, 2495, Curitiba, Paraná 80440-080, Brazil
[2]Universidade Federal do Paraná, Rua General Carneiro 181, Curitiba, Paraná 80060-900, Brazil

Background

The introduction of biologic drugs changed the treatment dramatically for patients with inflammatory rheumatic diseases [1] such as rheumatoid arthritis (RA), ankylosing spondylitis (AS) and psoriatic arthritis (PsA). Despite the increased number of biopharmaceutical options, a high proportion of patients is refractory to the available drugs [2]. A possible cause for the refractory treatment is the alterations in drug properties due to inadequate storage. It can compromise the stability and affect the characteristics of biopharmaceuticals, leading to human health risks. Conformational changes in the complex protein structure of biological products as a result of freezing-thawing or prolonged storage at high temperatures can lead to denaturation, irreversible formation of protein aggregates and loss of drug activity. Depending on the characteristics of the drug, the temperature and the duration of the exposure to this temperature can also cause significant economic losses to public health, given the high cost of these drugs [3, 4].

The presence of protein aggregates, which cause instability commonly observed in biopharmaceuticals or other protein drugs and are a major concern because they can influence the biodistribution and efficacy of the medication and may directly affect patient safety as the potential for adverse immune reactions is increased [5–7]. Protein aggregation can be induced by a wide variety of conditions, including temperature, mechanical stress, such as agitation and movement, freezing and/or thawing, and the drug formulation itself [3].

A likely explanation for the refractory treatment is immunogenicity, a complex phenomenon that depends on the interaction between several factors related to the drug and the patient. All biopharmaceuticals are potentially immunogenic and are also capable of inducing the production of anti-drug antibodies (ADAs) [2, 8, 9], which has been identified as an important (albeit not the only) contributor to treatment failure and increased risk of adverse events (AEs) in patients receiving biologic therapy [10–13].

Currently, all biologicals represent only 4% of the drugs distributed by the Unified Public System but cost 51% of the purchase budget [14]. The cold chain, a term used to describe the exact temperature conditions in which some products need to be kept during the storage, distribution and administration processes [15], is essential to ensure the quality of medicines. However, the cold chain is interrupted and sanitary control ceases at the time of dispensing the drug to the patient.

Considering this context, the objective of this study was to evaluate the domestic storage conditions in relation to the temperature range recommended by the manufacturer and to analyze possible variables that could influence the variation in refrigerator temperatures.

Methods

Study design and population

This was a prospective observational study.

The study population consisted of individuals ≥18 years old, diagnosed with RA, AS or PsA, who were using a biological drug (adalimumab, etanercept, golimumab, secukinumab, certolizumab or abatacept) dispensed exclusively by the Unified Public System. Patients who used intravenous biological drugs were excluded. The biological agents chosen to be part of this project must be stored, handled and administered correctly within the temperature range of 2 to 8 °C, according to the manufacturers' specifications. Patients were identified and recruited from a database of the Complex of the Clinical Hospital of the Federal University of Paraná (Portuguese acronym: CHC/UFPR), specifically in the Spondyloarthritis Outpatient Clinic and the Centro de Pesquisas Clínicas Edumed – Educação em Saúde S/S Ltda. (Edumed Clinical Research Center - Health Education).

A total of 131 patients were selected. Of these, 50 patients were excluded, 10 for not storing the biological medication in their household, 8 for no longer using biological medication, 8 because they resided in a region with difficult access, 14 patients due to communication difficulties, and 10 due to dropping out of the study. A total of 81 patients met the eligibility criteria.

Thermometers

The TagTemp Stick® is a small (78 × 23 × 10 mm), compact, robust and validated electronic temperature data logger that does not require the use of cables for operation and data collection. It connects directly to the USB interface of Windows computers for communication with LogChartII®, the configuration and data analysis software for TagTemp data loggers. It has an internal temperature sensor that has great accuracy. The temperature measurement range varies from − 20.0 °C to 70.0 °C and has a memory capacity of 32,000 (32 k) records [16].

Data collection

The researchers and the participants scheduled appointments for the implantation and removal of the thermometer in the refrigerator of the participant's home. Communication with participants was made by phone or electronic messages or in person. At each participant's residence, the informed consent form (ICF) was signed, and additional information was collected through questionnaires regarding socioeconomic level and habits regarding home medication storage. The variables on medication storage habits were collected through data of the refrigerator such as brand, model, volume and whether it had an alarm or not; number of people living at the same house as the patient, classified by sex and age group; time when the refrigerator door is most frequently opened; storage location of the biological drug within the refrigerator; occurrence of food stored in the same medication compartment; storage of warm food in the same refrigerator as the biological drug; how the patient was oriented to store the medication for the first time of use and which health professional transmitted this information; occurrence of electric power outage, for how long and what action patient took if it had happened. The socioeconomic variables were verified through level of education of the participant, monthly family income, employment status and employee job class (hours per week).

The thermometers were inserted inside the participant's refrigerator by the research team, and the participant was instructed to maintain the normal family routine regarding refrigerator use.

Thus, data were collected on temperature variations in each participant's refrigerator at home, in which he or she stored biological medication for 3 consecutive days next to the TagTemp Stick Novus®. The temperature was measured continuously for 3 consecutive days every 30 s. The total measurement time was the period between the first and the last temperature measurement. The time period was programmed by the team using the thermometer software.

A single temperature measurement outside the ideal storage range, which should be between 2 and 8 °C, was considered a temperature excursion. Cases with negative temperature readings were those that had at least one evaluation with a negative temperature during the follow-up period.

The period of data collection was from August 2017 to March 2019.

Statistical analyses

For the statistical analyses, Fisher's exact test was used to cross-reference the temperature data and the qualitative variables obtained using the questionnaires. For the description of quantitative variables, the statistics of mean, minimum and maximum values and standard deviation were considered. To evaluate the association between temperature excursion and the number of people in the house, the Mann-Whitney non-parametric test was considered. To evaluate the association between temperature excursion and the patient's age, Student's T test for independent samples was considered. A value of $p < 0.05$ was considered statistically significant.

Results

Temperatures measurements

Eighty one patients were included (Table 1). A total of 39 (48.14%) men and 42 (51.85%) women were selected. The mean age of the men was 48.38 years old, and the

mean age of the women was 54.10 years old. The mean time since diagnosis was 9.38 years for men and 12.74 years for women. Regarding the underlying disease, 7 (8.6%) men and 4 (4.9%) women had PsA; 4 (4.9%) men and 21 (25.9%) women had RA; and 28 (35%) men and 17 (21%) women had AS.

Of the 81 participants (Table 2), 67 (82.71%) recorded temperature excursions. The remaining 14 (17.29%) had no temperature excursions. Ten (12.3%) recorded at least one negative temperature measured during the period; among the cases with negative temperature readings, the mean was – 0.68 °C. For all measurements, the maximum and minimum temperatures were 15.5 °C and – 4.4 °C, respectively; the mean temperature was 5.6 °C. Standard deviation for mean temperature is 2.8 °C; 52 participants (64.2%) recorded temperatures > 8 °C; 23 participants (28.4%) recorded a temperature < 2 °C. The average duration of inadequate temperature for participants who had an inadequate temperature record was 8 h and 31 min. It was found that 64.2% of our sample recorded a temperature > 8 °C.

External variables versus temperature excursion

All variables described below were associated with a temperature excursion.

Regarding the storage of food in the same refrigerator as biopharmaceuticals, it was observed that all participants who stored their biopharmaceutical with food had at least one temperature excursion, but no statistically significant differences were found ($p > 0.05$).

Regarding the association between storage location of the medication in the refrigerator (Table 3), here was a greater chance of temperature excursion in some locations within the refrigerator, and this result was statistically significant ($p < 0.05$).

To evaluate the association between the storage location within the refrigerator and negative temperatures (Table 4), the results show that there may be a greater chance of negative temperatures, with statistical significance ($p < 0.05$), in some locations with the refrigerator.

Table 1 Profile of patients in the sample

Data	Male	Female
Number	39	42
Average age (years)	48.38	54.10
Standard deviation for age	10.69	15.27
Mean time since diagnosis (years)	9.38	12.74
Standard deviation for time since diagnosis	6.15	8.38
Psoriatic Arthritis Patients	7	4
Rheumatoid Arthritis Patients	4	21
Ankylosing Spondylitis Patients	28	17

Table 2 Patient proportion according to temperature measurements

Total number of patients	Patients who had temperature excursion	Patient who had at least one negative temperature measurement	Maximum temperature measured	Minimum temperature measured	Average temperature of all patients	Patients whose temperature was> 8 °C	Patients whose temperature was < 2 °C
81 (100%)	67 (82.71%)	10 (12.3%)	15.5 °C	−4.4 °C	5.6 °C	52 (64.2%)	23 (28.4%)

The mean temperature by subgroups of storage location within the refrigerator was evaluated (Table 5). It was found that sites 6 and 7 had a mean temperature above that recommended by the manufacturers.

Other factors that did not impact the storage of medication, i.e., those that were not statistically significant ($p > 0.05$), include sound alarm in the refrigerator, number of people in the house ($p = 0.891$), age of the patient ($p = 0.860$), ages of the household residents (p ranged from 0.280 to 1.000) and refrigerator model (p value ranged from 0.722 to 1.000). The association between age and gender [with temperature excursion] was not statistically significant. In addition, there was no association between food storage in the same refrigerator and temperature deviations ($p = 0.582$) and between temperature excursion and power outages ($p = 0.539$); there was no statistical significance regarding the level of education of the patient; family income was not associated with temperature excursion; there was no statistical significance regarding the person who advised the patient ($p = 0.954$); and finally, there was no association between the time the refrigerator was opened and the temperature excursion times.

Discussion

Our results address a relevant but little understood subject by health professionals, managers and patients. One of the most notable facts in our study is that patients do not perceive temperature deviations because, in the case of patients coming from the public health system, there are no financial means and resources available to patients to measure the exact temperature of their refrigerators using an accurate thermometer. Therefore, they do not know when to adjust the temperature of their refrigerator. Periods of inadequate drug storage usually go undetected. It was observed that inadequate storage by patients was unintentional.

Previous studies have shown that the conditions of domestic storage of thermolabile therapeutics are often not adequate since less than 50% of patients stored their biopharmaceutical within the recommended temperature range [1, 17, 18]. One study [1] revealed that the age of the refrigerator is an important factor, that is, the older the appliance, the greater the risk of inadequate storage and the greater the likelihood of drug instability due to temperature variation. So we can consider that there

Table 3 Association between storage of biological medication within a refrigerator and occurrence of temperature excursions

Storage location within the refrigerator		Temperature excursion		Total	"p" value
		Yes	No		
0 – Shelf/drawer just below the freezer	n	9	1	10	0.011*
	%	90.0%	10.0%		
1 - Shelves: back side, close to the wall	n	19	7	26	0.014*
	%	73.1%	26.9%		
2 - Shelves: front side	n	18	2	20	< 0.001*
	%	90.0%	10.0%		
3 - Shelves: side, close to the wall	n	10	2	12	0.019*
	%	83.3%	16.7%		
4 – Shelf/drawer above the lowest drawer (lower part of your refrigerator - lid of the vegetable drawer)	n	7	1	8	0.035*
	%	87.5%	12.5%		
5 - Refrigerator door	n	2	1	3	0.500
	%	66.7%	33.3%		
6 – In the can dispenser, if available, on the door	n	1	0	1	---**
	%	100.0%	0.0%		
7 - In the can dispenser, if available, below the freezer	n	1	0	1	---**
	%	100.0%	0.0%		

* Statistical significance
** Sites 6 and 7 were not considered in the table because only one case was observed and, therefore, the statistical test was not applicable

Table 4 Association between location of biological medications within a refrigerator and occurrence of negative temperatures

Storage location within the refrigerator		Negative temperature measured		Total	"p" value
		No	Yes		
0 – Shelf/drawer just below the freezer	n	8	2	10	0.055
	%	80.0%	20.0%		
1 - Shelves: back side, close to the wall	n	23	3	26	< 0.001*
	%	88.5%	11.5%		
2 - Shelves: front side	n	17	3	20	0.001*
	%	85.0%	15.0%		
3 - Shelves: side, close to the wall	n	11	1	12	0.003*
	%	91.7%	8.3%		
4 – Shelf/drawer above the lowest drawer (lower part of your refrigerator - lid of the vegetable drawer)	n	7	1	8	0.035*
	%	87.5%	12.5%		
5 - Refrigerator door	n	3	0	3	0.125
	%	100.0%	0.0%		
6 - In the can dispenser, if available, on the door	n	1	0	1	---**
	%	100.0%	0.0%		
7 - In the can dispenser, if available, below the freezer	n	1	0	1	---**
	%	100.0%	0.0%	1	---**

* Statistical significance
** Sites 6 and 7 were not considered in the table because only one case was observed and, therefore, the statistical test is not applicable

may be intrinsic characteristics of refrigerators involved in temperature deviations. However, these data were not addressed or evaluated in the present study because it would be necessary to assess technical parameters, such as the operation of home appliances, which was not the focus of our work. Patient perception and subjective reporting would be limitations of these data because of memory issues or uncertainty regarding refrigerator specifications.

Although it was not found statistically significant results regarding the aspects that could change storage, it was found that the location of the medication within the refrigerator is very important for proper storage. Storage in the refrigerator door exposes products to greater temperature variations. Our findings show that participants who stored their medication in the can dispenser on the door or below the freezer had a mean temperature of 9.0 °C, which is above that recommended by the manufacturers.

Products should be placed on shelves to allow air circulation; and for this reason, the boxes should be kept away from the wall and with a minimum spacing of 2 to 3 cm between them. Products that tolerate negative temperatures, which is not the case for biopharmaceuticals, should be placed on the upper shelf. To avoid freezing, these drugs should be stored on lower shelves [19]. Several authors recommend that biopharmaceuticals be stored on the middle shelf because it is believed that this

Table 5 Mean temperature by subgroups of storage location within the refrigerator

Storage location within the refrigerator	Patients included in analysis (n = 81)	Mean temperature	Standard deviation
0 – Shelf/drawer just below the freezer	10	5.6	3.0
1 - Shelves: back side, close to the wall	26	4.8	2.4
2 - Shelves: front side	20	5.8	3.6
3 - Shelves: side, close to the wall	12	5.6	2.2
4 – Shelf/drawer above the lowest drawer (lower part of your refrigerator - lid of the vegetable drawer)	8	6.7	2.9
5 - Refrigerator door	3	6.1	1.4
6 - In the can dispenser, if available, on the door	1	9.0	---*
7 - In the can dispenser, if available, below the freezer	1	9.1	---*

* Standard deviation in sites 6 and 7 was not considered because only one case was observed and, therefore, this is not applicable

is the best place in the refrigerator for maintaining the temperature between 2 and 8 °C. It was found that the majority (90%) of participants who stored medication at the front of the shelves recorded a temperature excursion, with statistical significance ($p < 0.001$). This may be due to the occurrence of exchanging hot and cold air in the opening of the refrigerator door, which causes the temperature to oscillate and, therefore, increase the incidence of temperature excursions.

For "duplex" and "frost-free" refrigerators, there must be communication between the freezing system and the storage chamber for better medication storage [19]. It was observed that 88.9% of the participants with a "duplex" refrigerator recorded a temperature excursion; however, this result was not statistically significant ($p = 0.722$). In the case of frost-free refrigerators, 76.9% recorded a temperature excursion, without statistical significance ($p = 0.687$). It was observed that some participants who stored their biopharmaceutical near the refrigerator wall, at the back part, recorded a negative temperature ($p < 0.001$), which may be because the cold air in the refrigerator may penetrate the walls, leading to freezing of items nearby.

Many participants had a sound alarm system in the refrigerator, which is activated when the refrigerator door remains open after a period of time, determined by each manufacturer, but this seems to be a nonrelevant factor for maintaining the appropriate temperature.

James et al. [20] found that many refrigerators around the world operate at temperatures higher than those recommended. Our findings show that 64.2% of our sample recorded a temperature > 8 °C.

The reasons for patients not complying with manufacturers' storage recommendations are, to a large extent, unknown. It is essential that patients receive information about the adequate storage of medications at the time of dispensing. Although most patients receive these guidelines, they expose the drugs to various unfavorable storage conditions. Patients are not always able to determine adequate storage in their homes and have problems independently administering their medications at home [21].

Because most patients did not store medications properly, in theory, it would be possible for physicians to adjust prescriptions so that they could be dispensed according to their treatment regimen (weekly, biweekly or monthly) and not for prolonged periods, as occurs with the Unified Public System, to minimize the storage time.

Another relevant factor is the existence of centers specialized in high-cost medication that aim to ensure the comprehensiveness of drug treatment at the outpatient level and, in addition, to perform the dispensing and administration of patient medication. According to the Brazilian Ministry of Health [22], the reference centers used for the administration of biological medications have greater rationality of use and monitor the effectiveness of these drugs. The rational use and monitoring of the effectiveness of these drugs can also avoid the incorrect use of these medications. Pharmacists can play a key role in promoting good storage practices, providing supervision and training patients. Since 2010, The High-Cost Medication Dispensing Center (CEDMAC for its Portuguese acronym) of the Clinics Hospital of the State University of Campinas (HC-UNICAMP for its Portuguese acronym), located in the state of São Paulo, has been a reference for treatment using immunobiological agents in rheumatologic diseases; when indicated, these agents are dispensed and applied at the center so that improper or incorrect use of these medications is avoided [23].

There are no data in the literature comparing inadequate storage with adverse events and there are no evidences that inadequate storage specifically increases failure or adverse events. A full discussion of if inadequate storage can change the outcome of the patient's treatment is beyond the scope of this article. It has been widely acknowledged that temperature fluctuations increase the formation of protein aggregates and this can enhance immunogenicity by inducing the production of ADA [24, 25]. Several studies have related the presence of ADA with adverse reaction. In other words, drug immunogenicity may also affect drug safety, increasing the risk of adverse events [26–31].

In this study, the temperature excursion was similar to that of developed countries, as it was found results similar to those of the studies discussed herein. Therefore, temperature excursion is not characterized as an independent cultural or socioeconomic factor.

It must bear in mind that patients have different levels of education and understanding; thus, one way to improve home storage would be through explanatory materials that can be provided to patients through clear and concise language, with illustrations and short text. This material may include explanations such as, the most appropriate place to store the medication within the refrigerator, the importance of keeping the medication in its primary packaging and guidelines on the medication conditions before applying it.

The strategies discussed above are very important and require mastery of the subject by the professionals involved through knowledge, training, development of new guidelines and implementation of innovations of storage systems (temperature monitoring devices). All this should be done to inform patients and ensure they can better control home storage conditions.

More research in home storage area is required to evaluate the relation between inadequate storage and the effectiveness of biologic treatment.

Conclusion

We concluded from this study that the majority of participants included (82.71%) did not maintain adequate home storage conditions for their biological medication and that intrinsic characteristics of home refrigerators may be involved in the temperature deviations. Temperature excursions cannot be characterized as a cultural or socioeconomic factor because our findings are similar to those of developed countries.

Abbreviations
ADA: Anti-drug antibodies; AS: Ankylosing spondylitis; CAPES: Coordenação de Aperfeiçoamento de Pessoal de Nível Superior; CEDMAC: High-Cost Medication Dispensing Center; CHC/UFPR: Complex of the Clinical Hospital of the Federal University of Paraná; HC-UNICAMP: Clinics Hospital of the State University of Campinas; ICF: Informed consent form; PsA: Psoriatic arthritis; RA: Rheumatoid arthritis; TNF: Tumor necrosis factor

Acknowledgments
To our patients who gently agreed to participate in this study.

Authors' contributions
VA and GS: Conception and study design; Manuscript preparation; Elaboration of article; Data analysis and interpretation; Elaboration of article and critical review; MS and W had some participation in the writing of the manuscript; All authors, except VA, performed data collection; GS had full access to all study data and takes responsibility for the integrity of the data. All authors read and approved the final manuscript to be published.

References
1. Vlieland ND, et al. The majority of patients do not store their biologic disease-modifying antirheumatic drugs within the recommended temperature range. Rheumatology. 2016;55(4):704–9. https://doi.org/10.1093/rheumatology/kev394.
2. Mócsai A, Kovács L, Gergely P. What is the future of targeted therapy in rheumatology: biologics or small molecules? BMC Med. 2014;12(1):1–9. https://doi.org/10.1186/1741-7015-12-43.
3. Wang W, Nema S, Teagarden D. Protein aggregation-pathways and influencing factors. Int J Pharm. 2010;390(2):89–99. https://doi.org/10.1016/j.ijpharm.2010.02.025 Epub 2010 Feb 24.
4. Ricote-Lobera I, et al. Estabilidad de los medicamentos termolabiles ante una interrupcion accidental de la cadena de frio. Farm Hosp. 2014;38(3): 169–92. ISSN 2171-8695. https://doi.org/10.7399/FH.2014.38.3.1164.
5. Moussa EM, et al. Immunogenicity of therapeutic protein aggregates. J Pharm Sci. 2016;105(2):417–30. https://doi.org/10.1016/j.xphs.2015.11.002.
6. Mahler HC, Friess W, Grauschopf U, Kiese S. Protein aggregation: pathways, induction factors and analysis. J Pharm Sci. 2009;98(9):2909–34. https://doi.org/10.1002/jps.21566.
7. Rosenberg AS. Effects of protein aggregates: an immunologic perspective. AAPS J. 2006;8(3):E501–7.
8. Vincent FB, Morand EF, Murphy K, Mackay F, Mariette X, Marcelli C. Antidrug antibodies (ADAb) to tumour necrosis fator (TNF)-specific neutralising agents in chronic inflammatory diseases: a real issue, a clinical perspective. Ann Rheum Dis. 2013;72:165–78. https://doi.org/10.1136/annrheumdis-2012-202545.
9. Deehan M, Garces S, Kramer D, Baker MP, Rat D, Roettger Y, et al. Managing unwanted immunogenicity of biologicals. Autoimmun Rev. 2015;14(7):569–74. https://doi.org/10.1016/j.autrev.2015.02.007 Epub 2015 Mar 2.
10. van Schouwenburg PA, Rispens T, Wolbink GJ. Immunogenicity of anti-TNF biologic therapies for rheumatoid arthritis. Nat Rev Rheumatol. 2013;9(3): 164–72. https://doi.org/10.1038/nrrheum.2013.4.
11. Jullien D, Prinz JC, Nestle FO. Immunogenicity of biotherapy used in psoriasis: the science behind the scenes. J Invest Dermatol. 2015;135(1):31–8. https://doi.org/10.1038/jid.2014.295.
12. Krieckaert C, Rispens T, Wolbink G. Immunogenicity of biological therapeutics: from assay to patient. Curr Opin Rheumatol. 2012;24(3):306–11. https://doi.org/10.1097/BOR.0b013e3283521c4e.
13. Garceˆs S, Demengeot J, Benito-Garcia E. The immunogenicity of anti-TNF therapy in immune-mediated inflammatory diseases: a systematic review of the literature with a meta-analysis. Ann Rheum Dis. 2013;72(12):1947–55. https://doi.org/10.1136/ annrheumdis-2012-202220.
14. Da Saúde M. Espondilite anquilosante. Brasil: Protocolo Clínico e Diretrizes Terapêuticas; 2017. http://portalarquivossaudegovbr/images/pdf/2017/agosto/03/PCDT- Accessed 18 July 2019.
15. Purssell E. Reviewing the importance of the cold chain in the distribution of vaccines. Br J Community Nurs. 2015;20(10):481–6. https://doi.org/10.12968/bjcn.2015.20.10.481.
16. NOVUS, Produtos eletrônicos. http://www.novus.com.br/produtos/732906. Accessed 18 July 2019.
17. Cuéllar MJ, et al. Calidad en la conservación de los medicamentos termolábiles en el ámbito domiciliario. Revista de Calidad Asistencial. 2010; 25(2):64–9. https://doi.org/10.1016/j.cali.2009.09.001.
18. De Jong MJ, et al. Exploring conditions for redistribution of anti-tumor necrosis factors to reduce spillage: a study on the quality of anti-tumor necrosis factor home storage. J Gastroenterol Hepatol. 2018;33(2):426–30. https://doi.org/10.1111/jgh.13920.
19. Rapkiewicz J, Grobe R. Cuidados no armazenamento de medicamentos sob refrigeração; 2014.
20. James SJ, Evans J, James C. A review of the performance of domestic refrigerators. J Food Eng. 2008;87(1):2–10.
21. Sino CGM, et al. Medication management capacity in relation to cognition and self-management skills in older people on polypharmacy. J Nutr Health Aging. 2014;18(1):44–9. https://doi.org/10.1007/s12603-013-0359-2.
22. Ministério da Saúde (2018). Enquete pública de medicamentos biológicos. http://portalarquivos2.saude.gov.br/images/pdf/2018/outubro/19/Resultado-Enquete-Problemas-Versao-Publica.pdf. .
23. Bértolo MB, et al. Manual de Processos de Trabalho do Centro de Dispensação de Medicação de Alto Custo (CEDMAC). Campinas: Série Manuais do Hospital de Clínicas da Unicamp; 2012. p. 16–23. https://intranet.hc.unicamp.br/manuais/cedmac.pdf. Accessed 05 September 2019.
24. Carpenter JF, Randolph TW, Jiskoot W, et al. Overlooking subvisible particles in therapeutic protein products: gaps that may compromise product quality. J Pharm Sci. 2009;98:1201–5. https://doi.org/10.1002/jps.21530.
25. Rosenberg AS. Effects of protein aggregates: an immunologic perspective. AAPS J. 2006;8:E501–7.
26. Baert F, Noman M, Vermeire S, Van Assche G. D' Haens G, Carbonez a, et al: influence of immunogenicity on the long-term efficacy of infliximab in Crohn's disease. N Engl J Med. 2003;348:601–8.
27. Pascual-Salcedo D, Plasencia C, Ramiro S, Nuno L, Bonilla G, Nagore D, et al. Influence of immunogenicity on the efficacy of long-term treatment with infliximab in rheumatoid arthritis. Rheumatology (Oxford). 2011;50:1445–52.
28. Wolbink GJ, Vis M, Lems W, Voskuyl AE, de Groot E, Nurmohamed MT, et al. Development of antiinfliximab antibodies and relationship to clinical response in patients with rheumatoid arthritis. Arthritis Rheum. 2006;54:711–5.
29. Vultaggio A, Matucci A, Nencini F, Pratesi S, Parronchi P, Rossi O, et al. Antiinfliximab IgE and non-IgE antibodies and induction of infusion-related severe anaphylactic reactions. Allergy. 2010;65:657–61. https://doi.org/10.1111/j.1398-9995.2009.02280.x Epub 2009 Nov 27.
30. Matucci A, Pratesi S, Petroni G, Nencini F, Virgili G, Milla M, et al. Allergological in vitro and in vivo evaluation of patients with hypersensitivity reactions to infliximab. Clin Exp Allergy. 2013;43:659–64. https://doi.org/10.1111/cea.12098.
31. Farrell RJ, Shah SA, Lodhavia PJ, Alsahli M, Falchuk KR, Michetti P, et al. Clinical experience with infliximab therapy in 100 patients with Crohn's disease. Am J Gastroenterol. 2000;95:3490–7.

7

Favorable rituximab response in patients with refractory idiopathic inflammatory myopathies

Fernando Henrique Carlos de Souza[1], Renata Miossi[1], Júlio Cesar Bertacini de Moraes[1], Eloisa Bonfá[2] and Samuel Katsuyuki Shinjo[2*]

Abstract

Background: Interpretation of rituximab efficacy for refractory idiopathic inflammatory myopathies (IIM) is hampered by the absence of a uniform definition of refractory myositis and clinical response. Therefore, rigorous criteria of refractoriness, together with a homogenous definition of clinical improvement, were used to evaluate rituximab one-year response.

Methods: A retrospective cohort study including 43 IIM (15 antisynthetase syndrome, 16 dermatomyositis, 12 polymyositis) was conducted. All patients had refractory disease (inadequate response to at least two immunosuppressives/immunomodulatories and no less than three months sequentially or concomitantly glucocorticoid tapering) criteria. Clinical/laboratory improvement at one-year was based on modified International Myositis Assessment & Clinical Studies Group (IMACS) core set measures. The patients received two infusions of rituximab (1 g each) at baseline, followed by repeated dose after 6 months. Baseline immunosuppressive therapy was maintained and glucocorticoid dose was tapered according to clinical/laboratory parameters.

Results: Five patients had side effects at the first rituximab application and were excluded. Therefore, 38 out of 43 patients completed the one-year follow up. Almost 75% of the patients attained clinical and laboratory response after one-year. A significant reduction in median glucocorticoid dose (18.8 vs. 6.3 mg/day) was achieved and 42% patients were able to discontinue prednisone. In contrast, young individuals and patients with dysphagia had a tendency to be non-responders to rituximab. No severe infections were observed.

Conclusion: This study provides convincing evidence that rituximab is an effective and safe therapy for refractory IIM.

Keywords: Antibodies, Dermatomyositis, Myositis, Polymyositis, Rituximab

Background

Idiopathic inflammatory myopathies (IIM) constitute a heterogeneous group of chronic systemic autoimmune diseases with a high rate of morbidity and disability [1–3]. Based on their clinical, laboratory, histopathological and progression features, IIM can be classified as polymyositis (PM), dermatomyositis (DM), antisynthetase syndrome (ASS), inclusion body myositis, and others [2, 3].

A number of studies have suggested rituximab efficacy for refractory IIM, with response rates ranging from 61 to 83% [4–11]. This high and wide range of response rate is partly explained by the lack of a standardized definition for refractoriness and/or use of heterogeneous response parameters. In fact, refractory myositis has several definitions including intolerance to or an inadequate response to glucocorticoids and at least one other immunosuppressive agent, but few studies provide a clear description of whether the maximum tolerated therapeutic dose was achieved [5–11].

With regard to rituximab response parameters, most reports are limited to serum level of creatine phosphokinase and muscle strength improvements [6–11]. However, creatine phosphokinase may be not the best parameter, particularly if the evaluation includes different types of myositis,

* Correspondence: samuel.shinjo@gmail.com
[2]Division of Rheumatology, Faculdade de Medicina FMUSP, Universidade de Sao Paulo, Sao Paulo, Brazil
Full list of author information is available at the end of the article

such as DM and ASS, in which other target organ involvement is more relevant than muscular involvement [2]. Of note, the disease activity core set measures validated by the International Myositis Assessment & Clinical Studies Group (IMACS) [12, 13] have not been previously used to evaluate refractory IIM response to therapy. These measures defined response as a > 20% improvement on three out of any 6 of the following core set measures: Health Assessment Questionnaire (HAQ); Manual Muscle Testing-8 (MMT-8); Physician Global Activity - Visual Analogue Scale (VAS); Patient Global Activity - VAS; serum muscle enzymes; Myositis Disease Activity Assessment Tool (MDAAT); with no more than two core set measures worsening by > 25%, which cannot include MMT.

Therefore, the aim of the present study was to evaluate the efficacy and predictors of clinical improvement of rituximab in a homogeneous population of refractory IIM cases, using a rigorous definition of refractory disease and modified IMACS core set measures to evaluate long-term response.

Methods
Study design
This retrospective single-center cohort study conducted from 2011 to 2016 included 43 consecutive adult patients with refractory IIM: 15 ASS (defined as myositis, arthritis, pulmonary disease, positive antisynthetase antibody, with or without mechanic's hands, fever and/or Raynaud's phenomenon) [14]; 16 DM and 12 PM according to the criteria of Bohan and Peter [15].

Patient data
Patients with clinically amyopathic DM, overlap myositis, neoplasia associated myositis, necrotizing myopathies, acute and/or chronic infections were excluded.

Data were included in an ongoing electronic database protocol. Demographic, clinical, laboratory and therapeutic data were obtained by electronic medical records, containing previously standardized and parameterized data. The following parameters were analyzed: current age, gender, ethnicity, time between diagnosis and symptom onset, disease duration, gastrointestinal (upper dysphagia), pulmonary (moderate dyspnea or computed tomography disclosing evidence of interstitial pneumopathy and/or "ground-glass" pneumopathy), joint (arthralgia and/or arthritis), previous and current drug treatment.

Refractory myositis was defined as an inadequate response to at least two immunosuppressant/immuno-modulatory drugs (cyclophophamide, azathioprine, methotrexate, cyclosporine, leflunomide, mycophenolate mofetil and/or intravenous human immunoglobulin, in their full-dose, for a minimum period of 3 months) given sequentially or concomitantly, hampering glucocorticoid tapering. Upper dysphagia and pulmonary involvement

were considered as disease severity parameters. Severe infection was defined as requiring hospitalization and/or intravenous antibiotic therapy.

Rituximab schedule
Rituximab treatment consisted of two infusions (1 g each, 2 weeks apart) and this same scheme was repeated 6 months after the first dose for patients showing no response or stable disease. The 6-month second dose was contraindicated for patients with recrudescent disease, hypogammaglobulinemia, side effects at first rituximab infusion and recurrent or severe infections. After starting on rituximab only one immunosuppressant was maintained at full-dose, and glucocorticoid tapering was started 2 months after initial rituximab treatment.

Disease activity
At the one-year evaluation, clinical and laboratory improvements were defined as > 20% improvement in at least three of the following modified IMACS core set measures: MMT-8 [12], physician' and patient' VAS [13], HAQ [16] and serum levels of muscle enzymes; with no more than two previous core set measures worsening by > 25%, which cannot include MMT.

Serum levels of creatine phosphokinase (normal range: 24–173 U/L) and aldolase (1.0–7.5 U/L) were evaluated. The following autoantibodies were investigated in this study: antinuclear factor (Hep2) and also anti-Jo-1, anti-OJ, anti-EJ, anti-PL-7, anti-PL-12, anti-Mi-2 and anti-SS-A/Ro-52. For the myositis-specific and myositis-associated autoantibodies' assessment, a commercially available line blot test kit (Myositis Profile Euroline Blot test kit, Euroimmun, Lübeck, Germany) was used according to the manufacturer's protocol and to the previously published study [17]. Reaction positivity was also defined according to a previously study [17].

Statistical analysis
The Kolmogorov-Smirnov test was used to evaluate the distribution of each parameter. The demographic and clinical features are expressed as mean ± standard deviation (SD) for the continuous variables or frequency (%) for the categorical variables. The median (25th - 75th interquartile range) was calculated for the continuous variables that were not normally distributed. Comparisons between different clinical, laboratory and treatment parameters at baseline and 12 months after rituximab infusion were performed using Student's t-test or the Mann-Whitney U-test for continuous variables, whereas the Chi-squared test or Fisher's exact test was used to evaluate the categorical variables. The 95% confidence interval (95% CI) of percentage was calculated by a binomial distribution. Age at Rituximab application sensitivity and specificity for identifying therapy responder were

calculated, and a receiver operating characteristic (ROC) curve was constructed. $P < 0.05$ was considered significant. All of the analyses were performed using the SPSS 15.0 statistics software (Chicago, USA).

Results

Five of the initial 43 patients were later excluded due to moderate allergic reactions to the first rituximab infusion ($N = 4$) or lost to follow-up ($N = 1$). There were no cases of patients with recrudescent disease, hypogammaglobulinemia or severe infections. Therefore, 38 patients remained in the study for 1 year: 15 (39.5%) patients with DM, 10 (26.3%) with PM, and 13 (34.2%) with ASS (Table 1).

Among the 38 patients assessed, mean current age was 42.6 ± 10.9 years, 84.2% were female gender and 68.4% had white ethnicity. Median disease time was 3.0 years, whereas median time between disease diagnosis and symptom onset was 4.5 months.

The antinuclear factor was present in 81.6% of patients with the following autoantibodies specificities: anti-Ro-52 (42.1%), anti Jo-1 (34.2%), anti-Mi-2 (10.5%), and no cases of anti-OJ, anti-EJ, anti-PL-7 or anti-PL-12 autoantibodies.

All 38 patients were in concomitant use of at least two immunosuppressive / immunomodulatory drugs, in their full-dose, for a minimum period of 3 months, hampering glucocorticoid tapering. Due to disease severity, 34 (89.5%) patients had also received methylprednisolone pulse therapy 1 g/day, for three consecutive days, and/or intravenous human immunoglobulin (1 g/kg/day, for 2 days, for two consecutive days). Moreover, immediately before the first dose of rituximab, 23 (60.5%) of 38 patients received again this same scheme (methylprednisolone and intravenous human immunoglobulin pulse therapies). At the time of rituximab application, median dose of prednisone was 18.8 mg/day.

Comparison of therapies at study entry vs. 12 months after rituximab application revealed a reduction in median glucocorticoid dose (18.8 vs. 6.3 mg/day; $P < 0.001$) (Table 2) and complete discontinuation of prednisone in 16 (42.1%) of the 38 patients.

Twenty-nine (72.5%) of the 38 patients achieved overall progress according to the modified core set of IMACS after 12 months of rituximab treatment.

With regard to adverse events in the 38 patients at one-year follow-up, none had severe infection, two (5.3%) patients had mild allergic reactions and one (2.6%) patient was diagnosed with non-Hodgkin's lymphoma (Table 2).

Further analysis of responders vs. non-responders at baseline identified younger age ($P = 0.008$) and higher frequency of dysphagia ($P = 0.038$) in non-responders (Table 3). The area under the ROC curve was 0.669 and age at 32 had 72% sensitivity and 67% specificity.

Female gender, ethnicity, disease duration and time between diagnosis and symptom onset were comparable between responder and non-responder groups. There was also no differences in myositis type (DM, PM or ASS), joint and pulmonary clinical symptoms, initial serum level of muscle enzymes, autoantibodies, or pre-treatment with methylprednisolone and intravenous human immunoglobulin pulse therapies ($P > 0.05$).

Discussion

In the present one-year study, long-term rituximab efficacy in refractory patients with IIM was demonstrated.

Rigorous criteria of refractoriness and also the modified IMACS disease activity response parameters were adopted in this research. Notably, due to disease severity, more than half of the patients also needed to receive methylprednisolone associated with intravenous human immunoglobulin pulse therapy to induce disease remission. In contrast, a less strict criterion of refractoriness was observed in previous studies and data on severe symptoms such as dysphagia were not reported hampering comparison with the present

Table 1 Demographic features, types of idiopathic inflammatory myopathies, autoantibody distribution and therapy of 38 patients immediately before rituximab application (Baseline)

Parameters	N = 38
Current age (years)	42.6 ± 10.9
Female gender	32 (84.2)
White ethnicity	26 (68.4)
Disease duration (years)	3.0 (2.0–6.5)
Duration time: diagnosis - symptom onset (months)	4.5 (3.9–9.0)
Idiopathic inflammatory myopathies	
Dermatomyositis	15 (39.5)
Polymyositis	10 (26.3)
Antisynthetase syndrome	13 (34.2)
Autoantibodies	
Antinuclear factor	31 (81.6)
Anti-Ro-52	16 (42.1)
Anti-Jo-1	13 (34.2)
Anti-Mi-2	4 (10.5)
Anti-OJ	0
Anti-EJ	0
Anti-PL-7	0
Anti-PL-12	0
Prednisone dose (mg/day)	18.8 (10.0–36.3)
Methylprednisolone + intravenous human immunoglobulin pulse therapy	23 (60.5)

Results expressed as mean ± standard deviation, median (25th - 75th interquartile range) or frequency (%)

Table 2 Evaluation at baseline, 6 and 12 months of 38 patients with idiopathic inflammatory myopathies after rituximab therapy

	Baseline	6 months	12 months	Δ% (12 months vs. Baseline)
Prednisone dose (mg/day)	18.8 (10.0–36.3)	8.8 (2.5–15.0)	6.3 (0.0–16.3)	–
MMT-8 (0–80)	68.5 (56.8–72.5)	72.0 (67.0–78.0)	74.0 (70.0–78.0)	+ 11.3
HAQ (0.00–3.00)	1.00 (0.50–1.51)	0.63 (0.25–1.00)	0.50 (0.03–1.16)	−53.0
Patient's VAS (0–10 cm)	5.0 (3.0–7.0)	3.0 (1.0–5.0)	2.0 (0.0–4.0)	− 57.0
Physician's VAS (0–10 cm)	5.0 (3.8–7.0)	3.0 (1.0–4.3)	2.0 (1.0–4.0)	−60.0
Creatine phosphokinase (U/L)	429 (123–971)	224 (83–527)	254 (83–551)	−8.6
Aldolase (U/L)	5.5 (4.0–10.6)	3.9 (3.2–6.9)	3.6 (3.2–7.0)	−29.0
Severe infections	–	0	0	–
Adverse events	–	0	2 (5.3)	–
Neoplasia	–	0	1 (2.6)	–

Results expressed as percentage (%), or median (25th - 75th). *VAS* Visual Analogue Scale, *MMT* Manual Muscle Testing, *HAQ* Healthy Assessment Questionnaire, Δ% percentage variation

Table 3 Frequency of rituximab response according to myositis type, clinical involvement, autoantibody profile and treatment

	Responders (N = 29)	Non-responders (N = 9)	P
Age at disease diagnosis (years)	39.6 ± 12.2	28.3 ± 9.0	0.008
Age at Rituximab application (years)	44.7 ± 11.0	35.8 ± 8.1	0.017
Female gender	24 (82.7)	8 (88.9)	1.000
White ethnicity	19 (65.5)	7 (77.8)	0.689
Disease duration (years)	3.0 (1.5–5.5)	3.0 (2.0–10.0)	0.919
Duration: diagnosis - symptoms (months)	5.0 (3.0–8.0)	4.0 (2.5–12.0)	0.589
Myositis			
Dermatomyositis	14 (48.3)	1 (11.2)	0.061
Polymyositis	6 (20.7)	4 (44.4)	0.205
Antisynthetase syndrome	9 (31.0)	4 (44.4)	0.389
Clinical and laboratory features			
Dysphagia	18 (62.1)	9 (100.0)	0.038
Articular	11 (37.9)	5 (55.6)	0.450
Pulmonary	11 (37.9)	3 (33.3)	1.000
Creatine phosphokinase (U/L)	5798 (2796–13,630)	9000 (4484–12,472)	0.457
Aldolase (U/L)	36.1(18.7–42.3)	28.2 (20.6–40.6)	0.664
Autoantibodies			
Anti-Ro-52	11 (37.9)	5 (55.6)	0.450
Anti-Jo-1	9 (31.0)	4 (44.4)	0.689
Anti-Mi-2	4 (13.8)	0	–
Anti-OJ	0	0	–
Anti-EJ	0	0	–
Anti-PL-7	0	0	–
Anti-PL-12	0	0	–
Antinuclear factor	23 (73.9)	8 (88.9)	1.000
Pre-RTX infusion protocol			
Methylprednisolone + intravenous human immunoglobulin pulse therapy	16 (55.2)	7 (77.8)	0.273

Results expressed as mean ± standard deviation, median (25th - 75th) or percentage (%)
RTX Rituximab

analysis [4–11]. In fact, among patients evaluated in the present study, more than two-thirds had dysphagia, a known serious problem in patients with IIM that can be associated with nutritional deficiency, aspiration pneumonia and poor prognosis [18].

The rituximab protocol was a more aggressive approach than others previously reported [4–11], and included pre-infusion of methylprednisolone and intravenous human immunoglobulin for the majority of the patients. In addition, the rituximab fixed dose retreatment protocol was chosen as opposed to on-demand retreatment [4–11], taking into account refractoriness.

The long-term IMACS modified response rate obtained with the present protocol was comparable to that reported for the RIM trial [5], a remarkable result taking into consideration the disease severity and refractoriness of the patients selected. Our data reveals that this outcome occurred for all patients at 6 months and the improvement persisted at 1 year. In this regard, a highly successful prednisone taper was obtained, with a significant early mean dose reduction at 6 months and a substantial number of patients (42%) able to completely discontinue prednisone at 12 months. Reinforcing these results, a parallel improvement in MMT-8, HAQ, physician and patient' VAS, as well as in muscle enzymes occurred at 12 months.

Autoantibodies, especially anti-Jo-1 and anti-Mi-2, proved predictors of clinical improvement in a cohort of rituximab-treated myositis' patients, whereas at lack of definable autoantibodies was a predictor of no improvement [5]. Although this association was not found in the present study, the majority of patients with anti-Jo-1 and all with anti-Mi-2 autoantibodies, responded to a rituximab.

During the follow-up, rituximab was well-tolerated with few adverse reactions. The most common side effects in literature are infections (mainly respiratory tract infections), of which 5% were severe, requiring hospitalization. Infusion reactions rarely occurred and these were often mild and easily controlled with glucocorticoid. Notably, there were no cases of severe infections requiring hospitalization in the present study. The intravenous human immunoglobulin pre-rituximab may be contributed for these data. However, sustained clinical and laboratory improvement may be due to rituximab, since there was no difference between responders and non-responders regarding previous use of intravenous human immunoglobulin.

As a limitation of the present study, a small sample was included, given the rarity of the IIM and the strict inclusion and exclusion criteria applied. Moreover, a sequential analysis of the dysphagia (i.e.: manometry) and pulmonary function were not performed. Finally, it should be emphasized that the concomitant use of methylprednisolone associated with intravenous human immunoglobulin for the majority of the patients might have affected the outcomes.

Conclusions

The present study provides convincing evidence that rituximab treatment is an effective and safe therapy for refractory IIM with a sustained 1 year response and significant tapering/discontinuation of glucocorticoid therapy. Moreover, young individuals and patients with dysphagia have a tendency to be more refractory to rituximab.

Abbreviations
ASS: Antisynthetase syndrome; CI: Confidence interval; DM: Dermatomyositis; HAQ: Health Assessment Questionnaire; IIM: Idiopathic inflammatory myopathies; IMACS: International Myositis Assessment & Clinical Studies Group; MDAAT: Myositis Disease Activity Assessment Tool; MMT: Manual muscle testing; PM: Polymyositis; ROC: Receiver operating characteristic; SD: Standard deviation; VAS: Visual analogue scale

Acknowledgments
Not applicable.

Authors' contributions
All authors contributed to write and review the manuscript. All authors read and approved the final manuscript.

Author details
[1]Division of Rheumatology, Hospital das Clinicas HCFMUSP, Faculdade de Medicina, Universidade de Sao Paulo, Sao Paulo, Brazil. [2]Division of Rheumatology, Faculdade de Medicina FMUSP, Universidade de Sao Paulo, Sao Paulo, Brazil.

References
1. Feldman BM, Rider LG, Reed AM, Pachman LM. Juvenile dermatomyositis and other idiopathic inflammatory myopathies of childhood. Lancet. 2008; 371:2201–12.
2. Dalakas MC. Polymyositis, dermatomyositis and inclusion-body myositis. N Engl J Med. 1991;325:1487–98.
3. Fasano S, Gordon P, Hajji R, Loyo E, Isenberg DA. Rituximab in the treatment of inflammatory myopathies: a review. Rheumatology (Oxford). 2017;56:26–36.
4. Oddis CV, Reed AM, Aggarwal R, Rider LG, Ascherman DP, Levesque MC, et al. Rituximab in the treatment of refractory adult and juvenile dermatomyositis and adult polymyositis: a randomized, placebo-phase trial. Arthritis Rheum. 2013;65:314–24.
5. Aggarwal R, Bandos A, Reed AM, Ascherman DP, Barohn RJ, Feldman BM, et al; RIM Study Group, Oddis CV. Predictors of clinical improvement in rituximab-treated refractory adult and juvenile dermatomyositis and adult polymyositis. Arthritis Rheum. 2014;66:740–9.
6. Marie I, Dominique S, Janvresse A, Levesque H, Menard JF. Rituximab therapy for refractory interstitial lung disease related to anti-synthetase syndrome. Respir Med. 2012;106:581–7.
7. Levie TD. Rituximab in the treatment of dermatomyositis: an open-label pilot study. Arthritis Rheum. 2005;52:601–7.
8. Noss EH, Hausner-Sypek DL, Weinblatt ME. Rituximab as therapy for refractory polymyositis and dermatomyositis. J Rheumatol. 2006;33:1021–6.
9. Brulhart L, Waldburger JM, Gabay C. Rituximab in the treatment of antisynthetase syndrome. Ann Rheum Dis. 2006;65:974–5.
10. Dinh HV, McCormack C, Hall S, Prince HM. Rituximab for the treatment of the skin manifestations of dermatomyositis: a report of 3 cases. J Am Acad Dermatol. 2007;56:148–53.
11. Frikha F, Rigolet A, Behin A, Fautrel B, Herson S, Benveniste O. Efficacy of rituximab in refractory and relapsing myositis with anti-Jo-1 antibodies: a report of two cases. Rheumatology. 2009;48:1166–8.

12. Rider LG, Koziol D, Giannini EH, Jain MS, Smith MR, Whitney-Mahoney K, et al. Validation of manual muscle testing and a subset of eight muscles for adult and juvenile idiopathic inflammatory myopathies. Arthritis Care Res (Hoboken). 2010;62:465–72.

13. Sultan SM, Allen E, Oddis CV, Kiely P, Cooper RG, Lundberg IE, et al. Reliability and validity of the myositis disease activity assessment tool. Arthritis Rheum. 2008;58:3593–9.

14. Mahler M, Miller FW, Fritzler MJ. Idiopathic inflammatory myopathies and the anti-synthetase syndrome: a comprehensive review. Autoimmun Rev. 2014;13:367–71.

15. Bohan A, Peter JB. Polymyositis and dermatomyositis (first of two parts). N Engl J Med. 1975;292:344–7.

16. Bruce B, Fries JF. The Stanford health assessment questionnaire: dimensions and practical applications. Health Qual Life Outcomes. 2003;1:20.

17. Cruellas MG, Viana V dos S, Levy-Neto M, Souza FH, Shinjo SK. Myositis-specific and myositis-associated autoantibody profiles and their clinical associations in a large series of patients with polymyositis and dermatomyositis. Clinics. 2013;68:909–14.

18. Daković Z, Vesić S, Tomović M, Vuković J. Oropharyngeal dysphagia as dominant and life-threatening symptom in dermatomyositis. Vojnosanit Pregl. 2009;66:671–4.

8

Adverse drug reactions associated with treatment in patients with chronic rheumatic diseases in childhood: A retrospective real life review of a single center cohort

Manar Amanouil Said[*] [iD], Liana Soido Teixeira e Silva, Aline Maria de Oliveira Rocha, Gustavo Guimarães Barreto Alves, Daniela Gerent Petry Piotto, Claudio Arnaldo Len and Maria Teresa Terreri

Abstract

Background: Adverse drug reactions (ADRs) are the sixth leading causes of death worldwide; monitoring them is fundamental, especially in patients with disorders like chronic rheumatic diseases (CRDs). The study aimed to describe the ADRs investigating their severity and associated factors and resulting interventions in pediatric patients with CRDs.

Methods: A retrospective, descriptive and analytical study was conducted on a cohort of children and adolescents with juvenile idiopathic arthritis (JIA), juvenile systemic lupus erythematosus (JSLE) and juvenile dermatomyositis (JDM). The study evaluated medical records of the patients to determine the causality and the management of ADRs. In order to investigate the risk factors that would increase the risk of ADRs, a logistic regression model was carried out on a group of patients treated with the main used drug.

Results: We observed 949 ADRs in 547 patients studied. Methotrexate (MTX) was the most frequently used medication and also the cause of the most ADRs, which occurred in 63.3% of patients, followed by glucocorticoids (GCs). Comparing synthetic disease-modifying anti-rheumatic drugs (sDMARDs) vs biologic disease-modifying anti-rheumatic drugs (bDMARDs), the ADRs attributed to the former were by far higher than the latter. In general, the severity of ADRs was moderate and manageable. Drug withdrawal occurred in almost a quarter of the cases. In terms of risk factors, most patients who experienced ADRs due to MTX, were 16 years old or younger and received MTX in doses equal or higher than 0.6 mg/kg/week. Patients with JIA and JDM had a lower risk of ADRs than patients with JSLE. In the multiple regression model, the use of GCs for over 6 months led to an increase of 0.5% in the number of ADRs.

Conclusions: Although the ADRs highly likely affect a wide range of children and adolescents with CRDs they were considered moderate and manageable cases mostly. However, triggers of ADRs need further investigations.

Keywords: Autoimmune rheumatic diseases, Pharmacosurveillance, Adverse drug reactions, Biological agents, Childhood

* Correspondence: manarmanar2@yahoo.com
Division of Pediatric Rheumatology, Department of Pediatrics, Federal University Sao Paulo (Unifesp), Rua Borges Lagoa, 802, Sao Paulo ZIP CODE: 04038-001, Brazil

Background

According to the World Health Organization (WHO), an adverse drug reaction (ADR) is any unfavorable and unintentional reaction due to the use of a medication in a normal dose used in humans for prophylaxis, diagnosis, or treatment of diseases or to modify a physiological function [1]. ADR is the sixth leading cause of death worldwide. Therefore, monitoring ADRs is vital to prevent their detrimental consequences among patients [1, 2].

Chronic rheumatic diseases (CRDs) are inflammatory diseases arising from changes in the immune system, and their symptoms involve joints and other organs. CRDs treatment includes synthetic or biological disease-modifying anti-rheumatic drugs (sDMARDs or bDMARDs) and these medications can cause several ADRs, ranging from mild to severe that may require other medications to treat the ADR, dose reductions or even suspending the suspected medication [3–5]. Severity and frequency of ADRs depend on the dose, route of administration and length of use, in addition to the presence or absence of other risk factors [6, 7].

Most studies that have examined the safety of medications were restricted to a few years of follow-up or were performed in a cross-sectional way. Registering ADRs and associated risk factors, particularly in chronic diseases, is essential for the health team to select the best procedures and to help with pharmacosurveillance. These data can be used to predict the ADRs in children and adolescents with CRDs. A better understanding of the ADRs of each medication used to control chronic diseases leads to better treatment adherence and thereby to a better prognosis.

The objective of this study was to evaluate the frequency, severity and associated factors of ADRs in children and adolescents with CRDs and to estimate the medical decisions made as a result of these events during treatment in a cohort of pediatric patients with juvenile idiopathic arthritis (JIA), juvenile systemic lupus erythematosus (JSLE) and juvenile dermatomyositis (JDM) at a tertiary medical center in Sao Paulo.

Methods

This was a descriptive and retrospective observational cohort that included children and adolescents with JIA, JSLE and JDM, who were diagnosed according to the classification criteria for their diseases [8–10]. This center serves approximately 2000 patients with rheumatic diseases a year. A total of 622 medical records were evaluated (391 JIA, 162 JSLE and 69 JDM).

Patients were included if they were up to 16 years old for patients with JIA and up to 18 years old for patients with JSLE or JDM at the first medical attendance in the center, according to the published criteria for the diseases [8–10]; if they were 21 years old or younger at the last follow-up visit; and if they had been seen in the pediatric unit for at least six months from January 1st 1985 until December 31st 2016.

The exclusion criteria were: patients taking higher doses of medication than prescribed; patients who were not treated or were only treated with nonsteroidal anti-inflammatory drugs (NSAIDs) or analgesic drugs, due to the irregular length and dosis of use, making data difficult to evaluate; patients with more than one CRDs that could present symptoms or complications that could interfere with the data interpretation; and patients without enough data.

Data collection

The study included all the ADRs attributed to the listed drugs in the selected patients, whether or not reported to the Brazilian Health Surveillance Notification System (NOTIVISA). The data were collected at the baseline: sex, age at disease onset, the incidence of ADRs, last follow-up visit and last consultation, medications utilized to treatment besides their dose, route of administration, length of treatment, previous and current drugs at the occurrence of ADR.

The ADRs registered by the specialized physicians during the routine medical appointments and observed in the medical record were coded and analyzed with the causative drug. The data were compiled into a standard questionnaire for each disease and each medication separately.

ADRs definitions and characterizations

This study adopted the cited WHO definition of adverse drug event. The causality of ADRs was defined as "the connection between the appearance of ADRs and the drug utilization. It requires solid medical judgment based on observations of its onset and patient's status" [1].

The analysis adopted the expert judgment made by a panel of pediatric rheumatologists at that center [11, 12]. In addition, the majority of the patients used various medications combined together to control the disease. To attribute an ADR to a specific drug the following roles were used: if the ADR appeared after using the drug, lasted as long as the drug was used; were no longer observed after if that drug was withdrawn. In case of use of more than one drug, the causality of ADRs was based on previous knowledge from the literature and the judgement of the attending physician.

According to the CTCAE (Common Terminology Criteria for Adverse Events), the severity of ADRs was classified as mild when patients did not need an intervention; moderate when patients needed an intervention; serious when patients required hospitalization or caused an inability or limited ability to perform daily activities; life-threatening when patients needed immediate intervention; and fatal if they resulted in the death of the patient directly or indirectly [13].

All of the procedures to address ADRs were evaluated: medication withdrawal by the patient or by his (her) physician, a reduction in the dose, change in the route of administration, an introduction of another treatment for the ADR or patient education.

The study was approved by the Research Ethics Committee of the Federal University of Sao Paulo. As it was a retrospective observational study, the requirement for informed consent and assent was waived. However, the confidentiality and anonymity of the patients were guaranteed once the name and other personal data in the records were sheltered.

Statistical methods

Initially, all the data were stored in Excel into two tables: conventional treatments with sDMARDs and bDMARDs. To detect risk factors associated with the ADRs, the statistical analysis concerned a main used drug and the most causative of ADRs as well. For categorical variables, absolute and relative frequencies were presented and for numerical variables, measures (mean, minimum, maximum and standard deviation) or median were used. The existence of association between two categorical variables was verified using the Chi-square test and Fisher's exact test in cases of small samples. The comparison of means between two groups was performed using the nonparametric Mann-Whitney test.

Only methotrexate (MTX) and glucocorticoids (GCs) were analyzed separately. To evaluate the effect of sex, age, disease type, dosage and administration route on the occurrence of ADRs due to MTX use, a logistic regression model was applied. To access the effect of disease (JIA, JDM, JSLE) adjusted by dose, time of use and the form of application of the medications (MTX and GCs) on the number of ADRs attributed to them (dependent variable) we used the model of Poisson multiple regression. Models were adjusted separately for each medication. For all analysis, the statistical software SPSS 20.0 was used; for all statistical tests, a significance level of 5% was adopted.

Results

Patients characteristics

After applying the exclusion criteria, a total of 547 patients were evaluated (334 patients with JIA, 151 with JSLE and 62 with JDM). Of these patients, 389 (71.1%) experienced ADRs, including 220 with JIA (65.9% of JIA), 131 with JSLE (86.7% of JSLE) and 38 with JDM (61.3% of JDM), with a total of 949 ADRs (mean 1.7 ADRs per patient).

The patients mean age was 7.9 ± 2.5 years at disease onset and 17.9 ± 1.5 years at last evaluation; the mean disease duration at follow-up was 8.0 ± 1.4 years, and 72.6% were females.

A minority (7.6%) of the patients was treated in monotherapy with MTX, GC or HCQ. The majority was treated with at least two drugs.

ADR characteristics

In total, there were 33 serious events, 604 moderate events and 310 mild events. In addition, there were two cases (0.2%) of life-threatening anaphylaxis after using infliximab (IFX). Allergic skin reactions occurred in 2 of 27 patients treated with intravenous immunoglobulin (IVIG) during infusion.

MTX was responsible for 29.4% of moderate ADRs, 12.5 and 0.6% of mild and severe cases, respectively. GCs caused 18.2, 15.1 and 0.7%, of moderate, mild and severe ADRs, respectively. The Fig. 1 illustrates the severity of ADRs of the medications.

MTX and GCs were the main used drugs among the patients. According to Table 1, more than 60% of the patients who utilized MTX suffered from ADRs; followed by GCs as a second used drug and causative drug of ADRs as well, especially Cushing Syndrome. One JDM patient presented vertebral fracture and one JIA patient presented osteonecrosis. In terms of cyclophosphamide (CPA), notwithstanding it was used by a few patients, it caused ADRs in approximately 40% of them.

Out of 165 patients (with JIA, JDM and SJLE patients) treated with bDMARDs, 30 (18.2%) suffered from ADRs. Among 33 cases of ADRs, 33.3% were caused by etanercept (ETN); 33.3% by infliximab (IFX) and 24.2% by adalimumab (ADA). The principal ADR was pain/local reaction due to the injection of the bDMARDs. Table 2 shows all ADRs of the bDMARDs.

Infections were present in 45 cases among all the patients of the study; almost 45% were using MTX, 51% using other sDMARDs and two patients treated with the bDMARDs. The most of those infections were upper respiratory tract infections, herpes-zoster and cellulitis. Table 3 illustrates data on the ADRs as a dependent variable; age, dose, admissions and the use of MTX were screened into multivariate analysis. The median length of MTX use in patients who had ADRs was 35.5 months. There was no predicted time for the incidence of ADRs due to the use of MTX. The significant factors associated with the incidence of ADRs were the younger age, higher dose and the disease type.

Regarding the GCs, the median length of GCs use in patients who had ADRs was 28.0 months. ADRs due to GCs appeared after a median of 6.5 months. We observed that the dose of GCs was higher in patients with

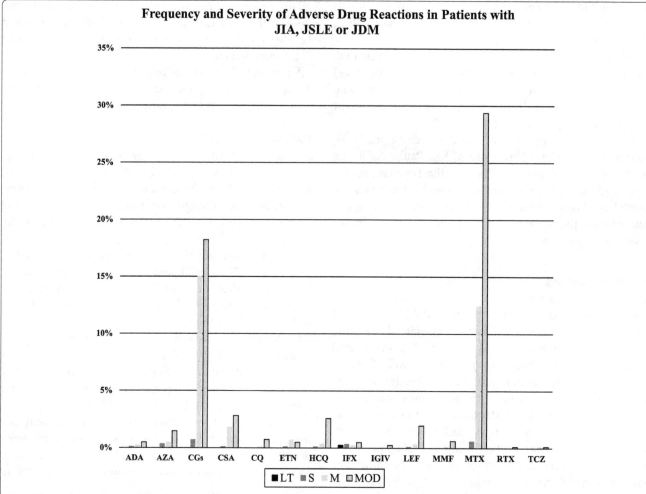

Fig. 1 Frequency and severity of adverse drug reaction. Frequency and severity of ADRs of medication used in patients with JIA, JSLE, and JDM. The vertical axis shows the percentage of adverse drug reactions of each medication. The horizontal axis shows the degree of severity of adverse drug reaction. ADR – adverse drug reaction. JIA – juvenile idiopathic arthritis. JSLE – juvenile systemic lupus erythematosus. JDM – juvenile dermatomyositis. LT – life threatening adverse event; S – severe adverse drug reaction; M – mild adverse drug reaction; MOD – moderate adverse drug reaction. % - percentage. ADA – adalimumab. AZA – azathioprine. CPA – cyclophosphamide. GCs – glucocorticoids. CSA – cyclosporine. CQ – diphosphate chloroquine. ETN – etanercept. HCQ – hydroxychloroquine. IFX – infliximab. IVIG – intravenous immunoglobulin. LEF – leflunomide. MMF – mycophenolate mofetil. MTX – methotrexate. RTX – rituximab. TCZ – tocilizumab

JDM than in patients with JSLE and JIA ($p = 0.001$). The patients with JSLE used GCs longer than patients with JIA ($p = 0.042$). Table 4 shows the characteristics of patients presented ADRs attributed to GCs. Females, younger age, patients with JSLE who used high doses of GCs demonstrated more ADRs.

Table 5 illustrates data on the risk factors associated with the ADRs. We observed that the odds ratio for experiencing an ADR in response to MTX in patients who were 16 years old or younger was 9.7-times higher than that in older patients. Additionally, patients who received MTX subcutaneously showed an odds ratio for experiencing an ADR that was 2.1 times higher than those who received MTX only orally. Higher doses of MTX were associated with the use of subcutaneous administration and with JIA. In addition, patients with JDM showed an odds ratio for experience an ADR that was 60% lower than

patients with JIA; no differences in the odds ratio among patients with JSLE and JIA were observed.

Patients with JIA and JDM showed odds ratios for experiencing an ADR that was 97 and 95% lower, respectively than patients with JSLE. In detail, the covariate analysis was multiple regression. There was no association between the number of ADRs in response to MTX ($p = 0.441$) and GCs ($p = 0.718$) and the diseases.

ADRs managements

In terms of the treatments for the ADRs, in 26.1% of the patients, other medications were introduced to minimize the ADRs, such as omeprazole, ranitidine, ondansetron and metoclopramide. Additionally, antibiotics and antiviral agents were indicated in cases of bacterial and viral infections, respectively.

Table 1 ADRs of glucocorticoids and synthetic DMARDs in patients with JIA, JSLE and JDM

Medications

	GCs	MTX	LEF	HCQ/CQ	CSA	MMF	AZA	CPA	TOTAL
Patients on MED	339	398	86	271	92	29	115	75	1405
Patients on MED with ADR	151	252	18	30	31	5	17	34	538
Patients on MED with ADR(%)	(44.5)	(63.3)	(20.9)	(11.1)	(33.7)	(17.2)	(14.8)	(45.3)	(38,3)
Infections	9	20	–	2	3	2	5	2	43
Blood and lymphatic system disorders:									
- Persistent anemia	–	1	–	–	–	–	–	–	1
- Leukopenia/Lymphopenia	–	–	–	–	–	–	6	4	10
- Pancytopenia/Neutropenia	–	–	–	–	–	–	1	–	1
Immune system disorders:									
- MAS	–	–	1	–	–	–	–	–	1
Endocrine disorders:									
- Cushing syndrome	122	–	–	–	–	–	–	–	122
- Obesity	3	–	–	–	–	–	–	–	3
Metabolism and nutrition disorders:									
-Osteoporosis*/ Low bone mineral density	51	9	–	–	–	–	–	–	60
Nervous system disorders:									
- Chronic headache/dizziness/discomfort	8	32	0	1	–	2	–	4	47
- Pseudotumor cerebri	2	–	–	–	–	–	–	–	2
-↓ convulsive threshold	–	–	1	–	–	–	–	–	1
Eye disorders:									
- Glaucoma	2	–	–	–	–	–	–	–	2
- Cataract	19	–	–	–	–	–	–	–	19
- Maculopathy	–	–	–	16	–	–	–	–	16
- Blurred vision	–	1	–	–	–	–	–	–	1
Cardiovascular disorders:									
- Arterial hypertension	42	–	–	–	3	–	–	–	45
- Arrhythmia	–	–	–	1	–	–	1	–	2
- Edema	4	–	–	–	–	–	–	–	4
Gastrointestinal disorders:									
- Nausea/vomiting	10	199	4	6	17	–	2	28	266
- Epigastric/abdominal pain	7	73	2	2	6	–	2	1	93
- Diarrhea	–	8	–	1	–	2	–	–	11
- Hyporexia	–	7	–	–	1	–	–	–	8
- Constipation	–	1	–	–	–	–	–	1	2
Hepatobiliary disorders:									
- ↑ liver enzymes	2	68	7	1	1	–	5	1	85
- Hepatic steatosis	1	–	–	–	–	–	–	–	1
- Jaundice	–	–	1	1	–	–	–	–	2
Oral disorders:									
- Mouth ulcers	–	3	1	–	–	–	–	–	4
- Mucositis	–	3	–	–	–	–	–	–	3
- Gingival hyperplasia	–	–	–	–	2	–	–	–	2
Skin and subcutaneous tissue disorders:									

Table 1 ADRs of glucocorticoids and synthetic DMARDs in patients with JIA, JSLE and JDM *(Continued)*

Medications	GCs	MTX	LEF	HCQ/CQ	CSA	MMF	AZA	CPA	TOTAL
- Striae	3	–	–	–	–	–	–	–	3
- Atopic dermatitis	–	–	–	1	–	–	–	–	1
- Alopecia	–	5	4	–	–	–	1	10	20
- Hypertrichosis	–	–	–	–	7	–	–	–	7
- Urticaria	4	5	1	2	2	–	–	–	14
Musculoskeletal and connective tissue disorders:									
-↑ muscle enzymes	–	–	–	1	–	–	–	–	1
- Myositis	–	–	–	1	–	–	–	–	1
- Myalgia	3	–	–	–	–	–	–	–	3
Renal and urinary disorders:									
-↑ urea	–	–	–	–	1	–	–	–	1
General disorders and administration site conditions:									
- Infusion reactions and pain	3	4	–	–	–	–	–	–	7
Total number of ADRs	295	439	22	36	43	6	23	51	915

ADR - adverse drug reaction, DMARDs - disease modifying antirheumatic drugs, JIA - juvenile idiopathic arthritis, JSLE - juvenile systemic lupus erythematosus, JDM - juvenile dermatomyosis, MED - Medication. Patients on MED- number of patients who used the medication. Patients on MED with ADR- number of patients who used the medication and experienced at least one adverse drug reaction. Patients on MED with ADR(%)- percentage of patients who used the medication and experienced at least one adverse drug reaction = N. P with ADR X 100/N.P on MED. ↑ liver enzymes - elevated liver enzymes. MAS - macrophagic activation syndrome. ↑ muscle enzymes - elevated muscle enzymes. ↓ convulsive threshold - reduction of the convulsive threshold. ↑ urea - elevated urea. MTX - methotrexate (median dose - 0.65 mg/kg/week and median length of treatment - 35.5 months). GCs - glucocorticoids (median dose - 0.64 mg/kg/day and median length of treatment - 28 months). CSA - cyclosporine (median dose - 4.2 mg/kg/day and median length of treatment - 35.3 months). LEF -leflunomide (median dose of 0.6 mg/kg/day and median length of treatment - 13.5 months). MMF - Mycophenolate mofetil (median dose - 32.2 mg/kg/day and median length of treatment - 19.8 months). HCQ-hydroxychloroquine (median dose - 5.5 mg/kg/day and median length of treatment - 30.7 months). CQ-diphosphate chloroquine (median dose - 4.7 mg/kg/day and median length of treatment - 28.3 months). CPA - cyclophosphamide (median dose of 734 mg/dose and median length of treatment - 5.9 months). AZA - azathioprine (median dose - 1.3 mg/kg/day and median length of treatment - 28.1 months). * one fracture

The withdrawal of the drug that caused the ADR (either by the medical staff or by the patient) occurred in 23.9% of the patients and 8.5% of the patients who used MTX had to interrupt the use. A reduction in the dose of the medication was required in 8.6% of all the patients and in 5.5% of patients who used MTX. In 6.3% of patients, there was a change in the route of administration.

Other procedures (2.9%) included patient education, such as taking MTX after breakfast or at night, or weekly dose administration at two different times on the same day. In 1.1% of the cases, we increased the interval between the doses of the medication. In 0.4% of cases, we did not increase the dose, even if there was a necessity due to disease activity.

Two patients (0.3%) suffered from pseudotumor cerebri caused by GCs that improved after lumbar puncture and the use of acetazolamide. No procedure was necessary in 30.4% of the patients because the ADRs were mild. Of the total of ADRs 64.5% remitted, 35.4% remained and 0.1% worsened despite treatment.

Discussion
More than two-thirds of the patients experienced at least one ADR, with a mean of 1.7 ADRs for each patient. We observed that some patients experienced up to 13 ADRs.

Patients with JIA constituted the major group in the study and MTX was the drug of choice. In terms of the ADRs, MTX was the most causative of ADRs among approximately 60% of the patients treated with it; followed by GCs and CPA, respectively.

The ADRs due to MTX have been found more common in our research than in literature, most of them were attributed to gastrointestinal events such as nausea and/or vomiting and elevated liver enzymes [14, 15].

Our study recorded a 17% of patients with increase in liver enzymes with the use of MTX, while Veld et al. [16] found that 8% of patients with JIA treated with MTX for a year showed an elevation in liver enzymes. The different lengths of treatment may have directly influenced the prevalence of the studied ADRs. Reducing dosis (5.5%) or withdrawal of MTX (8.5%) and monitoring levels of liver enzymes were the selected managements and we did not find any irreversible liver damage.

Infections attributed to MTX occurred in 20 patients (5%) mainly herpes zoster infections. Whilst, infections of the respiratory system (pneumonia and bacteremia) or septicemia were the main infections in hospitalized patients; exactly as it was mentioned in the literature [17]. Although mucositis and oral ulcers have been described during the use of MTX, the small number of our cases is

Table 2 ADRs of bDMARDs in patients with JIA, JSLE and JDM

	Medications						
	ETN	ADA	IFX	TCZ	ABA	RTX	TOTAL
Patients on MED	54	49	36	9	7	10	165
Patients on MED with ADR	10	6	11	2	–	1	30
Patients on MED with ADR(%)	18.5	12.2	30.5	22.2	–	10	18.2
Infections	–	–	1	–	–	1	2
Blood and lymphatic system disorders:							
- Thrombocytopenia	–	–	1	–	–	–	1
Nervous system disorders:							
- Headache/dizziness/discomfort	–	–	1	–	–	–	1
Eye disorders:							
- Uveitis	2	1	–	–	–	–	3
Gastrointestinal disorders:							
- Nausea/vomiting	2	3	1	–	–	–	6
- Epigastric pain	–	1	–	–	–	–	1
Hepatobiliary disorders:							
- ↑ liver enzymes	–	–	–	1	–	–	1
Skin and subcutaneous tissue disorders:							
- Atopic dermatitis	1	–	–	–	–	–	1
- Psoriasis	–	1	–	–	–	–	1
- Urticaria	–	–	3	1	–	–	4
Renal and urinary disorders:							
- Nephritis	1	–	–	–	–	–	1
- Hematuria	–	1	–	–	–	–	1
General disorders and administration site conditions:							
- Anaphylaxis	–	–	2	–	–	–	2
- Local reactions and pain	5	1	2	–	–	–	8
Total number of ADRs	11	8	11	2	–	1	33

ADR - adverse drug reaction, JIA - juvenile idiopathic arthritis, JSLE - juvenile systemic lupus erythematosus, JDM - juvenile dermatomyositis, MED - Medication. Patients on MED- number of patients who used the medication. Patients on MED with ADR- number of patients who used the medication and experienced at least one adverse drug reaction. Patients on MED with ADR(%)- percentage of patients who used the medication and experienced at least one adverse drug reaction = N. P with ADR X 100/N.P on MED. ↑ liver enzymes - elevated liver enzymes. ETN - etanercept (median dose - 1.1 mg/kg/week and median length of treatment - 8.4 months). ADA - adalimumab (median dose - 0.8 mg/kg/dose every 15 days and median length of treatment - 11 months). IFX - infliximab (median dose - 5.4 mg/kg/dose every 8 weeks and median length of treatment - 8.4 months). TCZ - tocilizumab (median dose - 9.7 mg/kg/dose monthly and median length of treatment - 7.5 months). ABA - abatacept (median dose - 10 mg/kg/dose monthly and median length of treatment - 12 months). RTX - rituximab (median dose 1 g/dose twice monthly every 6 months)

very likely due to the prophylactic routine use of folic acid and due to the MTX dose used to treat CRDs [18].

More ADRs attributed to MTX were found in younger patients. The need of high doses of MTX to control JIA may explain the association of this disease with a higher frequency of ADRs [19]. However, in the multiple regression model, the disease itself did not affect the number of ADRs, even with an adjusted using length, dose and route of administration of MTX. As also described in the literature, subcutaneous MTX has higher bioavailability and therefore can be more efficient [20]. Gastrointestinal intolerance and elevated liver enzymes are also associated with higher doses of MTX [21, 22] and the

eventual or continuous use of NSAIDs by JIA patients could exacerbate the ADRs [23].

Interestingly, patients with JDM experienced fewer ADRs than the group with JIA, although these patients used statistically similar doses of MTX for a similar length of time. This is maybe due to the frequent or long use of NSAIDs by patients with JIA that may exacerbate the incidence of ADRs. The lack of the evaluation of the use of NSAIDs precludes more accurate conclusions, characterizing a probable bias.

Among the 339 patients treated with GCs, approximately half experienced ADRs. These occurred mainly in patients with JSLE. Cushing's syndrome was the most

Table 3 Characteristics of patients who used methotrexate (MTX) and presented adverse drug reactions (ADRs)

Variable	ADRs of MTX (N = 398)		
	Yes	No	p*
	n = 252	n = 146	
Sex (%)			
Female	174 (63.3)	101 (36.7)	0.978
Male	78 (63.4)	45 (36.6)	
Age (years) – Cohort in median			
≤ 16	236 (72.6)	89 (27.4)	< 0.001
> 16	16 (21.9)	57 (78.1)	
Route of administration of MTX (%)			
Subcutaneous	40 (62.5)	24 (37.5)	0.882
Oral	212 (63.5)	122 (36.5)	
Dose of MTX (mg/kg/week)			
≥ 0.6	175 (69.7)	76 (30.3)	0.001
< 0.6	77 (52.4)	70 (47.6)	
Disease (%)			
JIA	207 (68.1)	97 (31.9)	0.001
JSLE	20 (57.1)	15 (42.9)	
JDM	25 (42.4)	34 (57.6)	

N - number of patients treated with MTX, JIA - juvenile idiopathic arthritis, JSLE - juvenile systemic lupus erythematosus, JDM - juvenile dermatomyositis
* Chi Pearson square or Fisher's exact. $P < 0.05$

Table 4 Characteristics of the patients who used glucocorticoids (GCs) and presented adverse drug reactions (ADRs)

Variable	ADRs of glucocorticoid (N = 339)		
	Yes n (151)	No n (188)	p*
Sex (%)			
Female	122 (48.2)	131 (51.8)	0.019
Male	29 (33.7)	57 (66.3)	
Age			
≤ 16	135 (56.3)	105 (43.7)	< 0.001
> 16 years	16 (16.2)	83 (83.8)	
Type of glucocorticoid			
Methylprednisolone	3 (12.5)	21 (87.5)	< 0,001
Prednisone	71 (100)	0 (0.0)	
Prednisone / Methylprednisolone**	77 (31.6)	167 (68.4)	
Dose of prednisone (mg/kg/day) ***			
≥ 0,5	91 (58.1)	65 (41.9)	< 0.001
< 0,5	57 (35.8)	102 (64.2)	
Disease			
JIA	18 (12.8)	123 (87.2)	< 0.001
JSLE	120 (82.8)	25 (17.2)	
JDM	13 (24.5)	40 (75.5)	

N - number of patients treated with GCs, JIA - juvenile idiopathic arthritis, JSLE - juvenile systemic lupus erythematosus, JDM - juvenile dermatomyositis
* Chi Pearson square or Fisher's exact $P < 0.05$
** Prednisone (oral) / Methyprednisolone (pulse therapy) indicates patients treated with GCs and who presented ADRs during the use of combined oral and pulse therapy. Three patients with ADRs and 21 patients in the group without ADRs did not use GCs orally but used pulse therapy only
*** The dose of 30 mg/kg/dose of pulse therapy was not considered in the calculation

observed ADR in patients treated with GCs, followed by low bone mineral density [24, 25].

Cushing syndrome was observed in 80.8% of patients who had ADRs using GCs and is characterized by growth failure, central obesity, facial plethora, headaches, hypertension, hirsutism, amenorrhea, delayed sexual development, virilization in pubertal children, acne, violaceous striae, bruising, or acanthosis nigricans [26]. Obesity was observed in 1.9% of patients who had ADRs using GCs and 1.4% of total of patients with JSLE and JDM in our study. Obesity is defined by World Health Organization for children age 0–5 years as body mass index (BMI) or weight for length/ height > +3SD and for children age 5–19 years as BMI > + 2 SD [27].

A recent systematic review about GCs use showed that the three most commonly observed ADRs associated with long-course oral corticosteroids in children were weight gain (ranging from 6 to 10%), growth retardation and cushingoid features, with respective incidence rates of 21.1, 18.1 and 19.4% of patients assessed for these ADRs [28]. The same review had found 21.5% of patients with decreased bone density [28].

Other ADRs, such as cataracts, arterial hypertension and psychiatric symptoms were observed in a few patients in our study. Two patients developed pseudotumor cerebri, which is associated with the use of GCs [29]. One patient with systemic JIA experienced hepatic steatosis, identified by ultrasonography, due to the need of high doses of the medication.

In terms of the risk factors associated with ADRs due to GCs, the ADRs occurred more frequently in females, younger age, oral use, higher doses and the presence of JSLE. Another study, however, showed that the administration of pulse therapy in association with oral doses of GCs is responsible for ADRs in 70% of treated patients [30]. A study emphasized that treatment with doses lower than 7.5 mg per day was safe during GC administration, whereas other studies showed that higher doses were associated with ADRs [31–33].

We observed that the dose of GCs was higher in patients with JDM than in JSLE and JIA patients. However, the JDM group did not show a higher frequency of

Adverse drug reactions associated with treatment in patients with chronic rheumatic diseases...   63

Table 5 Risk of ADRs in response to methotrexate (MTX) and glucocorticoids (GCs) based on logistic regression

Variable	Logistic regression to methotrexate			
	OR		Adjusted OR	
	(IC95%)	p	(IC95%)	p
Sex: male (ref-female)	1.01 (0.65–1.56)	0.978	1.04 (0.61–1.77)	0.882
Age (years)	0.84 (0.80–0.88)	< 0.001	–	–
Age ≤ 16 years (ref-more than 16 years)	9.45 (5.15–17.31)	< 0.001	9.68 (4.86–19.28)	< 0.001
Administration routes of methotrexate (ref-oral)				
Subcutaneous	1.92 (1.07–3.44)	0.028	2.10 (1.05–4.20)	0.036
Dose	5.14 (2.14–12.36)	< 0.001	1.21 (0.4–3.68)	0.737
Dose of methotrexate ≥ 0.6 mg/kg/week (ref-more than 0,6)	2.09 (1.37–3.19)	0.001	–	–
Disease (ref.- JIA)				
JSLE	0.62 (0.31–1.27)	0.195	2.4 (0.95–6.07)	0.064
JDM	0.34 (0.19–0.61)	< 0.001	0.40 (0.2–0.79)	0.008
Variable	Logistic regression to glucocorticoid			
	OR		Adjusted OR	
	(IC95%)	p	(IC95%)	p
Sex: male (ref.- female)	0.55 (0.33–0.91)	0.02	1.10 (0.50–2.38)	0.816
Age (years)	0.86 (0.81–0.91)	< 0.001	–	–
Age ≤ 16 years (ref.- more than 16 years)	6.67 (3.69–12.07)	< 0.001	9.92 (4.36–22.54)	< 0.001
Dose of glucocorticoid (oral)	5.63 (2,88-11,00)	< 0,001	–	–
Dose of glucocorticoid (oral) ≥ 0.5 mg/kg/day (ref.-less than 0.5)	2.51 (1.59–3.95)	< 0.001	1.88 (0.96–3.69)	0.067
30 mg/kg/dose (Pulse therapy)	0.26 (0.07–0.89)	0.033	0.54 (0.12–2.39)	0.42
Disease (ref.- JSLE)				
JIA	0.03 (0.02–0.06)	< 0.001	0.03 (0.01–0.06)	< 0.001
JDM	0.07 (0.03–0.14)	< 0.001	0.05 (0.02–0.11)	< 0.001

ADR - adverse drug reaction, OR - odds ratio, aOR - adjusted odd ratios, CI - confidence interval, p - probability of significance, Ref - reference, JIA - juvenile idiopathic arthritis, JSLE - juvenile systemic lupus erythematosus, JDM - juvenile dermatomyositis, MTX - methotrexate, mg/kg-milligrams per kilogram, GCs - glucocorticoids

ADRs; 14.5% of the JDM patients did not use GCs, because this was a mild disease with a favorable outcome. In the multiple regression model, every additional month of use of GCs led to an increase of 0.5% in the mean number of ADRs.

CPA was the medication that caused the second-most ADRs when the number of patients who used CPA was taken into account. Half of the patients experienced ADRs, which mainly included nausea and/or vomiting and alopecia. We observed, in contrast to what was described in the literature, a small percentage of myelotoxicity, which manifested as leukopenia and/or lymphopenia [34]. The routine use of 2-mercaptoethane sulfonate (Mesna) and hyperhydration probably prevented hemorrhagic cystitis. Although CPA is a potent immunosuppressant, infections directly associated with this drug occurred in only two JSLE patients.

The most frequent ADR related hydroxychloroquine (HCQ) / diphosphate chloroquine (CQ) was the maculopathy, that occurred in 5.9% of the patients in use. It was observed that median dose of HCQ was 5.5 mg/kg/d and the median length was 30.7 months. Previous study about toxic retinopathy related HCQ use showed that the overall prevalence of HCQ retinopathy was 7.5% although varied with daily intake and with duration of use [35]. For daily intake of 4.0 to 5.0 mg/kg, the prevalence of retinal toxicity remained less than 2% within the first 10 years of use and almost 20% after 20 years of use but is 2 to 3 times higher at use exceeding 5.0 mg/kg [35].

Thereby, the American Academy of Ophthalmology recommends that all patients using HCQ keep daily dosage less than 5.0 mg/kg and a baseline fundus examination should be performed to rule out preexisting maculopathy, followed by annual screening after 5 years for patients on acceptable doses and without major risk factors [36].

Biological DMARDs are medications indicated in refractory cases that have a great effect and have been used in our service for approximately 15 years; however, their ADRs are potentially important, including infectious and the possibility of cancer [37–39]. The evaluation of immunogenicity and neoplasia associated with bDMARDs was not the objective of this study.

Approximately 20% of patients who used bDMARDs experienced some ADRs. However, among the ADRs studied, reactions and pain at the injection site, allergic reactions and/or anaphylaxis and gastrointestinal intolerance were the predominant ADRs. Although infections and their complications are the most known ADRs related to bDMARDs in some studies, in our study, fortunately, it was found in approximately 1% of patients. A bacterial abscess after IFX use and a case of tuberculosis after rituximab (RTX) use were described.

Interestingly, a patient with JIA, treated with ETN, experienced features of the mixed-renal syndrome (with hematuria and nephrotic levels of proteinuria) and needed hospitalization. Some series of cases reports in literature describe the nephropathy as an uncommon ADR related to anti-TNF-alpha agents that can present with a range of asymptomatic microscopic or macroscopic hematuria and varying degrees of proteinuria [40].

The triggering of uveitis by ETN occurred in two patients in our study, as it has been described in the literature [41], and one case of uveitis was registered during treatment with ADA. IFX caused two cases of life-threatening anaphylaxis and three serious cases of allergic skin reactions, as mentioned in other studies [42]. A patient with JIA experienced thrombocytopenia while taking IFX; however, autoantibodies for JSLE were negative.

The conventional drugs (GCs, sDMARD) caused much more ADRs than the bDMARDs (96.4% × 3.6%). Additionally, when considering the total use of sDMARDs medications (1405), we observed 915 ADRs (65.1% of the cases), whereas when considering the use of bDMARDs (165 uses of these medications), we observed 33 ADRs (20% of the cases). The fact that the use of bDMARDs is more recent and sometimes they are used in combination and with similar ADR must be taken into account. However, two life-threatening events were caused by bDMARDs.

The management of the ADRs was substantially based on the severity. The usual attitude of the physicians who were attending these patients at the referral medical center in front of an ADR was to stop the suspected medication, what occurred in roughly a quarter of the cases.

In regard to the limitations of this study, the retrospective nature and the eventual omission of complaints or information by the patient, caregiver or even by the examiner, when completing the file should be mentioned. The lack of the evaluation of the disease activity and of the use of NSAIDs (due to the transient treatment with these medications and sometimes due to self-medication by the patient) is also a limitation.

NSAIDs and analgesic drugs (such as paracetamol and dipyrone) were used as adjuvant medications in case of pain and not regularly. A total of 251 (45.8%) of patients have ever used NSAIDs, especially JIA patients (244), with the objective of controlling symptoms and supporting the main drug. In 72.5% of the patients who used NSAIDs, it was associated with MTX (data not shown). As we said before, these data couldn't be measured due to the large variability of the length and posology of the use. The ADRs presented were attributed to each medication due to previous knowledge based on the literature and the judgement of the attending physician.

Due to the need to control disease, drug combination was inevitable, which prevented the detection of ADR causality separately or even the use of associated drugs in multivariate analysis. In addition, the socioeconomic status and the health system in Brazil with consequent limited use of bDMARDs in patients with CRDs means that ADRs may be different in other countries due to different treatment practices. The lack of history of allergy of patients or ADRs prior to the listed drugs retains the study to detect the possibility of preventing ADRs. The lack of patients' history of allergy or previous ADRs to the listed drugs withholds the study to detect the preventability of ADRs.

This study is the largest in the literature in a real-life setting that investigated all ADRs associated with the medical treatment in a large number of children and adolescents with CRDs, based on a 30 years data from a reference center in Brazil and transferred information about the ADRs management made by pediatric rheumatologist. This study provides a greater awareness of about the necessity of pharmacovigilance to monitor and manage the ADRs in health care centers, which treat children with CRDs to avoid their detrimental complications and it can be in the future, a model for a long-term prospective study with the drugs used in children with CRDs.

Conclusions

A wide range of children and adolescents with CRDs might suffer from ADRs. Nonetheless, they were considered as a moderate and manageable. Triggers of ADRs need further investigation. This study was the first step towards the self-censorship in a health care center to monitor ADRs.

Acknowledgments

The authors would like to thank the physicians, caregivers and administration staff at the Pediatric Rheumatology Center at Hospital Sao Paulo.

Authors' contributions

MAS performed the sample collection and processing, data analysis and drafted the manuscript. MTT participated in the design of the study, helped to data analysis and in drafting of the manuscript. LSST, AMOR and GGBA helped to data analysis and in drafting of the manuscript. DGPP and CAL participated in the design of the study, helped to data analysis and in drafting of the manuscript. All authors have read and approved the final manuscript.

Adverse drug reactions associated with treatment in patients with chronic rheumatic diseases...

65

References

1. WHO. National Pharmacovigilance Systems – country profiles and overview. Uppsala: The Uppsala Monitoring Centre; 1997.
2. Thomas S, Griffiths C, Smeeth L, Rooney C, Hall A. Burden of mortality associated with autoimmune diseases among females in the United Kingdom. Am J Public Health. 2010;100(11):2279–87.
3. Grevich S, Shenoi S. Update on the management of systemic juvenile idiopathic arthritis and role of IL-1 and IL-6 inhibition. Adolesc Health Med Ther. 2017;8:125–35.
4. Thakra A, Klein-Gitelman MS. An update on treatment and management of pediatric systemic lupus erythematosus. Rheumatol Ther. 2016;3(2):209–19.
5. Papadopoulou C, Wedderburn LR. Treatment of juvenile dermatomyositis: an update. Paediatr Drugs. 2017;19(5):423–34.
6. Mazaud C, Fardet L. Relative risk of and determinants for adverse events of methotrexate prescribed at a low dose: a systematic review and meta-analysis of randomized placebo-controlled trials. Br J Dermatol. 2017;177(4):978–86.
7. Alsufyani K, Ortiz-Alvarez O, Cabral DA, Tucker LB, Petty RE, Malleson PN. The role of subcutaneous administration of methotrexate in children with juvenile idiopathic arthritis who have failed oral methotrexate. J Rheumatol. 2004;31(1):179–82.
8. Petty RE, Southwood TR, Manners P, Baum J, Glass DN, Goldenberg J, et al. International league of associations for rheumatology classification of juvenile idiopathic arthritis: second revision. Edmonton 2001. J Rheumatol. 2004;31:390–2.
9. Hochberg MC. Updating the American College of Rheumatology revised criteria for the classification of systemic lupus erythematosus. Arthritis Rheum. 1997;40(9):1725.
10. Bohan A, Peter J. Polymyositis and dermatomyositis. N Engl J Med. 1975;292(7):344–7.
11. Mouton J, Mehta U, Rossiter D, Maartens G, Cohen K. Interrater agreement of two adverse drug reaction causality assessment methods. PLoS One. 2017;12(2):0172830.
12. Brown EG, Wood L, Wood S. The medical dictionary for regulatory activities (MedDRA). Drug Saf. 1999;20(2):109–17.
13. National Institutes of Health (US), National Cancer Institute, Department of health and human services. Common Terminology Criteria for Adverse Events (CTCAE). Version 5.0. 2017.
14. Dijkhuizen EHP, Wulffraat NM. Prediction of methotrexate efficacy and adverse events in patients with juvenile idiopathic arthritis: a systematic literature review. Ped Rheumatol. 2014;2:51.
15. Fráňová J, Fingerhutová Š, Kobrová K, Srp R, Němcová D, Hoza J, et al. Methotrexate efficacy, but not its intolerance, is associated with the dose and route of administration. Pediatr Rheumatol Online J. 2016;14(1):36.
16. Veld J, Wulffraat NM, Swart JF. Adverse events of methotrexate treatment in JIA. Pediatr Rheumatol Online J. 2011;9(1):203.
17. Beukelman T, Xie F, Chen L, Baddley JW, Delzell E, Grijalva CG, et al. Rates of hospitalized bacterial infection associated with juvenile idiopathic arthritis and its treatment. Arthritis Rheum. 2012;64(8):2773–80.
18. Ravelli A, Migliavacca D, Viola S, Ruperto N, Pistorio A, Martini A. Efficacy of folinic acid in reducing methotrexate toxicity in juvenile idiopathic arthritis. Clin Exp Rheumatol. 1999;17:625–7.
19. Klein A, Kaul I, Foeldvari I, Ganser G, Urban A, Horneff G. Efficacy and safety of oral and parenteral methotrexate therapy in children with juvenile idiopathic arthritis: an observational study with patients from the German methotrexate registry. Arthritis Care Res. 2012;64(9):1349–56.
20. Vena GA, Cassano N, Iannone F. Update on subcutaneous methotrexate for inflammatory arthritis and psoriasis. Ther Clin Risk Manag. 2018;14:105–16.
21. Attar SM. Adverse effects of low dose methotrexate in rheumatoid arthritis patients. A hospital-based study. Saudi Med J. 2010;31(8):909–15.
22. Becker M, Rosé CD, Cron RQ, Sherry DD, Bilker WB, Lautenbach E. Effectiveness and toxicity of methotrexate in juvenile idiopathic arthritis: comparison of 2 initial dosing regimens. J Rheumatol. 2010;37(4):870–5.
23. Ting TV, Hashkes PJ. Methotrexate/naproxen – associated severe hepatitis in a child with juvenile idiopathic arthritis. Clin Exp Rheumatol. 2007;25(6):928–9.
24. Schäcke H, Döcke WD, Asadullah K. Mechanisms involved in the side effects of glucocorticoids. Pharmacol Ther. 2002;96(1):23–43.
25. Eastell R, Reid DM, Compston J, Cooper C, Fogelman I, Francis RM, et al. A UK consensus group on management of glucocorticoid-induced osteoporosis: an update. J Int Med. 1998;244:271–92.
26. Stratakis CA. Cushing syndrome in pediatrics. Endocrinol Metab Clin N Am. 2012;41(4):793–803.
27. Aggarwal B, Jain V. Obesity in children: definition, etiology and approach. Indian J Pediatr. 2018;85(6):463–71.
28. Aljebab F, Choonara I, Conroy S. Systematic review of the toxicity of long-course oral corticosteroids in children. PLoS One. 2017;12(1):e0170259.
29. Raeeskarami S, Shahbaznejad L, Assari R, Aghighi Y. Pseudotumor cerebri as the first manifestation of juvenile systemic lupus erythematosus. Iran J Pediatr. 2016;26(5):5176.
30. Beleslin NB, Ciric J, Zarkovic M, Stojkovic M, Savic S, Knezevic M, et al. Efficacy and safety of combined parenteral and oral steroid therapy in Graves' orbitopathy. Hormones (Athens). 2014;13(2):222–8.
31. Ruiz-Irastorza G, Danza A, Khamashta M. Glucocorticoid use and abuse in SLE. Rheumatol. 2012;51(7):1145–53.
32. Da Silva JA, Jacobs JW, Kirwan JR, Boers M, Saag KG, Inês LB, et al. Safety of low dose glucocorticoid treatment in rheumatoid arthritis: published evidence and prospective trial data. Ann Rheum Dis. 2006;65(3):285–93.
33. Stuart FA, Segal TY, Keady S. Adverse psychological effects of corticosteroids in children and adolescents. Arch Dis Child. 2005;90:500–6.
34. Hu SC, Lin CL, Lu YW, Chen GS, Yu HS, Wu CS, et al. Lymphopaenia, anti-Ro/anti-RNP autoantibodies, renal involvement and cyclophosphamide use correlate with increased risk of herpes zoster in patients with systemic lupus erythematosus. Acta Derm Venereol. 2013;93(3):314–8.
35. Melles RB, Marmor MF. The risk of toxic retinopathy in patients on long-term hydroxychloroquine therapy. JAMA Ophthalmol. 2014;132(12):1453–60.
36. Marmor MF, Kellner U, Lai TY, Melles RB, Mieler WF. American Academy of ophthalmology. Recommendations on screening for Chloroquine and Hydroxychloroquine retinopathy (2016 revision). Ophthalmology. 2016;123(6):1386–94.
37. Viswanathan V, Murray KJ. Management of children with juvenile idiopathic arthritis. Indian J Ped. 2016;83(1):63–70.
38. Stoll ML, Cron RQ. Treatment of juvenile idiopathic arthritis: a revolution in care. Pediatr Rheumatol Online J. 2014;12:13.
39. Pastore S, Naviglio S, Canuto A, Lepore L, Martelossi S, Ventura A, et al. Serious adverse events associated with anti-tumor necrosis factor alpha agents in pediatric-onset inflammatory bowel disease and juvenile idiopathic arthritis in a real-life setting. Pediatr Drugs. 2017;6:1–7.
40. Lernia VD. IgA nephropathy during treatment with TNF-alpha blockers: could it bepredicted? Med Hypotheses. 2017;107:12–3.
41. Horneff G, Klein A, Klotsche J, Minden K, Huppertz HI, Weller-Heinemann F, et al. Comparison of treatment response, remission rate and drug adherence in polyarticular juvenile idiopathic arthritis patients treated with etanercept, adalimumab or tocilizumab. Arthritis Res Ther. 2016;18(1):272.
42. Barbosa CMPL, Terreri MTRA, Oliveira SKF, Rodrigues MCF, Bica B, Sacchetti S, et al. Adverse events during the infusion of infliximab in children and adolescents: a multicenter study. Rev Bras Reumatol. 2008;48(5):278–82.

9

Antiphospholipid Syndrome Committee of the Brazilian Society of Rheumatology position statement on the use of direct oral anticoagulants (DOACs) in antiphospholipid syndrome (APS)

Gustavo Guimarães Moreira Balbi[1][*] , Marcelo de Souza Pacheco[2], Odirlei Andre Monticielo[3], Andreas Funke[4], Adriana Danowski[2], Mittermayer Barreto Santiago[5], Henrique Luiz Staub[6], Jozelia Rêgo[7] and Danieli Castro Oliveira de Andrade[8]

Abstract

Background: The term Direct Oral Anticoagulants (DOACs) refers to a group of drugs that inhibit factor Xa or thrombin. Even though their use for treating different thrombotic or prothrombotic conditions is increasing recently, there is no compelling evidence indicating that those medications are safe in all antiphospholipid syndrome (APS) patients.

Methodology: To address this issue, specialists from the Antiphospholipid Syndrome Committee of the Brazilian Society of Rheumatology performed a comprehensive review of the literature regarding DOACs use in APS to answer the three following questions: (1) potential mechanisms of action of these drugs that could be relevant to APS pathogenesis, (2) DOACs interference on lupus anticoagulant testing, and (3) the efficacy of DOACs in APS.

Position statement: After critically reviewing the relevant evidence, the authors formulated 8 Position Statements about DOACs use in APS.

Conclusion: DOACs should not be routinely used in APS patients, especially in those with a high-risk profile (triple positivity to aPL, arterial thrombosis, and recurrent thrombotic events). In addition, DOACs interferes with LA testing, leading to false-positive results in patients investigating APS.

Keywords: Antiphospholipid syndrome, Factor Xa inhibitors, Rivaroxaban, Apixaban, Edoxaban, Antithrombins, Dabigatran

Background

Direct oral anticoagulants (DOACs) are medications used for treating different thrombotic or prothrombotic conditions, such as non-valvular atrial fibrillation (AFib) [1–5], deep vein thrombosis (DVT) [6–9], and pulmonary embolism (PE) [10], as well as for

thromboprophylaxis after elective lower limb orthopedic surgery [11] and for acutely ill medical patients [12–14]. Until now, this class of medication comprises five different drugs, dabigatran, rivaroxaban, apixaban, endoxaban and betrixaban (not discussed in this review, since it is not available in Brazil at this time), each of them with different half-life, pharmacokinetics, pharmacodynamics, and even clinical indications. Table 1 provides summarized information regarding those drugs [15–19].

In the pivotal trials, DOACs were non-inferior to the standard-of-care warfarin, with a good safety profile.

* Correspondence: ggmbalbi@gmail.com
[1]Serviço de Reumatologia, Hospital Universitário, Universidade Federal de Juiz de Fora (UFJF), Av. Eugênio do Nascimento, s/n - Dom Bosco, Juiz de Fora, MG 36038-330, Brazil
Full list of author information is available at the end of the article

Table 1 Characteristics of DOACs. Adapted from references [15–19]

Drugs	Mechanism of action	Brand name	Clinical indications	Half-life	Elimination	Drug interactions (see Table 2)
Dabigatran	Direct thrombin inhibitor	Pradaxa	- Non-valvular AFib; - Treatment of DVT and PE; - Reduction in the risk of recurrence of DVT and PE.	12–14 h	Renal (80%)	- P-gp inducers - P-gp inhibitors
Rivaroxaban	Factor Xa inhibitor	Xarelto	- Non-valvular AFib; - Treatment of DVT and PE; - Reduction in the risk of recurrence of DVT and PE; - Prophylaxis of DVT following hip or knee replacement surgery; - Prophylaxis of DVT and PE in acutely ill medical patients; - Risk reduction of major cardiovascular events in stable atherosclerotic vascular disease (in combination with ASA).	5–13 h	Renal (67%)	- Combined P-gp and strong CYP3A4 inhibitors and inducers
Apixaban	Factor Xa inhibitor	Eliquis	- Non-valvular AFib; - Treatment of DVT and PE; - Prophylaxis of DVT following hip or knee replacement surgery.	12 h	Faecal (56%)	- Strong dual inhibitors of P-gp and CYP3A4
Edoxaban	Factor Xa inhibitor	Savaysa (USA) / Lixiana (Brazil)	- Non-valvular AFib; - Treatment of DVT and PE following 5–10 days of initial parenteral anticoagulation.	10–14 h	Renal (50%)	- P-gp inducers and inhibitors.

AFib atrial fibrillation, *ASA* acetylsalicylic acid, *BID* twice daily, *CrCl* creatinine clearance, *DVT* deep vein thrombosis, *PE* pulmonary embolism, *P-gp* P-glycoprotein, *QD* once daily

More recently, after the results of the COMPASS trial [24], the U.S. Food and Drug Administration (FDA) approved rivaroxaban (2.5 mg twice daily in association with acetylsalicylic acid [ASA]) to reduce the risk of major cardiovascular events (myocardial infarction, stroke and/or cardiovascular death) in patients with stable atherosclerotic vascular disease (i.e. chronic coronary artery disease and peripheral artery disease).

In addition to the increasing number of indications, DOACs present some appealing advantages over vitamin K antagonists (VKA), such as: (1) rapid onset of the anticoagulant effect after drug initiation, shortening hospitalization time and often obviating the need of in-hospital treatment; (2) no need of laboratory monitoring of the anticoagulant effect, being therefore more convenient for the patients, (3) fixed therapeutic dosage, and (4) fewer interactions with dietary components and other drugs, which translates into a more stable anticoagulant effect, irrespective to the patient's diet and commonly prescribed medications [25–28].

Nevertheless, some potentially serious drug interaction between different DOACs and other frequently used medications, such as cyclosporine, tacrolimus, imidazole and triazole derivatives, antiretroviral therapies (especially ritonavir and telaprevir), amiodarone, anticonvulsants (carbamazepine, phenobarbital, phenytoin), selective serotonin reuptake

inhibitors and rifampicin, have been recently described and may increase the risk of bleeding or decrease the efficacy of DOACs [20–23] (Table 2). In addition, DOACs should not be prescribed to pregnant woman and to patients with severely impaired renal function (estimated GFR < 30 mL/min/1.73 m2 of body surface area), since these groups of patients were excluded from pivotal trials.

Of note, despite being increasingly employed in the management of other prothrombotic states, the use of DOACs in patients with antiphospholipid syndrome (APS) was not extensively evaluated in the pivotal trials (namely, RE-COVER, RE-SONATE, RE-MEDY, EINSTEIN, EINSTEIN-PE, AMPLIFY, and HOKUSAI-VTE trials) [6–10]. In fact, it is expected that around 10% of patients with venous thrombosis will test positive for antiphospholipid antibodies (aPL) [29]. Even though, in post-hoc studies of phase 3 DOACs trials, only a fraction of the expected patients were reported. Goldhaber et al. described the post-hoc analysis of dabigatran trials. They identified 43 APS patients (1.7%) treated with dabigatran in RE-COVER/RE-COVER II trials (vs. 43 warfarin patients) and 38 (2.7%) in RE-MEDY trial (vs. 54 warfarin patients) [30]. The authors stated that the incidence of VTE/VTE-related deaths in aPL positive patients did not differ between groups [30], but this study was underpowered to draw definite conclusions on the use of

Table 2 Drug-drug and food-drug interactions of DOACs. Adapted from references [20–23]

Pharmacokinetic interaction		Pharmacodynamic interaction
Can decrease DOAC concentration	Can increase DOAC concentration	Can increase risk of bleeding
Carbamazepine	Amiodarone	Aspirin
Phenobarbital	Clarithromycin	ADP receptor (P2Y$_{12}$) inhibitors (clopidogrel, prasugrel, ticarelor)
Phenytoin	Cyclosporin A	Fibrinolytics (alteplase, tenecteplase)
Rifampin	Diltiazem	Heparins
St John's Wort	Dronedarone	NSAIDs
	Grapefruit components (p.e. furanocoumarins)	SNRIs/SSRIs
	Itraconazole	Warfarin
	Ketoconazole	
	Nelfinavir	
	Quinidine	
	Ritonavir	
	Tacrolimus	
	Verapamil	

DOAC Direct oral anticoagulants, *NSAIDs* non-steroidal anti-inflammatory drugs, *SNRIs* serotonin norepinephrine reuptake inhibitors, *SSRIs* selective serotonin reuptake inhibitors

dabigatran in this subgroup of patients [31]. In AMPLIFY study [7], 74 patients (2.85%) in the apixaban arm were diagnosed with thrombophilia (vs. 59 in enoxaparin + warfarin arm), but no specific analysis of APS patients was provided [7, 31]. In the EINSTEIN and EINSTEIN-PE trials, 6.2% patients in the rivaroxaban group (vs. 6.8% in warfarin group) and 5.7% (vs. 5.0% in warfarin group), respectively, had a known thrombophilia. Efficacy and safety endpoints were consistent with the overall observed effect; however, again, there was no specific analysis of APS patients [6, 10, 31]. Moreover, published trials on the use of rivaroxaban in APS failed to demonstrate non-inferiority of rivaroxaban when compared to warfarin (one using intermediate/laboratory and 2 using clinical outcomes – please see Randomized clinical trials (RCT) section below) [32–34].

This position statement will cover the published data regarding the use of DOACs in APS patients and will discuss the potential uses and contraindications of this class of drugs in this very specific group.

Questions to explore

The authors will explore the published data about DOACs use in APS, especially regarding their potential mechanisms of action that may influence APS treatment, their impact on lupus anticoagulant (LA) testing, and their efficacy in this subset of patients.

Methodology

Specialists from the Antiphospholipid Syndrome Committee of the Brazilian Society of Rheumatology performed a comprehensive review of the literature regarding DOACs use in APS to address the three following questions: (1) potential mechanisms of action of these drugs that could be relevant to APS pathogenesis, (2) DOACs interference on LA testing, and (3) the efficacy of DOACs in APS.

MEDLINE, EMBASE, Cochrane, and BIREME databases were searched up until March 20th, 2020. No language restriction was applied. We divided MeSH terms in two groups and combined each term of group 1 with each term of group 2, as following: (1) "antiphospholipid syndrome", "antiphospholipid antibodies", "lupus anticoagulant", "anticardiolipin antibodies", "beta 2 glycoprotein I"; and (2) "dabigatran", "rivaroxaban", "apixaban", "edoxaban". All retrieved articles were screened according to its title, abstract and full-text (if title and abstract were appropriate) and our group selected the most relevant ones to answer the proposed questions.

After critically reviewing the relevant evidence, the authors formulated a Position Statement on the use of DOACs in APS. All participants had the opportunity to express their opinion and contributed to the final document.

Literature review and analysis
Mechanism of action

DOACs exert their anticoagulant effects by directly inhibiting either factor Xa (rivaroxaban, apixaban, edoxaban) or thrombin (dabigatran). This inhibition occurs in a reversible, competitive, highly selective and dose-dependent way [25, 35, 36].

Factor Xa and thrombin play very important roles in normal hemostasis. The primary physiologic trigger of clotting event (initiation) is the interaction between tissue factor and activated factor VII (VIIa). Factor VIIa then activates factor X in factor Xa, which in turn generates thrombin from prothrombin. The initial small amount of thrombin activates factor V, factor VIII, factor XI, and platelets, resulting in an explosive thrombin generation (amplification). Then, the high thrombin levels convert fibrinogen into fibrin, forming and stabilizing the clot (propagation) [37, 38].

Artang et al. studied the effects of rivaroxaban, apixaban, and dabigatran on thrombin generation measurements using the Calibrated Automated Thrombogram (CAT) in 10 healthy male volunteers. Lag time was the thrombin generation assay (TGA) parameter most strongly associated with DOACS levels in all drugs. Endogenous thrombin potential (ETP) and thrombin peak height were significantly reduced for both rivaroxaban and apixaban, but not for dabigatran, with moderate and strong correlation, respectively, with factor Xa inhibitors levels. The authors demonstrated that thrombin peak height was superior to ETP in predicting factor Xa inhibitors concentrations. It also showed nonlinear exponential decay pattern, what may suggest it may be a useful parameter to monitor factor Xa inhibitors effect at lower concentrations [39].

Tripodi et al. performed a similar analysis using apixaban and the results were consistent with those previously reported. Apixaban altered all paramenters of CAT, increasing lag time and decreasing ETP, thrombin peak height, and velocity index. They also found that those effects were more prominent in the presence of thrombomodulin, an endothelial protein C activator [40].

Even though, when those parameters were tested in APS patients randomized to receive rivaroxaban or warfarin, rivaroxaban did not reach the noninferiority threshold for the percentage change in ETP at day 42. Nonetheless, peak thrombin generation was significantly lower in rivaroxaban group, when compared to warfarin, and no episode of recurrent thrombosis was observed during the short follow-up period. The details of Cohen et al. publication will be presented in the section "Randomized Clinical Trials" below in this paper [32].

Some authors have proposed that DOACs may also modulate inflammatory response. Both factor Xa and thrombin cleave PARs (protease-activated receptor), which are protein G-associated thrombin receptors activated by proteolysis, resulting in signal transduction, inflammation and thrombosis [41]. By inhibiting factor Xa and thrombin, DOACs may block those pathologic processes universally present in APS patients and therefore exert anti-inflammatory, anti-fibrotic and anti-angiogenic effects [42].

In addition, Arachchillage et al. found that patients taking rivaroxaban presented lower levels of C3a, C5a and SC5b-9 than those taking warfarin. There was no difference between Bb fragment levels between groups.

These findings suggest that rivaroxaban may reduce complement activation, especially in the classic pathway. As complement activation plays a significant pathogenic role in APS, the authors hypothesized that APS patients may benefit from rivaroxaban beyond its anticoagulating effect [43], which needs confirmation in prospective clinical trials.

Investigating the presence of lupus anticoagulant in patients using DOACs

It is widely known that different anticoagulants, such as warfarin and other VKA, unfractionated heparin (UFH), argatroban, lepirudin, and even some low-molecular-weight heparins (LMWH) may interfere with the detection of LA, as they interfere with clot formation [44–46].

Merriman et al. identified that many subjects taking rivaroxaban presented a positive LA test. Of the 32 patients randomized to rivaroxaban in their center, twenty-one were tested for LA and 19 presented a positive screening test. Dilute Russel's viper venom time (dRVVT) ratio was the test most affected by rivaroxaban. In contrast, only two out of twenty-one had an abnormal Kaolin clotting test, and only five out of fifteen had an abnormal aPTT (activated partial thromboplastin time) (Triniclot). An aPTT phospholipid correction test (STA-Clot method), which would be expected to be positive in the presence of true LA, was performed in twelve of the 19 positive LA subjects, with negative results in all of them; anti-beta-2-glycoprotein I (aßGPI) and anticardiolipin (aCL) antibodies were within the normal range in 10 of the 12 patients. Finally, thirteen of the 19 subjects were retested for the presence of LA after discontinuation of rivaroxaban and only one tested positive. The authors concluded that rivaroxaban might lead to false positive LA tests, especially for dRVVT ratio, as Russel's viper venom is a protease that cleaves factor X into Xa and rivaroxaban targets the factor Xa [45, 47].

The study by van Os et al. tested LA in the presence and in the absence of an in vitro preparation of rivaroxaban using three different assays: aPTT (screen PTT-LA and confirm Actin FS), dRVVT (screen LA-1 and confirm LA-2), and snake venom assay (screen Taipan snake venom time and confirm Ecarin venom time). The addition of rivaroxaban prolonged all conventional assays (PTT-LA, Actin FS, LA-1 and LA-2) in all groups, including normal pooled plasma of healthy subjects, leading to false-positive results. While dRVVT ratio was the most affected, aPTT ratio was only minimally influenced, as both PTT-LA and Actin FS had comparable prolongations. Rivaroxaban did not influence either Taipan venom time or Ecarin time [48].

Since then, different reports evaluated the impact of DOACs in the interpretation of LA assays. In summary, because of the higher prolongation of the screen dRVVT when compared with the confirm dRVVT, dRVVT ratio was the most affected assay, with high rates of false-positive results, both in in vitro and in ex vivo studies. It is noteworthy that, among factor Xa inhibitors, false-positive LA rates were less frequent with apixaban than with rivaroxaban (highest rates) and edoxaban. Additionally, screen Taipan snake venom time (TSVP) and confirm Ecarin clotting time (ECT) do not seem to be affected by the use of rivaroxaban, representing a possible alternative to dRVVT in this setting. Dabigatran induced high rates of false-positive LA, similar to those observed with rivaroxaban. Table 3 summarizes data regarding effect of different DOACs on different LA testing [45, 46, 48–65].

In order to provide a more accurate LA analysis in patients on DOACs, Exner et al. tested an activated charcoal product (DOAC Stop™) intended to extract DOACs from test plasmas. They found that DOAC Stop™ was capable of removing all types of DOACs (rivaroxaban, apixaban, edoxaban, and dabigatran) and it corrected false-positive dRVVT (screen, confirm and ratio) caused by the presence of those medications [66, 67]. Other authors performed similar studies with comparable results [56, 68]. The use of the antidotes idarucizumab (monoclonal antibodies against dabigatran) and adexanet alfa (recombinant human coagulation factor Xa for rivaroxaban and apixaban) may be considered for testing LA in patients using those medications, but difficulty of access and high costs could limit this approach [47]. Góralczyk et al. suggested another option based on their findings: as LA was corrected after > 24 h of discontinuation of rivaroxaban, they recommended that blood should be drawn at least 24 h after the last dose of the drug [62]. In this matter, Douxfils et al. suggested that LA testing should be performed preferably at trough level (C_{TROUGH}) (i.e. 12 or 24 h after last drug intake for bid [dabigatran, apixaban] or qd [rivaroxaban, edoxaban] drugs, respectively). Since invalid results may still happen, the authors state the real need for LA testing should be carefully evaluated in these scenarios and results should be interpreted with caution [65]. Favaloro et al. reported false positive (especially with rivaroxaban) and false negative (especially with apixaban) LA results in patients using DOACs [69], leading to a mistaken diagnosis of APS.

Current evidence on the efficacy of DOACs in APS patients

Randomized clinical trials (RCT)

To date, six trials on the use of DOACs in APS were registered in ClinicalTrials.gov and only three of them have been fully published.

The first published trial was the RAPS trial (Rivaroxaban in AntiPhospholipid Syndrome – NCT02116036), a prospective, randomized, controlled, non-inferiority, phase 2/3 study of rivaroxaban 20 mg once daily vs. warfarin (INR target 2.0–3.0) in thrombotic primary or secondary APS patients. Patients with arterial events and recurrent venous thrombosis were excluded. The authors decided to use percentage change in the ETP as the primary efficacy outcome, rather than clinical evidence of thrombosis. Nonetheless, after 6 weeks, rivaroxaban did not reach the non-inferiority laboratory threshold, when compared to warfarin [32]. No thrombotic episodes were registered during the follow-up period of 6 months, even though triple positivity (defined as positive aCL and β2GPI antibodies greater than the 99th percentile and a positive LA) was present in 20% vs. 12% of the warfarin and rivaroxaban groups, respectively. Rivaroxaban did not reach non-inferiority threshold for ETP [32, 70].

Pengo et al. recently published the results of TRAPS trial (Rivaroxaban in Thrombotic AntiphosPholipid Syndrome – NCT02157272). It was a randomized, open-label, multicenter, non-inferiority trial designed to evaluate the efficacy of rivaroxaban 20 mg once daily (or 15 mg once daily in case of moderate renal insufficiency) vs. warfarin INR target 2.0–3.0 in preventing thromboembolic events, risk of major bleeding and vascular death in high-risk APS patients, that is the presence of triple positivity for LA, aCL and aß2GPI (aCL and aß2GPI ELISA tests had to be positive for the same isotype). Past history of arterial events was not an exclusion criterium. After a mean follow up of 569 days, the study was prematurely terminated due to an excess of arterial thrombotic events in the rivaroxaban arm (4 ischemic strokes and 3 myocardial infarctions vs. none in the warfarin arm). Additionally, the number of major bleeding events was numerically higher in the rivaroxaban group (4 vs. 2). The authors concluded that the use of rivaroxaban in high-risk APS patients showed no benefits, as it leads to an excessive risk of events [33].

ASTRO-APS (Apixaban for the Secondary Prevention of Thrombosis Among Patients With APS – NCT02295475) is a prospective, randomized, open-label, blinded event, phase 4 pilot trial, comparing the efficacy of apixaban (vs. warfarin – target INR 2.0–3.0) in the secondary prevention of thrombosis in APS patients. Exclusion criteria included previous history of arterial events, recurrent thrombosis while receiving warfarin at a target INR of 2–3 or history of catastrophic APS (CAPS) [71]. After the study design was published, its protocol was modified due to an unanticipated excessive risk of arterial events during the first months of the trial in the apixaban group. To address this issue, apixaban dose was increased from 2.5 mg twice a day to 5 mg

Table 3 Effect of different DOACs in commonly used LA assays. Adapted from references [45, 46, 48–64]

Reference	DOAC	Tests analyzed	Results
Merriman (2010)	Rivaroxaban	aPTT (Triniclot), aPTT (STAClot), dRVVT (screen, confirm and ratio), Kaolin, DTT	False positive dRVVT ratio (88.9%) - all other tests negative / normalization of LA after discontinuation in all but one patient
van Os (2011)	Rivaroxaban	aPTT (screen PTT-LA and confirm Actin FS), dRVVT (screen LA-1 and confirm LA-2), and snake venom assays (screen TSVT and confirm ECT)	False positive dRVVT ratio (40% of SLE w/o aPL became LA positive after rivaroxaban mixing)
Halbmayer (2012)	Dabigatran	dRVVT (screen, confirm, standard ratio, and normalized ratio)	Higher frequency of false positive dRVVT ratio with increasing dabigatran concentrations
Martinuzzo (2014)	Rivaroxaban, dabigatran	aPTT, dRVVT (screen, confirm, ratio), SCT (screen, confirm, ratio)	False positive dRVVT ratio (76.5–100%)
Hillarp (2014)	Apixaban	aPTT, dRVVT (screen, confirm and ratio)	Apixaban did not cause false-positive results
Kim (2014)	Dabigatran	aPTT (PTT-LA, STAClot-LA)	False positive aPTT ratio (50% borderline and 40% positive)
Arachchillage (2015)	Rivaroxaban	Textarin time, dPT, dRVVT (3 methods: Siemens LA-1/LA-2, HemosIL dRVVT screen and confirm, and in-house dRVVT), TSVT/ECT	In vitro: false positive dRVVT ratio by conventional assays, but not in-house assay (90% normal controls and 92% LA-negative APS patients) Ex vivo: false-positive dRVVT ratio (100%) - remained false-positive at 18 h after the last dose of rivaroxaban
Bonar (2015)	Dabigatran	dRVVT (screen, STAClot confirm and ratio)	False positive dRVVT ratio (in vivo and ex vivo)
Góralczyk (2015)	Rivaroxaban	aPTT (PTT-LA screen and STAClot confirm), dRVVT (2 methods: HemosIL screen and confirm, and LA-1/LA-2)	False positive dRVVT ratio (patients were retested and became LA negative after 24 h of rivaroxaban discontinuation)
Bonar (2016)	Rivaroxaban, apixaban	dRVVT (screen, STAClot confirm and ratio)	False positive dRVVT ratio (rivaroxaban, but not apixaban, caused increased dRVVT ratio ≥ 1.2)
Gosselin (2016)	Rivaroxaban, apixaban, and edoxaban	dRVVT (3 methods: Siemens LA-1/LA-2, CRYOCheck LA-1/LA-2, dRV-LS/dRV-LR), hexagonal phase (STAClot-LA)	False positive dRVVT ratio (for all DOACs)
Pouplard (2016)	Rivaroxaban	dRVVT (STAClot DRVVT), TSVT/ECT	False positive dRVVT ratio; TSVT/ECT was not influenced by rivaroxaban
Ratzinger (2016)	Rivaroxaban, apixaban, and dabigatran	aPTT, dRVVT	False positive dRVVT ratio: - Dabigatran: 43.3%; - Rivaroxaban: 30%; - Apixaban: 20.7% (w/o dose dependent increase).
Antovic (2017)	Rivaroxaban, apixaban, and dabigatran	aPTT, dRVVT	False positive dRVVT ratio (≥1.2): - Dabigatran: 73%; - Rivaroxaban: 75%; - Apixaban: 76%.
Seheult (2017)	Rivaroxaban, apixaban, and dabigatran	aPTT, dRVVT, TII + PT	False positive dRVVT ratio and TTI + PT (aPTT was less affected); Apixaban was less affected than rivaroxaban; After rivaroxaban discontinuation, LA positivity dropped from 83 to 26%.
Flieder (2018)	Rivaroxaban, apixaban, and	aPTT, dRVVT (HemosIL and STAClot)	False positive dRVVT ratio: - Dabigatran: 20% (HemosIL) and 71% (STAClot);

Table 3 Effect of different DOACs in commonly used LA assays. Adapted from references [45, 46, 48–64] *(Continued)*

Reference	DOAC	Tests analyzed	Results
	dabigatran		- Rivaroxaban: 70% (IL) and 100% (STAClot): - Apixaban: no influence. Less important change in aPTT in all DOACs.
Hillarp (2018)	Edoxaban	dRVVT (Technoclot and STAClot)	False positive dRVVT ratio on Technoclot, but not with STAClot
Martinuzzo (2018)	Rivaroxaban	dRVVT (HemosIL and STAClot)	False positive dRVVT ratio (89.2% with HemosIL and 86.2% with STAClot)
Platton (2018)	Rivaroxaban and apixaban	dRVVT (Siemens LA1 and LA2)	dRVVT screen and confirm were falsely increased for both rivaroxaban and apixaban groups. After treatment with DOAC Stop, both dRVVT screen and confirm decreased to normal values.

aPTT activated partial thromboplastin time, *DOAC* direct oral anticoagulant, *dRVVT* dilute Russell's viper venom time, *LA* lupus anticoagulant, *TII* + *PT* thromboplastin inhibition index with prothrombin time, *TSVT* Taipan snake venom time, *ECT* Ecarin clotting time

twice a day and the Data Safety Monitoring Board recommended researchers to obtain a brain magnetic resonance imaging (MRI) for all patients, excluding from randomization those with prior silent stroke or white matter changes disproportionate to the patient's age [72].

The Canadian RAPS trial (NCT02116036) is a pilot phase 4 single-arm feasibility study evaluating, as a secondary outcome, the rates of bleeding and thrombosis in APS patients receiving rivaroxaban 20 mg once daily for the secondary prevention of thrombosis. Patients with arterial thrombosis and recurrent events while taking adjusted warfarin, rivaroxaban or dabigatran were excluded. This protocol was last update in ClinicalTrials. gov in 2017 and its complete results were not published to date [73]. However, in a written communication quoted elsewhere [74], the authors state that there were 2 arterial (cerebrovascular) and 2 venous events in 129.8 patients-year of follow-up after rivaroxaban initiation ($N = 82$ patients, no triple positivity included, 5 had previous history of venous thromboembolism [VTE]). While the authors claimed that these event rates were similar to previous warfarin studies, the absence of a control arm and the lack of population comparability data prevent a definitive conclusion to be obtained [74].

NCT02926170 was a randomized, prospective, open-label phase 3 trial, designed to investigate the efficacy and safety of rivaroxaban 20 mg once daily (or 15 mg once daily, if estimated GFR 30–49 mL/min) vs. acenocumarol (INR target 2.0–3.0 or 2.5–3.5 in those with recurrent thrombotic episodes) for secondary thrombosis prophylaxis in APS patients. Patients with previous arterial events and recurrent thrombosis were allowed to participate [75]. Ninety-five patients were assigned to receive rivaroxaban and 95 to receive warfarin. Around 6% of patients in each group dropped out early. The mean follow-up time for rivaroxaban group was 33.1 months vs. 34.1 for warfarin group. Global AntiPhospholipid Syndrome Score (GAPSS) was similar between groups, but migraine and livedo racemosa were more frequent in patients treated with rivaroxaban; 13.7% of rivaroxaban patients were taking concomitant ASA (vs. 11.7% in warfarin). Mild to moderate mitral thickening was slightly more frequent in the rivaroxaban group (22.1 vs. 14.7%). In the per protocol analysis, overall recurrent thrombosis rates were 11.6% in rivaroxaban arm vs. 6.3% in warfarin arm (risk ratio [RR] 1.83 [95%CI 0.71–4.76]; p for noninferiority = 0.29; p for VKA superiority = 0.20). Stroke occurred in 9 (9.5%) patients taking rivaroxaban vs. 0 taking VKA (RR 19; 95%CI 1.12–321.9; p = < 0.001). In the intention to treat analysis, overall recurrent thrombosis rates were 12.6% in rivaroxaban group vs. 6.3% in warfarin group (RR 2 [95%CI 0.78–5.11]; p for noninferiority = 0.57; p for VKA superiority = 0.13).

Both overall arterial events (RR 3.67 [95%CI 1.06–12.73]; $p = 0.040$) and stroke (RR 21 [95%CI 1.25–353.3]; $p = 0.001$) were more frequent in rivaroxaban group. Regarding safety outcomes, any bleeding, major bleeding, nonmajor clinically relevant bleeding, and minor bleeding did not differ between groups, in the as-treated analysis. In rivaroxaban-treated patients with previous arterial events, livedo racemosa or APS-related valvopathy, post hoc analysis suggested an increased risk of new thrombotic event during follow-up. In conclusion, rivaroxaban could not demonstrate its non-inferiority to VKAs in the secondary thrombosis prevention [34].

RISAPS (RIvaroxaban for Stroke patients with Anti-Phospholipid Syndrome – NCT03684564) is a recently registered randomized, controlled, phase 2/3, noninferiority trial on the use of rivaroxaban (vs. warfarin) for the secondary prevention of stroke in APS patients who have had previous stroke or other ischemic brain manifestations. Rivaroxaban dose will be 15 mg twice a day and warfarin will be administered to achieve a target INR of 3.5 (range 3.0 to 4.0). The primary efficacy outcome will be the rate of change in brain white matter hyperintensity (WMH) volume on MRI, assessed on the 3D FLAIR sequence, between baseline and 24 months. The estimated completion date is October 2022 [76].

A summary of the most relevant aspects of the clinical trials cited above can be found in Table 4.

Observational studies

Martinelli et al. enrolled consecutively 28 APS patients (13 treated with rivaroxaban and 15 with VKA) retrieved from 672 patients with venous thrombosis referred to their clinics. When patient switched between treatment groups, the authors recorded both treatments as periods (i.e., one patients accounted for 1 period of rivaroxaban and 1 period of warfarin), what led to 13 periods of rivaroxaban and 20 periods of VKA. During follow-up, one patient taking warfarin (incidence rate of 2.4 [95%CI 0.2–11.3] per 100 patient years) developed acute myocardial infarction and 4 taking rivaroxaban (incidence rate of 19.4 [95%CI 6.5–46.2] per 100 patient years) had recurrent thrombosis (1 stroke, 2 acute myocardial infarction, and 1 cerebral vein thrombosis). All of those were triple positive. The cumulative incidence at 24 months was 42% (95% 8.3–75.7) for rivaroxaban vs. 7.1% (95%CI 1–41) for warfarin, with a HR of 7.53 (95%CI 0.84–67.6). After 24 months, no episodes of recurrent thrombosis were observed. The authors concluded that there was an increased risk of recurrent thrombosis in triple positive patients using rivaroxaban and that the limited experience on the use of DOACs in treating APS cannot establish their safety in this subset of patients [77].

Table 4 Summary of completed and ongoing clinical trials of the use of DOACs in APS. Adapted from references [32, 70–76]

Trial	Design	Patient Population	Intervention	Comparison	Primary Outcome	Results/ ECD
RAPS (NCT02116036)	Prospective, controlled, phase 2/3, non-inferiority RCT	Primary or secondary thrombotic APS with previous isolated venous thromboembolism	Rivaroxaban 20 mg once daily	Warfarin (INR 2.0–3.0)	Endogenous thrombin potential (ETP)	Rivaroxaban did not reach the non-inferiority threshold
TRAPS (NCT02157272)	Phase 3, open-label, multicenter, non-inferiority RCT with blinded end-point	Triple positive thrombotic APS patients	Rivaroxaban 20 mg once daily (CrCl> 50) or 15 mg daily (if CrCl 30–50)	Warfarin (INR 2.0–3.0)	Cumulative incidence of thromboembolic events, major bleeding and vascular death	Terminated prematurely due to an excess of events in rivaroxaban arm
ASTRO-APS (NCT02295475)	Prospective, open-label, blinded event, phase 4 pilot RCT	Primary or secondary thrombotic APS. Exclusion: previous arterial events and recurrent venous thromboembolism when taking warfarin with INR of 2.0–3.0.	Apixaban 2.5 mg twice a day (increased to 5 mg twice a day + brain MRI after protocol modification)	Warfarin (INR 2.0–3.0)	Rates of thrombosis and deaths caused by thrombosis/ major bleeding plus clinically relevant non-major bleeding over 1 year	Protocol modification (2017): unanticipated excessive risk of arterial events during the first months in apixaban group. ECD: December 2019.
Canadian RAPS (NCT02116036)	Pilot phase 4, open-label RCT	Primary or secondary thrombotic APS (history of arterial thrombosis allowed). Exclusion: arterial thrombosis or recurrent venous events while on anticoagulation.	Rivaroxaban 20 mg daily	None (single-arm)	Rates of venous and arterial thrombosis and rates of minor, major and fatal bleeding	Single-arm feasibility study; Rates of thrombosis similar to warfarin studies
NCT02926170	Prospective, open-label, phase 3 RCT	APS patients with previous arterial events and recurrent thrombosis	Rivaroxaban 20 mg once daily (CrCl> 50) or 15 mg daily (if CrCl 30–50)	Acenocoumarol (INR 2.0 to 3.0 or 2.5 to 3.5 if recurrent thrombosis)	New thrombotic event or incidence of major bleeding (time frame: 36 months)	Rivaroxaban did not reach the non-inferiority threshold
RISAPS (NCT03684564)	Prospective, controlled, phase 2/3, non-inferiority RCT	Primary or secondary thrombotic APS with previous stroke or other ischemic brain manifestations	Rivaroxaban 15 mg twice a day	Warfarin (INR between 3.0–4.0)	Rate of chance in brain white matter hyperintensity volume on MRI (baseline and 24 months)	ECD: October 2022

APS antiphospholipid syndrome, *CrCl* creatinine clearance, *DOACs* Direct oral anticoagulants, *ECD* estimated completion date, *INR* international normalized ratio, *RCT* randomized clinical trial

Dufrost et al. have recently performed a patient-level data meta-analysis and found 447 APS patients that were treated with DOACs (290 with rivaroxaban, 114 with dabigatran, and 13 with apixaban). Of those, 319 patients were derived from observational studies, including cases series ($N = 14$), case reports ($N = 21$) and abstracts ($N = 9$). Seventy-three (16%) patients experienced at least one episode of recurrent thrombotic event (28 VTE, 31 arterial thromboses, and 13 small vessels thromboses) during DOACs use, with a mean duration until thrombosis of 12.5 months. When triple positive patients were analyzed separately, recurrence rate was 56% (mean duration until thrombosis: 16.1 months); triple positivity (OR = 4.3; 95%CI 2.3–7.7; $p < 0.001$) was associated with a higher risk of recurrent thrombosis. A higher number of clinical APS classification criteria and the positivity for aCL or aβ2GPI were also associated with a significantly higher recurrence risk. In the anti-Xa subgroup analysis, male gender ($p = 0.026$), history of arterial (OR = 2.8; 95%CI 1.4–5.7; $p = 0.006$), small vessels thrombosis (OR = 5.3; 95%CI 1.2–23.2; $p = 0.028$), and triple positivity (OR = 6.9; 95%CI 3.4–13.9; $p < 0.001$) were associated with higher rates of recurrence. In the dabigatran subgroup analysis, no differences regarding previous events or antibodies profile were observed between groups [78].

One relevant finding that must be stressed is that patients with recurrence of thrombosis on DOACs were more likely to have a past history of recurrence during VKA treatment, maybe representing a subgroup of APS that has a higher probability of recurrence, irrespective of the anticoagulant therapy prescribed. Due to the aforementioned data, the authors concluded that DOACs are not effective in all APS patients and should not be routinely prescribed to this subset of patients [65].

Additional relevant studies have been published since this meta-analysis was performed. Sato et al. reported the results of a longitudinal cohort that included 206 APS patients, with 18 patients who were treated with anti-factor Xa therapy (5 rivaroxaban, 12 edoxaban, 1 apixaban). When compared to warfarin, event-free survival (thrombotic and hemorrhagic events) was significantly shorter in the anti-Xa therapy group (HR 12.1; 95%CI 1.73–248; $p = 0.01$). When compared to control group (warfarin patients selected from the same cohort, matched by age, gender, SLE coexistence, and concomitant antiplatelet therapy), event-free survival was also significantly shorter in anti-Xa patients (HR 4.62; 95%CI 1.54–13.6; $p = 0.0075$). In the multivariate analysis, results remained unchanged (HR 11.9; 95%CI 2.93–56; $p = 0.0005$) [79] Malec et al. investigated 82 APS patients (56 have previously been reported) who used DOACs (36 rivaroxaban, 42 apixaban, and 4 dabigatran), which

were initiated after at least 3 months of anticoagulant therapy. Median follow-up was 45 [29–55] months (vs. 62 [50–63, 65–67] in warfarin group). DOACs group was compared with 94 patients using warfarin, regarding thrombotic and hemorrhagic events. Patients treated with DOACs had an increased risk of recurrent thromboembolic events and recurrent VTE alone. No differences were found when filtered by DOACs type (rivaroxaban and apixaban) or aPL status (single, double or triple positivity). Thrombotic events were associated with older age and higher GAPSS. The authors also reported an increased risk of bleeding in the DOACs group, but statistically significant difference was lost when excluded heavy menstrual bleeding or when analyzed only gastrointestinal bleeding [80]. Both studies aforementioned concluded that DOACs are, overall, less safe than warfarin in APS patients.

Regarding costs, Ciampa et al. performed a comparison between warfarin and a hypothetical use of rivaroxaban. Taking into account number of visits, number of laboratory tests for monitoring warfarin and the direct cost of both anticoagulants, the authors concluded that switching to rivaroxaban would increase the costs in 48%, for a 69% of time in therapeutic range. There are limitations related with indirect costs, time to target therapeutic range and differences in recurrent thrombosis or bleeding episodes on warfarin versus rivaroxaban during follow up [81].

Another APS subgroups that need consideration in this review are those with APS-related cardiac valvular disease and patients with microthrombotic disease. To date, we do not have studies in these specific subsets of disease. Extrapolating data on AFib, DOACs are not approved to treat valvular AFib [1–5]. Additionally, there is one letter that reported a 39 year-old female patient that developed CAPS after switching from warfarin to rivaroxaban [82].

All major DOAC trials excluded pregnant patients. There are evidences that these drugs can cross the placenta, raising concerns of embryopathy and adverse effects on fetal and neonatal coagulation [83]. There are no clinical trials of DOACs in APS pregnant patients.

Regarding the use of rivaroxaban during breastfeeding, three observational studies have been published to date, only one with an APS patient. In all of them, rivaroxaban concentrations in breast milk were quite low, but caution should be taken until clearer safety data are published [84–86]. Studies about dabigatran, apixaban or edoxaban concentrations in breast milk are still lacking.

APS treatment guidelines

European League Against Rheumatism (EULAR) recommendations for the treatment of APS were recently published and incorporated guidance on the use of DOACs in APS patients. The authors stated that rivaroxaban should not be used in triple-positive patients (Level of evidence 1b/Grade of recommendation B). However, it may be considered in cases that INR target is not achieved despite good adherence to VKA or in the presence of contraindications (allergy or intolerance) (Level of evidence 5/Grade of recommendation D). This latter recommendation was based in two aforementioned studies [30, 32] in this review, that reported no excessive risk of recurrent thrombosis, but samples were small, high-risk patients were under-represented, and follow-up was short. Overall level of agreement for this recommendation was 9.1 (range 0–10) [87].

American Society of Hematology (ASH) and American College of Chest Physicians (ACCP) recommendations for the treatment of venous thromboembolism made no specific recommendation regarding DOACs use in APS [88, 89].

Comments on switching DOACs to VKA

ASH guidelines provided some insights on how patients should be transitioned from DOACs to VKA. The recommendations were based on AFib, not DVT/PE, studies [88].

In patients with low-risk of recurrent VTE, VKA should be initiated on top of DOAC use. VKA dose should be titrated until target INR is achieved and, after that, DOAC should be withdrawn and VKA maintained in the same dose, until new INR evaluation. As DOACs may lead to spurious INR elevations, INR should be tested at DOAC-specific drug trough levels (i.e., 12 h after last dose of dabigatran or apixaban or 24 h after last dose of rivaroxaban or edoxaban). This can be easily accomplished by measuring INR right before next DOAC dose [88].

On the other hand, in patients with high-risk of recurrent VTE, DOAC should be replaced by LMWH or UFH bridging therapy. Then, VKA should be overlapped with LMWH or UFH until INR target is achieved. Patient's preference and ability to afford injections should be taken into account when opting for this strategy [88].

Position statement

- As both dRVVT and aPTT ratios may be influenced by the presence of DOACs, LA testing during DOACs use may lead to false-positive results, except if screen Taipan snake venom time and confirm Ecarin clotting time are available. The need for LA testing should be evaluated carefully in patients using DOACs. If LA is performed, blood collection should be performed at trough level (i.e., minimum concentration before next dose), which means 12 h after last dabigatran and apixaban dose and 24 h

after last rivaroxaban or edoxaban dose. If a patient tests positive for LA during the use of DOACs, it may represent a false-positive result and the diagnosis of APS should rely on clinical features and aCL and aß2GPI immunoassays;

- aCL and aß2GPI immunoassays are not expected to be influenced by DOACs use and, therefore, are preferred for diagnosing APS in patients on DOACs;

- Based on the presented data, the gold standard treatment for APS patients is still VKA and these patients should not be routinely treated with rivaroxaban. Our opinion is that dabigatran, apixaban and edoxaban also should not be routinely used to treat APS patients, since no efficacy and safety data are available to date;

- APS patients with triple positivity and/or a history of arterial events should not be treated with rivaroxaban. These statements may also be applicable for dabigatran, apixaban or edoxaban, since no efficacy and safety data are available to date;

- In the setting of low recurrence risk (single venous event and absence of triple positivity/low risk antibody profile), DOACs may be considered for secondary prophylaxis in patients who refuse to take VKA, are allergic or intolerant to VKA compounds or have difficult or poor anticoagulant control despite good adherence.

- In patients with APS-related cardiac valvular disease or microthrombotic disease, we believe warfarin is the most appropriate treatment, and dabigatran, rivaroxaban, apixaban and edoxaban should not be used, since there is no efficacy data available and there is a report of possible harm;

- There are no published studies considering the efficacy of DOACs in primary thromboprophylaxis of APS (i.e., in patients with positive antiphospholipid antibody testing but without thrombotic manifestations of the syndrome) or in pregnant APS patients. We do not recommend the use of DOACs in these scenarios;

- Currently, we consider good practice switching APS patients taking DOACs to VKA compounds, provided no intolerance or contraindications exist for the later. In general, this can be achieved by overlapping warfarin with DOAC until the INR is in the therapeutic range. In patients receiving direct factor Xa inhibitors (rivaroxaban, apixaban, edoxaban), it is important to test the INR right before the next dose (trough levels) to minimize the risk of spurious INR elevations. In high-risk patients, one can consider a transient switch from DOAC to LMWH or UFH as a "bridging therapy" while the initial VKA treatment is adjusted and until the target INR is achieved.

Conclusion

DOACs should not be routinely used in APS patients, especially in those with a high-risk profile (triple positivity to aPL, arterial thrombosis, and recurrent thrombotic events). In addition, DOACs interferes with LA testing, leading to false-positive results in patients investigating APS.

Abbreviations

aßGPI: anti-beta-2-glycoprotein I; aCL: anticardilipin; AFib: atrial fibrillation; aPL: antiphospholipid antibodies; APS: antiphospholipid syndrome; aPTT: activated partial thromboplastin time; ASTRO-APS: Apixaban for the Secondary Prevention of Thrombosis Among Patients With APS; BID: twice daily; CAPS: catastrophic antiphospholipid syndrome; DOACs: direct oral anticoagulants; dRVVT: dilute Russel's viper venom time; DVT: deep vein thrombosis; ECT: Ecarin clotting time; FDA: Food and Drug Administration; GFR: glomerular filtration rate; INR: international normalized ratio; LA: lupus anticoagulant; LMWH: low-molecular-weight heparin; MRI: magnetic resonance imaging; PAR: protease-activated receptor; PE: pulmonary embolism; QD: once daily; RAPS: Rivaroxaban in AntiPhospholipid Syndrome; RISAPS: Rivaroxaban for Stroke patients with AntiPhospholipid Syndrome; TRAPS: Rivaroxaban in Thrombotic Antiphospholipid Syndrome; TSVP: Taipan snake venom time; UFH: unfractionated heparin; VKA: vitamin K antagonists; VTE: venous thromboembolism; WMH: white matter hyperintensity

Acknowledgements

None.

Authors' contributions

All of the authors provided critical review, relevant edits, and feedback to direct content during multiple rounds of review. In addition, all authors have read and approved the final version of this manuscript.

Authors' information

All authors of this position statement are members of the Antiphospholipid Syndrome Committee of the Brazilian Society of Rheumatology. DA is also a member of the Antiphospholipid Syndrome Alliance for Clinical Trials & International Networking (APS ACTION).

Author details

[1]Serviço de Reumatologia, Hospital Universitário, Universidade Federal de Juiz de Fora (UFJF), Av. Eugênio do Nascimento, s/n - Dom Bosco, Juiz de Fora, MG 36038-330, Brazil. [2]Serviço de Reumatologia, Hospital Federal dos Servidores do Estado (HFSE), Rio de Janeiro, RJ, Brazil. [3]Serviço de Reumatologia, Departamento de Medicina Interna, Hospital de Clínicas de Porto Alegre (HCPA), Universidade Federal do Rio Grande do Sul (UFGRS), Porto Alegre, RS, Brazil. [4]Serviço de Reumatologia, Hospital de Clínicas, Universidade Federal do Paraná (UFPR), Curitiba, PR, Brazil. [5]Serviço de Reumatologia, Universidade Federal da Bahia (HUPES) e Escola Baiana de Medicina e Saúde Pública, Salvador, BA, Brazil. [6]Serviço de Reumatologia, Escola de Medicina, Pontifícia Universidade Católica do Rio Grande do Sul (PUCRS), Porto Alegre, RS, Brazil. [7]Serviço de Reumatologia, Faculdade de Medicina, Universidade Federal de Goiás (UFG), Goiânia, GO, Brazil. [8]Disciplina de Reumatologia, Faculdade de Medicina, Universidade de São Paulo (USP), São Paulo, SP, Brazil.

References

1. Connolly SJ, Ezekowitz MD, Yusuf S, Eikelboom J, Oldgren J, Parekh A, et al. Dabigatran versus warfarin in patients with atrial fibrillation. N Engl J Med. 2009;361:1139–51.
2. Connolly SJ, Eikelboom J, Joyner C, Diener H-C, Hart R, Golitsyn S, et al. Apixaban in patients with atrial fibrillation. N Engl J Med. 2011;364:806–17.
3. Patel MR, Mahaffrey KW, Garg J, Pan G, Singer DE, Hacke W, et al. Rivaroxaban versus warfarin in nonvalvular atrial fibrillation. N Engl J Med. 2011;365:883–91.
4. Giugliano RP, Ruff CT, Braunwald E, Murphy SA, Wiviott SD, Halperin JL, et al. Edoxaban versus warfarin in patients with atrial fibrillation. N Engl J Med. 2013;369:2093–104.
5. Granger CB, Alexander JH, McMurray JJ, Lopes RD, Hylek EM, Hanna M, et al. Apixaban versus warfarin in patients with atrial fibrillation. N Engl J Med. 2011;365:981–92.
6. Bauersachs R, Berkowitz SD, Brenner B, Buller HR, Decousus H, Gallus AS, et al. Oral rivaroxaban for symptomatic venous thromboembolism. N Engl J Med. 2010;363:2499–510.
7. Agnelli G, Büller HR, Cohen A, Curto M, Gallus AS, Johnson M, et al. Oral apixaban for the treatment of acute venous thromboembolism. N Engl J Med. 2013;369:799–808.
8. Büller HR, Decousus H, Grosso MA, Mercuri M, Middeldorp S, Prins MH, et al. Edoxaban versus warfarin for the treatment of symptomatic venous thromboembolism. N Engl J Med. 2013;369:1406–15.
9. Schulman S, Kearon C, Kakkar AK, Schellong S, Eriksson H, Baanstra D, et al. Extended use of dabigatran, warfarin, or placebo in venous thromboembolism. N Engl J Med. 2013;368:709–18.
10. Büller HR, Prins MH, Lensing AW, Decousus H, Jacobson BF, Minar E, et al. Oral rivaroxaban for the treatment of symptomatic pulmonary embolism. N Engl J Med. 2012;366:1287–97.
11. Turpie AGG, Lassen MR, Davidson BL, Bauer KA, Gent M, Kwong LM, et al. Rivaroxaban versus enoxaparin for thromboprophylaxis after total knee arthroplasty (RECORD4): a randomised trial. Lancet [Internet]. 2009; 373: 1673–80. Available from: https://doi.org/10.1016/S0140-6736(09)60734-0.
12. Goldhaber SZ, Leizorovicz A, Kakkar AK, Haas SK, Merli G, Knabb RM, et al. Apixaban versus enoxaparin for thromboprophylaxis in medically ill patients. New Engl J Med. 2011;365:2167–77.
13. Cohen A, Spiro TE, Büller HR, Haskell L, Hu D, Hull R, et al. Rivaroxaban for thromboprophylaxis in acutely ill medical patients. N Engl J Med. 2013;368: 513–23.
14. Cohen AT, Harrington RA, Goldhaber SZ, Hull RD, Wiens BL, Gold A, et al. Extended thromboprophylaxis with betrixaban in acutely ill medical patients. N Engl J Med. 2016;375:534–44.
15. Gosselin RC, Adcock DM, Bates SM, Douxfils J, Favaloro EJ, Gouin-Thibault I, et al. International Council for Standardization in Haematology (ICSH) recommendations for laboratory measurement of direct oral anticoagulants. Thromb Haemost. 2018;118:437–50.
16. Boehringer-Ingelheim. Pradaxa [package insert]. Available in: https://docs.boehringer-ingelheim.com/Prescribing%20Information/PIs/Pradaxa/Pradaxa.pdf. Last update: Nov 2019. Accessed 19 Mar 2020.
17. Janssen Pharmaceutica. Xarelto [package insert]. Available in: http://www.janssenlabels.com/package-insert/product-monograph/prescribing-information/XARELTO-pi.pdf. Last update: Marc 2020. Accessed 19 Mar 2020.
18. Bristol-Myers-Squibb. Eliquis [package insert]. Available in: https://packageinserts.bms.com/pi/pi_eliquis.pdf. Last update: Nov 2019. Accessed 19 Mar 2020.
19. Daiichi Sankyo. Savaysa [package insert]. Available in: https://dsi.com/prescribing-information-portlet/getPIContent?productName=Savaysa&inline=true. Last update: Aug 2019. Accessed 19 Mar 2020.
20. Vazquez SR. Drug-drug interactions in an era of multiple anticoagulants: a focus on clinically relevant drug interactions. Blood. 2018;132:2230–9.
21. Vranckx P, Valgimigli M, Heidbuchel H. The significance of drug – drug and drug – food interactions of oral anticoagulation. Arrhythmia Electrophysiol Rev. 2018;7:55–61.
22. Chang S-H, Chou I-J, Yeh Y-H, Chiou M-J, Wen M-S, Kuo C-T, et al. Association between use of non–vitamin K oral anticoagulants with and without concurrent medications and risk of major bleeding in nonvalvular atrial fibrillation. JAMA. 2017;318:1250–9.
23. Barr D, Epps QJ. Direct oral anticoagulants: a review of common medication errors. J Thromb Thrombolysis [Internet] 2018;47:146–54. Available from: https://doi.org/10.1007/s11239-018-1752-9.
24. Eikelboom JW, Connolly SJ, Bosch J, Dagenais GR, Hart RG, Shestakovska O, et al. Rivaroxaban with or without aspirin in stable cardiovascular disease. N Engl J Med. 2017;377:1319–30.
25. Chighizola C, Moia M, Meroni P. New oral anticoagulants in thrombotic antiphospholipid syndrome. Lupus. 2014;23:1279–82.
26. Arachchillage DJ, Cohen H. Use of new oral anticoagulants in antiphospholipid syndrome. Curr Rheumatol Rep. 2013;15:331.

27. Sciascia S, Lopez-Pedrera C, Cecchi I, Pecoraro C, Roccatello D, Cuadrado MJ. Non-vitamin K antagonist oral anticoagulants and antiphospholipid syndrome. Rheumatology. 2016;55:1726–35.

28. Signorelli F, Balbi GGM, Domingues V, Levy RA. New and upcoming treatments in antiphospholipid syndrome: a comprehensive review. Pharmacol Res. 2018;133.

29. van Es N, Büller HR. Using direct oral anticoagulants (DOACs) in cancer and other high-risk populations. Hematol Am Soc Hematol Educ Progr. 2015; 2015:125–31.

30. Goldhaber SZ, Eriksson H, Kakkar A, Schellong S, Feuring M, Fraessdorf M, et al. Efficacy of dabigatran versus warfarin in patients with acute venous thromboembolism in the presence of thrombophilia: findings from RE-COVER, RE-COVER II, and RE-MEDY. Vasc Med. 2016;21:506–14.

31. Cohen H, Efthymiou M, Isenberg DA. Use of direct oral anticoagulants in antiphospholipid syndrome. J Thromb Haemost. 2018;16:1028–39.

32. Cohen H, Hunt BJ, Efthymiou M, Arachchillage DRJ, Mackie IJ, Clawson S, et al. Rivaroxaban versus warfarin to treat patients with thrombotic antiphospholipid syndrome, with or without systemic lupus erythematosus (RAPS): a randomised, controlled, open-label, phase 2/3, non-inferiority trial. Lancet Haematol [Internet] 2016;3:e426–36. Available from: https://doi.org/10.1016/S2352-3026(16)30079-5.

33. Pengo V, Denas G, Zoppellaro G, Jose SP, Hoxha A, Ruffatti A, et al. Rivaroxaban vs warfarin in high-risk patients with antiphospholipid syndrome. Blood. 2018;132:1365–71.

34. Ordi-Ros J, Sáez-Comet L, Pérez-Conesa M, Vidal X, Riera-Mestre A, Castro-Salomó A, et al. Rivaroxaban versus vitamin K antagonist in antiphospholipid syndrome. A randomized noninferiority trial. Ann Intern Med. 2019. Online ahead of print. https://doi.org/10.7326/M19-0291.

35. Andrade D, Tektonidou M. Emerging therapies in antiphospholipid syndrome. Curr Rheumatol Rep. 2016;18:22.

36. Carvalho JF, Andrade DCO, Levy RA. Direct oral anticoagulants in antiphospholipid syndrome. Rev Bras Reumatol (English Ed [Internet]. 2016; 56:469–70. Available from: https://doi.org/10.1016/j.rbre.2016.09.006.

37. Leung LLK. Overview of hemostasis. In: UpToDate, Post, TW (Ed), UpToDate, Waltham, MA, 2020.

38. Rapaport SI, Rao LV. The tissue factor pathway: how it has become a "prima ballerina". Thromb Haemost. 1995;74:7.

39. Artang R, Anderson M, Riley P, Nielson JD. Assessment of the effect of direct oral anticoagulants dabigatran, rivaroxaban, and apixaban in healthy male volunteers using a thrombin generation assay. Res Pract Thromb Haemost. 2017;1:194–201.

40. Tripodi A, Padovan L, Chantarangkul V, Scalambrino E, Testa S, Peyvandi F. How the directo oral anticoagulants apixaban affects thrombin generation parameters. Thromb Res. 2015;135:1186–90.

41. Willis R, Cohen H, Giles I, Knight J, Krilis S, Rahman A, et al. Mechanisms of antiphospholipid antibody-mediated thrombosis. In: Erkan D, Lockshin M, editors. Antiphospholipid syndrome current research highlights and clinical insights. New York: Springer International Publishing AG; 2017. p. 77–116.

42. Alberio L. The new direct oral anticoagulants in special indications. Rationale and preliminary data in cancer, mechanical heart valves, APS, HIT, and beyond. Semin Hematol [Internet]. 2014;51:152–6. Available from: https://doi.org/10.1053/j.seminhematol.2014.03.002.

43. Arachchillage DRJ, Mackie IJ, Efthymiou M, Chitolie A, Hunt BJ, Isenberg DA, et al. Rivaroxaban limits complement activation compared with warfarin in antiphospholipid syndrome patients with venous thromboembolism. J Thromb Haemost. 2016;14:2177–86.

44. Miyakis S, Lockshin MD, Atsumi T, Derksen RHWM, Groot PGDE, Koike T, et al. International consensus statement on an update of the classification criteria for definite antiphospholipid syndrome. J Thromb Haemost. 2006; 4(2):295–306.

45. Merriman E, Kaplan Z, Butler J, Malan E, Gan E, Tran H. Rivaroxaban and false positive lupus anticoagulant testing. Thromb Haemost. 2011;105:385–6.

46. Halbmayer W-M, Weigel G, Quehenberger P, Tomasits J, Haushofer AC, Aspoeck G, et al. Interference of the new oral anticoagulant dabigatran. Clin Chem Lab Med. 2012;50:1601–5.

47. Favaloro EJ. The Russell viper venom time (RVVT) test for investigation of lupus anticoagulant (LA). Am J Hematol. 2019;94:1290–6.

48. van Os G, de Laat B, Kamphuisen P, Meijers J, de Groot P. Detection of lupus anticoagulant in the presence of rivaroxaban using Taipan snake venom time. J Thromb Haemost. 2011;9:1657–9.

49. Gosselin R, Grant RP, Adcock DM. Comparison of the effect of the anti-Xa direct oral anticoagulants apixaban, edoxaban, and rivaroxaban on coagulation assays. Int J Lab Hematol. 2016;38:505–13.

50. Pouplard C, Vayne C, Berthomet C, Guery E, Delahousse B, Gruel Y. The Taipan snake venom time can be used to detect lupus anticoagulant in patients treated by rivaroxaban. Int J Lab Hematol. 2017;39:e60–3.

51. Ratzinger F, Lang M, Belik S, Jilma-stohlawetz P, Schmetterer KG, Haslacher H, et al. Lupus-anticoagulant testing at NOAC trough levels. Thromb Haemost. 2016;116:235–40.

52. Antovic A, Norberg E, Berndtsson M, Rasmuson A, Malmström RE, Skeppholm M. Effects of direct oral anticoagulants on lupus anticoagulant assays in a real-life setting. Thromb Haemost. 2017;117:1700–4.

53. Seheult JN, Meyer MP, Bontempo FA, Chibisov I. The effects of indirect- and direct-acting anticoagulants on lupus anticoagulant assays a large , retrospective study at a coagulation reference laboratory. Am J Clin Pathol. 2017;147:632–40.

54. Flieder T, Weiser M, Eller T, Dittrich M, von Bargen K, Alban S, et al. Interference of DOACs in different DRVVT assays for diagnosis of lupus anticoagulants. Thromb res [internet]. 2018;165:101–6. Available from: https://doi.org/10.1016/j.thromres.2018.03.009.

55. Hillarp A, Strandberg K, Baghaei F, Blixter IF, Gustafsson KM, Lindahl TL, et al. Effects of the oral, direct factor Xa inhibitor edoxaban on routine coagulation assays, lupus anticoagulant and anti-Xa assays. Scand J Clin lab invest [internet]. 2018;78:575–83. Available from: https://doi.org/10.1080/00365513.2018.1522664.

56. Platton S, Hunt C. Influence of DOAC stop on coagulation assays in samples from patients on rivaroxaban or apixaban. Int J Lab Hematol. 2019;41:227–33.

57. Martinuzzo M, Forastiero R, Duboscq C, Barrera L, López M, Ceresetto J, et al. False-positive lupus anticoagulant results by DRVVT in the presence of rivaroxaban even at low plasma concentrations. Int J Lab Hematol. 2018. https://doi.org/10.1111/ijlh.12865. [Epub ahead of print].

58. HIllarp A, Gustafsson K, Faxalv L, Strandberg K, Bachaei F, Fagerberg Blixter I, et al. Effects of the oral, direct factor Xa inhibitor apixaban on routine coagulation assays and anti-FXa assays. J Thromb Haemost. 2014;12:1545–53.

59. Kim Y, Gosselin R, van Cott E. The effects of dabigatran on lupus anticoagulant diluted plasma thrombin time, and other specialized coagulation assays. Int J Lab Hematol. 2015;37:e81–4.

60. Arachchillage D, Mackie I, Efthymiou M, Isenberg D, Machin S, Cohen H. Interactions between rivaroxaban and antiphospholipid antibodies in thrombotic antiphospholipid syndrome. J Thromb Haemost. 2015;13:1264–73.

61. Bonar R, Favaloro EJ, Mohammed S, Pasalic L, Sioufi J, Marsden K. The effect of dabigatran on haemostasis tests: a comprehensive assessment using in vitro and ex vivo samples. Pathology. 2015;47:355–64.

62. Góralczyk T, Iwaniec T, Wypasek E, Undas A, Go T. False-positive lupus anticoagulant in patients receiving rivaroxaban : 24 h since the last dose are needed to exclude antiphospholipid syndrome. Blood Coagul Fibrinolysis. 2015;26:473–5.

63. Bonar R, Favaloro EJ, Mohammed S, Ahuja M, Pasalic L, Sioufi J, et al. The effect of the direct factor Xa inhibitors apixaban and rivaroxaban on haemostasis tests: a comprehensive assessment using in vitro and ex vivo samples. Pathology. 2016;48:60–71.

64. Martinuzzo ME, Barrera LH, D'Adamo MA, Otaso JC, Gimenez MI, Oyhamburu J. Frequente false-positive results of lupus anticoagulant tests in plasma of patients receiving the new oral anticoagulants and enoxaparin. Int J Lab Hematol. 2014;36:144–50.

65. Douxfils J, Ageno W, Samama C-M, Lessire S, Ten Cate H, Verhamme P, et al. Laboratory testing in patients treated with direct oral anticoagulants: a practical guide for clinicians. J Thromb Haemost. 2018;16:209–19.

66. Exner T, Michalopoulos N, Pearce J, Xavier R, Ahuja M. Simple method for removing DOACs from plasma samples. Thromb Res. 2018;163:117–22.

67. Exner T, Ahuja M, Ellwood L. Effect of an activated charcoal product (DOAC stop™) intended for extracting DOACs on various other APTT-prolonging anticoagulants. Clin Chem Lab Med. 2019;57:690–6.

68. Ząbczyk M, Kopytek M, Natorska J, Undas A. The effect of DOAC-stop on lupus anticoagulant testing in plasma samples of venous thromboembolism patients receiving direct oral anticoagulants. Clin Chem Lab Med. 2019;57:1374 81.

69. Favaloro EJ, Mohammed S, Curnow J, Pasalic L. Laboratory testing for lupus anticoagulant (LA) in patients taking direct oral anticoagulant (DOACs): potential for false positives and false negatives. Pathology. 2019;51:292–300.

70. Urbanus RT. Rivaroxaban to treat thrombotic antiphospholipid syndrome. Lancet Haematol [Internet]. 2016;3:e403–4. Available from: https://doi.org/10.1016/S2352-3026(16)30107-7.

71. Woller SC, Stevens SM, Kaplan DA, Branch DW, Aston VT, Wilson EL, et al. Apixaban for the secondary prevention of thrombosis among patients with antiphospholipid syndrome: study rationale and design (ASTRO-APS). Clin Appl Thromb Hemost. 2016;22:239–47.

72. Woller SC, Stevens SM, Kaplan DA, Rondina MT. Protocol modification of apixaban for the secondary prevention of thrombosis among patients with antiphospholipid syndrome study. Clin Appl Thromb Hemost. 2018;24:192.

73. Legault KJ, Crowther MA. Rivaroxaban for antiphospholipid antibody syndrome (RAPS) [Internet]. [cited 2019 Aug 14]. Available from: https://clinicaltrials.gov/ct2/show/NCT02116036.

74. Skeith L. Anticoagulating patients with high-risk acquired thrombophilias. Blood. 2018;132:2219–30.

75. Cortes J. Rivaroxaban for patients with antiphospholipid syndrome (NCT02926170) [Internet]. [cited 2019 Aug 14]. Available from: https://clinicaltrials.gov/ct2/show/NCT02926170.

76. Cohen H. Rivaroxaban for stroke patients with antiphospholipid syndrome (RISAPS) [Internet]. [cited 2019 Aug 14]. Available from: https://clinicaltrials.gov/ct2/show/NCT03684564?te.

77. Martinelli I, Abbattista M, Bucciarelli P, Tripodi A, Artoni A, Gianniello F, et al. Recurrent thrombosis in patients with antiphospholipid antibodies treated with vitamin K antagonists or rivaroxaban. Haematologica. 2018;103:e317.

78. Dufrost V, Risse J, Reshetnyak T, Satybaldyeva M, Du Y, Yan X, et al. Increased risk of thrombosis in antiphospholipid syndrome patients treated with direct oral anticoagulants. Results from an international patient-level data meta-analysis. Autoimmun rev [internet]. 2018;17:1011–21. Available from: https://doi.org/10.1016/j.autrev.2018.04.009.

79. Sato T, Nakamura H, Fujieda Y, Ohnishi N, Abe N, Kono M, et al. Factor Xa inhibitors for preventing recurrent thrombosis in patients with antiphospholipid syndrome: a longitudinal cohort study. Lupus. 2019;28:1577–82.

80. Malec K, Broniatowska E, Undas A. Direct oral anticoagulants in patients with antiphospholipid syndrome: a cohort study. Lupus. 2020;29:37–44.

81. Ciampa A, Salapete C, Vivolo S, Ames PRJ. Oral anticoagulation cost in primary antiphospholipid syndrome: comparison between warfarin and hypothetical rivaroxaban. Blood Coagul Fibrinolysis. 2018;29:135–8.

82. Crowley MP, Cuadrado MJ, Hunt BJ. Catastrophic antiphospholipid syndrome on switching from warfarin to rivaroxaban. Thromb Res. 2017;153:37–9.

83. Bapat P, Pinto L, Lubetsky A, Berger H, Koren G. Rivaroxaban transfer across the dually perfused isolated human placental cotyledon. Am J Obstet Gynecol. 2015;213:710.e1–6.

84. Saito J, Kaneko K, Yakuwa N, Kawasaki H, Yamatani A, Murashima A. Rivaroxaban concentration in breast milk during breastfeeding: a case study. Breastfeed Med. 2019;14:748–51.

85. Muysson M, Marshall K, Datta P, Rewers-Felkins K, Baker T, Hale TW. Rivaroxaban treatment in two breastfeeding mothers: a case series. Breastfeed Med. 2020;15:41–3.

86. Wiesen MHJ, Blaich C, Müller C, Streichert T, Pfister R, Michels G. The direct factor Xa inhibitor rivaroxaban passes into breast milk. Chest. 2016;150:e1–4.

87. Tektonidou MG, Andreoli L, Limper M, Amoura Z, Cervera R, Costedoat-Chalumeau N, et al. EULAR recommendations for the management of antiphospholipid syndrome in adults. Ann Rheum Dis. 2019;78:1296–304.

88. Witt DM, Nieuwlaat R, Clark NP, Ansell J, Holbrook A, Skov J, et al. American Society of Hematology 2018 guidelines for management of venous thromboembolism: optimal management of anticoagulation therapy. Blood Adv. 2019;2(22):3257–91.

89. Kearon C, Akl EA, Ornelas J, Blaivas A, Jimenez D, Bounameaux H, et al. Antithrombotic therapy for VTE disease. CHEST guideline and expert panel report. Chest. 2016;149:315–52.

10

Higher rate of rheumatic manifestations and delay in diagnosis in Brazilian Fabry disease patients

Nilton Salles Rosa Neto[*] ⓘ, Judith Campos de Barros Bento and Rosa Maria Rodrigues Pereira

Abstract

Background: Fabry disease (FD) is an X-linked lysosomal disorder due to mutations in the *GLA* gene resulting in defective enzyme alpha-galactosidase A. FD patients are frequently misdiagnosed, commonly for rheumatic diseases. Determining pathogenicity of a mutation depends of in silico predictions but mostly on available clinical information and interpretation may change in light of evolving knowledge. Similar signs and symptoms in carriers of *GLA* gene genetic variants of unknown significance or of benign variants may hamper diagnosis. This study reviews rheumatic and immune-mediated manifestations in a cohort of Brazilian FD patients with classic mutations and also in subjects with *GLA* gene A143T and R118C mutations. Misdiagnoses, time to correct diagnosis or determination of GLA gene status, time to treatment initiation and reasons for treatment prescription in A143T and R118C subjects are reviewed.

Methods: Genotype confirmed classic FD patients ($n = 37$) and subjects with GLA gene mutations A143T and R118C ($n = 19$) were referred for assessment. Subjects with R118C and A143T mutations had been previously identified during screening procedures at hemodialysis units. All patients were interviewed and examined by a rheumatologist with previous knowledge of disease and/or mutation status. A structured tool developed by the authors was used to cover all aspects of FD and of common rheumatic conditions. All available laboratory and imaging data were reviewed.

Results: Thirty-seven consecutive FD patients were interviewed – 16 male / 21 female (mean age: 43.1 years) and 19 consecutive subjects with *GLA* gene mutations R118C and A143T were evaluated – 8 male / 11 female (mean age: 39.6 years); 15 [R118C] / 4 [A143T]. Misdiagnosis in FD patients occurred in 11 males (68.8%) and 13 females (61.9%) of which 10 males and 9 females were previously diagnosed with one or more rheumatic conditions, most frequently rheumatic fever or "rheumatism" (unspecified rheumatic disorder). Median time for diagnosis after symptom onset was 16 years (range, 0–52 years). Twenty-two patients were treated with enzyme replacement therapy (ERT) – 13 male and 9 female. Median time to ERT initiation after FD diagnosis was 0.5 years (range, 0–15 years). Rheumatic manifestations occurred in 68.4% of R118C and A143T subjects. Two subjects had been prescribed ERT because of renal disease [R118C] and neuropsychiatric symptoms [A143T].

Conclusion: Misdiagnoses occurred in 64.8% of FD patients, most frequently for rheumatic conditions. Median time for correct diagnosis was 16 years. Rheumatic manifestations are also frequent in subjects with *GLA* gene R118C and A143T mutations. These results reinforce the need to raise awareness and increase knowledge about Fabry disease among physicians, notably rheumatologists, who definitely have a role in identifying patients and determining disease burden. Decision to start treatment should consider expert opinion and follow local guidelines.

Keywords: Fabry disease, *GLA* gene, Misdiagnosis, Diagnostic delay, Rheumatology, Genetic variants of unknown significance

* Correspondence: nsalles@yahoo.com
Rheumatology Division, Faculdade de Medicina da Universidade de São, Paulo, São Paulo, Brazil

Background

Fabry disease (FD) is an X-linked lysosomal disorder due to mutations in the *GLA* gene and where defective enzyme alpha-galactosidase A contributes to accumulation of substrate in numerous organs, with varying degrees of severity and subsequent loss of organ functions. Early diagnosis is the clue to better treatment outcomes [1, 2].

FD patients are commonly misdiagnosed [3, 4]. Incorrect diagnoses are often related to rheumatologic conditions, since patients may present with different rheumatic and immune-mediated manifestations [5–13]. Inappropriate diagnosis may lead to improper therapies and delay in FD recognition and adequate treatment initiation, thus hampering prognosis.

Fabry disease in males is characteristically linked to low or absent residual enzyme activity and elevated lyso-Gb3 (globotriaosylsphingosine) – a biomarker of substrate storage. In females, serum levels of residual enzyme activity and of lyso-Gb3 may fall within normal range even in symptomatic probands and thus molecular analysis is required. Diagnosis of Fabry disease requires, therefore, a compatible clinical history with X-linked inheritance associated with altered alpha-galactosidase A assay in male probands, elevated lyso-Gb3 (serum or urinary), and GLA gene analysis depicting a pathogenic mutation. Definition of pathogenicity of a mutation may change in light of evolving knowledge about the pathophysiology of the disease alongside improvement of genetic testing, analysis and interpretation. Whenever possible target-organ tissue portraying storage material should be obtained [14, 15].

Some *GLA* gene mutations, however, have little interference on enzyme activity and consequently normal or near normal enzyme and lyso-Gb3 levels are found, what is not fully compatible with the pathophysiology of Fabry disease. Hence, it is not reasonable to diagnose probands with such mutations as having Fabry disease.

Nevertheless, the question of pathogenicity remains as in silico analysis might classify some of them as pathogenic and laboratories may disclose results as class I mutations (definitely pathogenic) as recommended by the American College of Clinical Genetics Standards and Guidelines [16].

Probands with questionable mutations are commonly identified in large screening protocols in patients with unspecified kidney failure or cryptogenic cerebrovascular accident or cardiomyopathy. Because of similar signs and symptoms not otherwise explained by another disease, those patients might end up being considered as having Fabry disease. Whenever possible, clinical and pathological data may allow classification as benign mutations. When current available information on a specific mutation is insufficient to determine pathogenicity or benignity, it should be regarded as a genetic variant of unknown significance (GVUS) [14–16].

This is the case with subjects with *GLA* gene A143T and R118C mutations. Once considered to be pathogenic, there have been important studies disregarding their roles as disease-causing mutations whereas numerous recent publications relate their presence to evident disease [17–24]. In this sense, carriers of those mutations around the world may receive prescriptions of enzyme replacement therapies or oral chaperone therapy based on degree of symptoms and organ damage. However, it is not clear what other factors might interfere with the presenting phenotype, whether there is a real impact of the *GLA* gene mutation per se and whether subjects are affected by other undiagnosed disease. Nevertheless, the presence of specific rheumatic manifestations and rheumatological misdiagnosis in subjects with *GLA* gene A143T and R118C mutations have never been consistently evaluated.

Objectives

To review rheumatic and immune-mediated manifestations in a cohort of Brazilian FD patients with classic mutations. To review rheumatic and immune-mediated manifestations in subjects with *GLA* gene A143T and R118C mutations. To review diagnostic errors in those patients, time to correct diagnosis or determination of *GLA* gene status, and time to treatment initiation when indicated. To review reasons for treatment prescription in A143T and R118C subjects.

Methods

Genotype confirmed classic FD patients ($n = 37$) and subjects with GLA gene mutations A143T and R118C ($n = 19$) were referred for assessment. Subjects with R118C and A143T mutations had been previously identified during screening procedures at hemodialysis units. All patients were interviewed and examined by a rheumatologist (NSRN) with previous knowledge of disease and/or mutation status. A structured tool developed by the authors was used to cover all aspects of FD and of common rheumatic conditions. All available laboratory and imaging data was reviewed including lyso-Gb3 analysis. All patients and subjects had had at least one analysis of lyso-Gb3 performed by Centogene, Germany as result of programs of access to diagnosis or treatment follow-up sponsored by the pharmaceutical industry.

Clinical characteristics related to rheumatic or immune-mediated signs and symptoms and previous rheumatic diagnosis are described. Attention was given to information about age at first symptoms, age at correct FD diagnosis and age at ERT initiation.

Statistical analysis

Results are presented as mean and standard deviation for continuous variables and percentages for categorical variables. A p-value < 0.05 was required for statistical significance.

Results

Fabry disease

Thirty-seven consecutive patients were interviewed – 16 male / 21 female with a mean age of 43.1 years (range, 12–72). Thirty-three were considered to be symptomatic with symptoms associated with FD. All patients had classic mutations which are described in Table 1. Index cases in this cohort were diagnosed because of the following reasons: renal failure – kidney biopsy (Y264SX; L180F); nephrotic syndrome – kidney biopsy (P293S); family screening after screening at hemodialysis unit (R227X; C142R); angiokeratoma (A156D); lymphedema + angiokeratoma + acroparesthesia (W262X); recurrent fever + Fabry crises + acroparesthesia (G271A).

Misdiagnosis occurred in 11 males (68.8%) and 13 females (61.9%) of which 10 males and 9 females were previously diagnosed with one or more rheumatologic conditions, most frequently rheumatic fever or "rheumatism" (unspecified rheumatic disorder). Ten of those misdiagnosed patients had angiokeratomas (8 male [72.7%] and 2 [15.4%] female) that could aid medical reasoning and bring about Fabry disease as a possible diagnosis. Table 2 summarizes previous rheumatic and non-rheumatic diagnosis.

Median/mean age at first symptoms were 13.0/20.0 years (range, 5–66) overall; 12.0/17.6 years (range, 5–55) for males and 16.5 and 22.1 years (range, 9–66) for females, $p > 0.05$. Mean age at diagnosis (including asymptomatic patients) was 35.7 years (range, 4–71) overall; 35.5 years for males (range, 8–55) and 35.9 years for females (range, 4–71) $p > 0.05$. Median/mean time for

diagnosis after symptom onset was 16.0/18.6 years (range, 0–52) overall; 20.5/21.6 years (range, 1–42) for males; 14.0/17.9 years (range, 0–52) for females, $p > 0.05$.

Twenty-two patients were being treated with ERT – 13 male and 9 female and median/mean time to ERT initiation after FD diagnosis was 0.5/2.4 years (range, 0–15) overall; 1.0/3.7 years (range, 0–15) for males; 0/0.4 year (range, 0–1) for females, $p > 0.05$. As for the remaining 3 male patients, two had been recently diagnosed and awaited treatment initiation and the other had started treatment after approximately 6 months of diagnosis but had the delivery of medication interrupted more than 1 year before assessment due to governmental administrative reasons.

Rheumatic manifestations – signs and symptoms – were present in 36 patients (97.3%) which are listed in Table 3. The only patient who did not present any rheumatic symptoms at the time of study was the youngest female at age 12.

Pain in the extremities (nociceptive and/or neuropathic) was present in 26 patients (70.3%). This symptom may account not only for classic acroparesthesia but also for arthralgia and myalgia.

Past or present Fabry crises were referred by 16 patients (43.2%) – all mutations in this cohort had, at least, one male patient with typical Fabry crises. Interestingly, fibromyalgia, a condition characterized by widespread chronic pain, could be diagnosed after thorough rheumatologic assessment in 16 patients (43.2%). Before FD diagnosis, 2 patients had been misdiagnosed with fibromyalgia.

Bone mineral density abnormalities, which include osteopenia, osteoporosis and low bone mineral density for age, were present in 24 patients (64.8%). Lymphedema was present in 8 patients (21.6%). Only one male

Table 1 List of mutations in this cohort of Fabry disease patients

# of patients	Exon	Molecular	Mutation	Type	Description	ACMG Classification [16]	Clinical Classification	Amenability
8	3	c. 424 C > T (p. Cys142Arg)	C142R	missense	Topaloglu et al. 1999 [25]	1	Pathogenic	No
8	3	c. 467 C > A (p.Ala156Asp)	A156D	missense	Turaça et al. 2012 [26]	1	Pathogenic	No
3	3	c. 540 G > T (p. Leu180Phe)	L180F	missense	Serebrinsky et al. 2012 [27]	1	Pathogenic	Yes
2	5	c. 679 C > T (p. Arg227*)	R227X	nonsense	Davies et al. 1993 [28]	1	Pathogenic	No
3	5	c. 785 G > A (p. Trp262*)	W262X	nonsense	Shabbeer et al. 2006 [29]	1	Pathogenic	No
5	6	c. 812 G > C (p. Gly271Ala)	G271A	missense	Rosa Neto 2014 [30]	1	Pathogenic	Yes
1	6	c. 877 C > T (p. Pro293Ser)	P293S	missense	Cooper et al. 2000 [31]	1	Pathogenic	No
7	7	c. 1235_1236delCT (p. Tyr264Serfs*)	Y264SX	deletion	Blaydon et al. 2001 [32]	1	Pathogenic	No

ACMG American College of Medical Genetics

Table 2 Misdiagnosis in Fabry disease patients

	Total N = 37	Males N = 16	Females N = 21	Mutations	p-value
Misdiagnosis – overall, n (%)	24 (64.8%)	11 (68.8%)	13 (61.9%)		0.68
Patients diagnosed with any rheumatologic condition before Fabry Disease diagnosis, n (%)	19 (51.4%)	10 (62.5%)	9 (42.9%)		0.25
Rheumatic fever, n (%)	7 (18.9%)	4 (25%)	2 (9.5%)	A156D P293S Y264SX (5)	–
"Rheumatism" (unspecified rheumatic disorder), n (%)	8 (21.6%)	4 (25%)	4 (19%)	A156D (3) C142R (3) Y264SX (2)	–
Rheumatoid arthritis, n (%)	1 (2.7%)	0	1 (4.8%)	W262X	–
Fibromyalgia, n (%)	2 (5.4%)	1 (6.3%)	1 (4.8%)	G271A	–
Growing pains, n (%)	3 (8.1%)	2 (12.5%)	1 (4.8%)	A156D (2) G271A	–
Systemic sclerosis, n (%)	1 (2.7%)	1 (6.3%)	0	Y264SX	–
Tendinopathy, n (%)	1 (2.7%)	0	1 (4.8%)	G271A	–
Carpal tunnel syndrome, n (%)	1 (2.7%)	0	1 (4.8%)	G271A	–
Patients diagnosed with other conditions before Fabry Disease diagnosis, n (%)	9 (24.3%)	3 (18.8%)	6 (28.6%)		0.50
Heart murmur, n (%)	1 (2.7%)	1 (6.3%)	0	Y264SX	–
Diabetes mellitus, n (%)	1 (2.7%)	0	1 (4.8%)	L180F	–
Ischemic cardiomyopathy, n (%)	1 (2.7%)	0	1 (4.8%)	C142R	–
Migraine, n (%)	3 (8.1%)	0	3	C142R G271A W262X	0.13
Fever of unknown origin, n (%)	1 (2.7%)	0	1 (4.8%)	A156D	–
Focal and segmental glomerulosclerosis, n (%)	1 (2.7%)	1 (6.3%)	0	L180F	–
Dysmenorrhea, n (%)	1 (2.7%)	0	1 (4.8%)	W262X	–
Ulcerative colitis, n (%)	1 (2.7%)	1 (6.3%)	0	P293S	–

Patients may have been misdiagnosed more than once – percentage of the total number of diagnoses is not equal to 100%

Table 3 Rheumatic manifestations in Fabry disease patients

Signs/Symptoms/Diagnosis	Total N (%)	Males N (%)	Females N (%)	p-value
Pain in the extremities (nociceptive and/or neuropathic)	26 (70.3%)	13 (81.3%)	13 (61.9%)	0.21
Fabry crises (past/present)	15 (40.5%)	10 (62.5%)	5 (23.8%)	**0.02**
Osteopenia/osteoporosis/ low bone mineral density for age	24 (64.8%)	13 (81.3%)	11 (52.4%)	0.07
Fibromyalgia	16 (43.2%)	6 (37.5%)	10 (47.6%)	0.55
Lymphedema	8 (21.6%)	7 (43.8%)	1 (4.8%)	**0.003**
Neuropathic osteoarthropathy (Charcot foot) (2 patients = toe amputation)	4 (10.8%)	3 (18.8%)	1 (4.8%)	0.18
Chronic low back pain	5 (13.5%)	1 (6.3%)	4 (19%)	0.27
Hip/knee osteoarthritis	5 (13.5%)	3 (18.8%)	2 (9.5%)	0.43
Gout	1 (2.7%)	0	1 (4.8%)	–
Clinodactyly	1 (2.7%)	1 (6.3%)	0	–
HyperCKemia	1 (2.7%)	1 (6.3%)	0	–
Carpal tunnel syndrome	3 (8.1%)	0	3 (14.3%)	0.12

Data in bold means that the difference of frequencies between males and females was statistically significant

patient presented with bilateral upper and lower limbs lymphedema, and a history of recurrent cellulitis.

Neuropathic osteoarthropathy (Charcot foot) was present in four patients (3 male / 1 female). The mutations related were L180F, A156D, C142R, Y264SX. Only one patient had concurrent diabetes mellitus (the female patient), with kidney biopsy, in addition, showing signs of Kimmestiel-Wilson lesions and who eventually required toe amputation. All men had been submitted to kidney transplantation and were on immunosuppressive drugs but none had history of glucose imbalance. One male patient required toe amputation and another had been already indicated for toe surgery. Of note, all three patients who required or were indicated for surgery had lymphedema.

Other diagnosis included chronic low back pain in five patients; hip and/or knee osteoarthritis in five patients; gout in one patient; clinodactyly in one patient; unspecific hyperCKemia in one patient; and clinical carpal tunnel syndrome in two patients.

Six immune-related diseases were diagnosed in 4 patients (10.8%), all female:

a) biopsy-proven and autoantibody positive celiac disease, in a patient with HLA-DQ8 and autoantibody positive hypothyroidism (mutation G271A);
b) autoantibody positive hyperthyroidism (mutation G271A);
c) biopsy-proven IgA nephropathy and psoriasis (mutation L180F);
d) vitiligo (mutation C142R).

Worth mentioning that not all patients underwent autoantibody tests, what might account for underestimation of immune-mediated phenomena.

R118C and A143T subjects
Nineteen consecutive subjects were evaluated – 8 male and 11 female, with a mean age of 39.6 years (range, 9–

66). R118C was detected in 15 patients and A143T in 4. Lyso-Gb3 (Centogene, Germany) levels were normal in all subjects.

Two patients were on Enzyme Replacement Therapy following decision of their treating physician. Application of the Mainz Severity Score Index (MSSI) [33] for FD depicted those 2 patients as "Moderate" severity, which was accounted for:

a) renal (subnephrotic proteinuria/kidney transplantation) [R118C]; and.
b) neuropsychiatric symptoms [A143T].

Thirteen subjects (68.4%) presented rheumatic manifestations which are listed in Table 4.

Pain in the extremities in 10 patients (52.6%); fibromyalgia in 7 patients (36.8%). Of note, four patients [3 A143T/ 1 R118C] referred past/present pain crises comparable to FD.

Osteopenia/osteoporosis in 11 patients (57.9%);

Other diagnosis included chronic low back pain (3), osteoarthritis (3); trigger finger (1); leg cramps (1).

Interestingly, 4 patients had been previously diagnosed with a rheumatic disease: rheumatoid arthritis (R118C male), rheumatic fever (2 patients – A143T female), and "rheumatism" (A143T female). Three of those patients were affected by pain crises comparable to FD crises. Both patients currently being treated with ERT are included in this group.

Discussion
The evidence from this study reinforces that Fabry disease is still frequently misdiagnosed. Data from the medical literature have repeatedly shown that many of those patients present unspecific signs and symptoms, but nevertheless require specialized assessment [1, 2]. Our results show that almost 65% of patients were diagnosed with one or more rheumatological conditions before the correct diagnosis, the higher incidence

Table 4 Rheumatic manifestations in A143T and R118C subjects

Signs/Symptoms/Diagnosis	Total N (%)	Males N (%)	Females N (%)	p-value	A143T N (%)	R118C N (%)	p-value
Pain in the extremities (nociceptive and/or neuropathic)	10 (52.6%)	4 (50%)	6 (54.5%)	0.86	2 (50%)	8 (53.3%)	0.34
Fabry-like crises (past/present)	4 (21.1%)	0	4 (36.4%)	0.06	3 (75%)	1 (6.7%)	**0.001**
Osteopenia/osteoporosis/ low bone mineral density for age	11 (57.9%)	5 (62.5%)	6 (54.5%)	0.75	3 (75%)	8 (53.3%)	0.46
Fibromyalgia	7 (36.8%)	1 (12.5%)	6 (54.5%)	0.07	3 (75%)	4 (26.7%)	0.08
Chronic low back pain	3 (15.8%)	1 (12.5%)	2 (18.2%)	0.38	2 (50%)	1 (6.7%)	**0.04**
Hip/knee osteoarthritis	3 (15.8%)	2 (25%)	1 (9.1%)	0.38	0	3 (20%)	0.36
Trigger finger	1 (5.3%)	1 (12.5%)	0	–	0	1 (6.7%)	–
Cramps	1 (5.3%)	1 (12.5%)	0	–	0	1 (6.7%)	–

Data in bold means that the difference of frequencies between males and females was statistically significant

reported in the literature [3, 13, 34]. Gender did not seem to impact in the occurrence of wrong diagnoses.

Furthermore, FD patients also manifest several rheumatic signs and symptoms and may present with immune-mediated illnesses irrespective of disease pathophysiology and increase the chances of requiring a pediatric or adult rheumatologist consultation. Median time to FD diagnosis is somewhere between one and two decades after symptoms onset what is similar to what is reported in the literature [2]. In our cohort female patients had a lower median time to diagnosis after symptom onset than males.

Unfortunately, lack of knowledge about the disease from physicians brings about delayed diagnosis and prescription of incorrect treatments [3]. It is important to review classification and diagnostic criteria or clinical characteristics of rheumatic conditions to avoid misdiagnosis. For example, rheumatic fever and growing pains, that are among the most frequent rheumatic misdiagnoses [3, 34], have specific features such as age of incidence, family history, pattern of pain, response to medication and usually neuropathic pain is not present [35, 36]. It is important to say that FD patients do present with arthralgia and myalgia as part of the disease itself, but not true arthritis [11].

Cimaz et al. [37] assessed awareness of rheumatologists about Fabry disease and results highlight that they are not well acquainted with the disease characteristics or with the appropriate workup. In fact, that observation put emphasis on the inclusion of FD and other lysosomal disorders in the differential when investigating multisystemic diseases [38].

Nonetheless, there are rheumatologists who have been interested in finding those rare patients amidst rheumatic patients and investigating specific features such as pain or Raynaud's phenomenon [39–41]. Routine screening of early arthritis, juvenile idiopathic arthritis and fibromyalgia patients have been performed to identify those patients but the yield to definite pathogenic mutations was low [42–44]. Vordenbäumen et al. [45] suggest that regular rheumatology care to early arthritis patients will not overlook patients with FD but reinforce the lack of familiarity of physicians with FD signs and symptoms.

All patients diagnosed with FD in this study had classical mutations and most of them were prescribed ERT. In Brazil, only ERT preparations are approved for use but are not available in the Public Health System and coverage is not expected from insurance companies. Oral chaperone therapy was not available at the time of the study. For the time being, access to ERT depends on judicial request or compassionate use. In this cohort, patients waited a median time of 6 months to start treatment after initial prescription.

In regard to subjects with R118C and A143T *GLA* gene mutations, identification occurred after screening

protocols in dialysis clinics. A143T and R118C subjects were enrolled because they are or were followed by physicians under the label of Fabry disease because of genetic reports confirming pathogenicity of their mutation.

Remarkably, two patients were receiving ERT in arrangement with their attending physician. No histopathological sample was obtained from those patients. All patients had normal levels of Lyso-Gb3 what is in accordance to the literature [15]. However, many of them present signs and symptoms that could be attributed to rheumatic conditions as well as to Fabry disease itself.

When categorized by severity by the MSSI, the patients were classified as "Moderate". Despite the fact that current understanding may not be sufficient to establish a relation between genotype and phenotype, there exist information in the medical literature in support of treatment of some of those patients. It is believed that physicians who choose to treat them do it in the best interest of their patients but constant updates on information regarding pathogenicity should be sought. Noteworthy, those two subjects under ERT had been previously misdiagnosed with a rheumatic disease.

It is important to recognize that some patients with those variants present typical findings of Fabry disease, including angiokeratoma. Our study showed that symptoms that could be defined or described as Fabry-like crises, were present in 4 women, three with A143T and one with R118C. This information may be strongly connected to the occurrence of misdiagnoses with rheumatological conditions.

A lot of controversy exists when those patients are evaluated. It is difficult and expensive to have thorough investigations to include or exclude a diagnosis. It is also difficult and expensive to give such drugs to whom may not need or benefit entirely from them. As stated by Ferreira et al. in the European study [23], R118C variant is frequent in Portugal. Brazil colonization was much influenced by the Portuguese, what may have interfered with the frequency of this variant in our population. It is important to remind that medicine and genetics are constantly evolving disciplines and diagnosis and treatment should be reappraised and readjusted whenever needed.

This paper has several limitations. Despite thorough assessment by a rheumatologist, data is subject to memory bias since not all patients had easy access to health services or regular medical follow-up since childhood. Also, not all patients had autoantibodies assessed, what might underestimate our findings.

Conclusion

Misdiagnoses occurred in 64.8% of FD patients, most frequently for rheumatological conditions. Median time for correct diagnosis in this cohort was 16 years.

Rheumatic manifestations are very frequent in FD, related or not to the pathophysiology of the disease, and some patients may present with concomitant immune-mediated diseases.

Rheumatic manifestations are also frequent in subjects with *GLA* gene R118C and A143T mutations. FD-like pain crises might account for misdiagnosis, and whether the symptoms derive from the gene mutation itself is yet to be determined. In this cohort renal and neuropsychiatric manifestations directed the choice of ERT in 2 of them - one of each mutation. Nonetheless, numerous diseases may present with the same findings. Subjects with questionable mutations warrant further investigation to exclude other diagnosis and, preferably, target biopsy–proven storage accumulation before choosing to initiate FD specific treatment.

Delay in diagnosis in this cohort overall was similar to what is reported in the medical literature with the exception that females had a lower median time to diagnosis than males.

These results reinforce the need to raise awareness and increase knowledge about Fabry disease among physicians, notably rheumatologists, who definitely have a role in identifying patients and determining disease burden. Decision to start treatment should consider expert opinion and follow local guidelines.

Abbreviations

ERT: Enzyme replacement therapy; F: Female; FD: Fabry disease; GVUS: Genetic variant of unknown significance; M: Male; MSSI: Mainz severity score index

Acknowledgements

The authors would like to acknowledge Rachel Sayuri Honjo Kawahira, Jaelson.
Guilhem Gomes, Ana Carolina de Paula and Rosiane Lacerda for referral of. patients.

Authors' contributions

NSRN designed the study, collected, analyzed and interpreted the data, wrote and reviewed the manuscript. JCBB collected, analyzed and interpreted the data, and reviewed the manuscript. RMRP analyzed and interpreted the data, and reviewed the manuscript. All authors read and approved the final manuscript.

References

1. Schiffmann R. Fabry disease. Handb Clin Neurol. 2015;132:231–48.
2. Germain DP. Fabry disease. Orphanet J Rare Dis. 2010;5:30.
3. Marchesoni CL, Roa N, Pardal AM, Neumann P, Cáceres G, Martínez P, et al. Misdiagnosis in Fabry disease. J Pediatr. 2010;156(5):828–31.
4. Lidove O, Kaminsky P, Hachulla E, Leguy-Seguin V, Lavigne C, Marie I, et al. FIMeD investigators. Fabry disease 'The new great Imposter': results of the French Observatoire in Internal Medicine Departments (FIMeD). Clin Genet. 2012;81(6):571–7.
5. Paira SO, Roverano S, Iribas JL, Barceló HA. Joint manifestations of Fabry's disease. Clin Rheumatol. 1992;11(4):562–5.
6. Michels H, Mengel E. Lysosomal storage diseases as differential diagnoses to rheumatic disorders. Curr Opin Rheumatol. 2008;20(1):76–81.
7. Manger B, Menge E, Schaefer R, Haase C, Seidel J, Michels H. Gaucher disease, Fabry disease and mucopolysaccharidosis type I--how can the rheumatologist recognize these patients? Z Rheumatol. 2006;65(1):32 34–43.
8. Manger B, Mengel E, Schaefer RM. Rheumatologic aspects of lysosomal storage diseases. Clin Rheumatol. 2007;26(3):335–41.
9. James RA, Singh-Grewal D, Lee SJ, McGill J, Adib N. Australian Paediatric rheumatology group. Lysosomal storage disorders: a review of the musculoskeletal features. J Paediatr Child Health. 2016;52(3):262–71.
10. Lidove O, Zeller V, Chicheportiche V, Meyssonnier V, Sené T, Godot S, et al. Musculoskeletal manifestations of Fabry disease: a retrospective study. Joint Bone Spine. 2016;83(4):421–6.
11. Politei J, Remondino G, Heguilen R, Wallace E, Durand C, Schenone A. When arthralgia is not arthritis. Eur J Rheumatol. 2016;3(4):182–4.
12. Pagnini I, Borsini W, Cecchi F, Sgalambro A, Olivotto I, Frullini A, et al. Distal extremity pain as a presenting feature of Fabry's disease. Arthritis Care Res (Hoboken). 2011;63(3):390–5.
13. Moiseev S, Karovaikina E, Novikov PI, Ismailova D, Moiseev A, Bulanov N. What rheumatologist should know about Fabry disease. Ann Rheum Dis. 2019. https://doi.org/10.1136/annrheumdis-2019-215476 [Epub ahead of print].
14. Van der Tol L, Smid BE, Poorthuis BJ, Biegstraaten M, Deprez RH, Linthorst GE, et al. A systematic review on screening for Fabry disease: prevalence of individuals with genetic variants of unknown significance. J Med Genet. 2014;51(1):1–9.
15. Duro G, Zizzo C, Cammarata G, Burlina A, Burlina A, Polo G, et al. Mutations in the *GLA* Gene and LysoGb3: Is It Really Anderson-Fabry Disease? Int J Mol Sci. 2018;19(12):E3726. https://doi.org/10.3390/ijms19123726.
16. Richards S, Aziz N, Bale S, Bick D, Das S, Gastier-Foster J, et al. Standards and guidelines for the interpretation of sequence variants: a joint consensus recommendation of the American College of Medical Genetics and Genomics and the Association for Molecular Pathology. Genet Med. 2015; 17(5):405–24.
17. Hauth L, Kerstens J, Yperzeele L, Eyskens F, Parizel PM, Willekens B. Galactosidase Alpha p.A143T Variant Fabry Disease May Result in a Phenotype With Multifocal Microvascular Cerebral Involvement at a Young Age. Front Neurol. 2018;9:336.
18. Lenders M, Weidemann F, Kurschat C, Canaan-Kühl S, Duning T, Stypmann J, et al. Alpha-Galactosidase A p.A143T, a non-Fabry disease-causing variant. Orphanet J Rare Dis. 2016;11(1):54.
19. Corry A, Feighery C, Alderdice D, Stewart F, Walsh M, Dolan OM. A family with Fabry disease diagnosed by a single angiokeratoma. Dermatol Online J. 2011;17(4):5.
20. De Brabander I, Yperzeele L, Ceuterick-De Groote C, Brouns R, Baker R, Belachew S, et al. Phenotypical characterization of α-galactosidase a gene mutations identified in a large Fabry disease screening program in stroke in the young. Clin Neurol Neurosurg. 2013;115(7):1088–93.
21. Smid BE, Hollak CE, Poorthuis BJ, van den Bergh Weerman MA, Florquin S, Kok WE, et al. Diagnostic dilemmas in Fabry disease: a case series study on *GLA* mutations of unknown clinical significance. Clin Genet. 2015;88(2):161–6.
22. Talbot A, Nicholls K. Elevated Lyso-Gb3 suggests the R118C *GLA* mutation is a pathological Fabry variant. JIMD Rep. 2019;45:95–8.
23. Ferreira S, Ortiz A, Germain DP, Viana-Baptista M, Caldeira-Gomes A, Camprecios M, et al. The alpha-galactosidase a p.Arg118Cys variant does not cause a Fabry disease phenotype: data from individual patients and family studies. Mol Genet Metab. 2015;114(2):248–58.
24. Caetano F, Botelho A, Mota P, Silva J, Leitão MA. Fabry disease presenting as apical left ventricular hypertrophy in a patient carrying the missense mutation R118C. Rev Port Cardiol. 2014;33(3):183.e1–5.
25. Topaloglu AK, Ashley GA, Tong B, Shabbeer J, Astrin KH, Eng CM, et al. Twenty novel mutations in the alpha-galactosidase a gene causing Fabry disease. Mol Med. 1999;5(12):806–11.
26. Turaça LT, Pessoa JG, Motta FL, Muñoz Rojas MV, Müller KB, Lourenço CM, et al. New mutations in the *GLA* gene in Brazilian families with Fabry disease. J Hum Genet. 2012;57(6):347–51.
27. Serebrinsky GP, Migueles R, Politei JM. Personal communication of mutation L180F. Available at www.fabry-database.org/mutants. Accessed 13 Feb 2019.
28. Davies JP, Winchester BG, Malcolm S. Mutation analysis in patients with the typical form of Anderson-Fabry disease. Hum Mol Genet. 1993;2(7):1051–3.
29. Shabbeer J, Yasuda M, Benson SD, Desnick RJ. Fabry disease: identification of 50 novel alpha-galactosidase a mutations causing the classic phenotype and three-dimensional structural analysis of 29 missense mutations. Hum Genomics. 2006;2(5):297–309.
30. Rosa Neto NS. Identification and clinical characterization of a novel alpha-Galactosidase a mutation. J Inborn Errors Metab Screen. 2014;2. https://doi. org/10.1177/2326409814554700

31. Cooper A, Cooper JA, Wraith JE. Human gene mutations in *GLA*. Hum Genet. 2000;107:535–6.

32. Blaydon D, Hill J, Winchester B. Fabry disease: 20 novel *GLA* mutations in 35 families. Hum Mutat. 2001;18(5):459.

33. Whybra C, Kampmann C, Krummenauer F, Ries M, Mengel E, Miebach E, et al. The Mainz severity score index: a new instrument for quantifying the Anderson-Fabry disease phenotype, and the response of patients to enzyme replacement therapy. Clin Genet. 2004;65(4):299–307.

34. Mehta A, Ricci R, Widmer U, Dehout F, Garcia de Lorenzo A, Kampmann C, et al. Fabry disease defined: baseline clinical manifestations of 366 patients in the Fabry outcome survey. Eur J Clin Investig. 2004;34(3):236–42.

35. Carapetis JR, Beaton A, Cunningham MW, Guilherme L, Karthikeyan G, Mayosi BM, et al. Acute rheumatic fever and rheumatic heart disease. Nat Rev Dis Primers. 2016;2:15084.

36. Lehman PJ, Carl RL. Growing pains. Sports Health. 2017;9(2):132–8.

37. Cimaz R, Guillaume S, Hilz MJ, Horneff G, Manger B, Thorne JC, et al. Awareness of Fabry disease among rheumatologists—current status and perspectives. Clin Rheumatol. 2011;30(4):467–75.

38. Cimaz R. Lysosomal storage diseases: underrecognized by rheumatologists? Ann Rheum Dis. 2010;69(suppl 3):27.

39. Lidove O, Noel E, Hachulla E, Gaches F, Douillard C, Darne B, et al. Characteristics of Pain in Fabry Disease. (abstract #256). Presented at the 2014 American College of Rheumatology/Association of Rheumatology Health Professionals Annual Meeting, November 14-19, in Boston, Massachusetts.

40. Kaminsky P, Barbey F, Jaussaud R, Gaches F, Leguy-Seguin V, Hachulla E et al. Pain As Predictor of Organ Involvement in Fabry Disease. (abstract #255). Presented at the 2014 American College of Rheumatology/Association of Rheumatology Health Professionals Annual Meeting, November 14-19, in Boston, Massachusetts.

41. Deshayes S, Jaussaud R, Imbert B, Lidove O, Parienti JJ, Triclin N et al. Prevalence of Raynaud's Phenomenon and Nailfold Capillaroscopic Abnormalities in Fabry's Disease: A Cross-Sectional Study. (abstract #2193). Presented at the 2014 American College of Rheumatology/Association of Rheumatology Health Professionals Annual Meeting, November 14-19, in Boston, Massachusetts.

42. Vordenbäumen S, Brinks R, Richter JG, Albrecht K, Schneider M. Clinical characteristics of patients with alpha-galactosidase a gene variants in a German multicenter cohort of early undifferentiated arthritis. Ann Rheum Dis. 2019. https://doi.org/10.1136/annrheumdis-2019-215223 [Epub ahead of print].

43. Gonçalves MJ, Mourão AF, Martinho A, Simões O, Melo-Gomes J, Salgado M, et al. Genetic Screening of Mutations Associated with Fabry Disease in a Nationwide Cohort of Juvenile Idiopathic Arthritis Patients. Front Med (Lausanne). 2017;4:12.

44. Hasunuma T, Araki N, Nakamura K, Shikano K, Momosaki K, Kawai S, et al. Significance Of Measuring Alpha-Galactosidase A In Fibromyalgia Patients: Possibility Of Fabry disease In Fibromyalgia Patients. Ann Rheum Dis. 2015; 74(suppl 2):1217.

45. Vordenbäumen S, Brinks R, Richter JG, Albrecht K, Schneider M. Response to 'what rheumatologist should know about Fabry disease' by Moiseev et al. Ann Rheum Dis. 2019. https://doi.org/10.1136/annrheumdis-2019-215516 [Epub ahead of print].

11

The Brazilian Society of Rheumatology recommendations on investigation and diagnosis of systemic autoimmune myopathies

Fernando Henrique Carlos de Souza[1], Daniel Brito de Araújo[2], Verônica Silva Vilela[3], Ricardo Santos Simões[1], Wanderley Marques Bernardo[1], Thais Amanda Frank[4], Bernardo Matos da Cunha[5] and Samuel Katsuyuki Shinjo[6*]

Abstract

Background: This research is recommended by the Myopathy Committee of the Brazilian Society of Rheumatology for the investigation and diagnosis of systemic autoimmune myopathies.

Body: A systematic literature review was performed in the Embase, Medline (PubMed) and Cochrane databases, including studies published until October 2018. PRISMA was used for the review, and the articles were evaluated, based on the Oxford levels of evidence. Ten recommendations were developed addressing different aspects of systemic autoimmune myopathy investigation and diagnosis.

Conclusions: The European League Against Rheumatism/ American College of Rheumatology (EULAR/ACR) classification stands out for the diagnosis of systemic autoimmune myopathies. Muscular biopsy is essential, aided by muscular magnetic resonance images and electroneuromyography in complementary research. Analysis of the factors related to prognosis with the evaluation of extramuscular manifestations, and comorbidities and intense investigation regarding differential diagnoses are mandatory.

Keywords: Autoantibodies, Electroneuromyography, Magnetic resonance, Muscle biopsy, Systemic autoimmune myopathies

Background

Systemic autoimmune myopathies (SAM) are rare systemic muscle diseases that include dermatomyositis (DM), juvenile dermatomyositis, clinically amyopathic dermatomyositis, polymyositis (PM), juvenile myositis, antisynthetase syndrome, inclusion body myositis, immune-mediated necrotizing myopathies, overlapped myositis syndrome, cancer-associated myopathies, and among others [1, 2].

Among the several diagnostic criteria proposed, convergence was observed in the evaluation of the following aspects: muscle weakness, observation of inflammatory infiltrate in muscle biopsy, electroneuromyography evaluation, serum muscle enzymes with special emphasis on creatine phosphokinase (CPK), and specific myositis antibodies. Comorbidities should be investigated, highlighting the presence of neoplasia, and a thorough investigation must always be carried out with regard to differential diagnoses [3, 4].

The purpose of these recommendations is to guide the investigation and diagnosis of SAM patients according to the current evidence in the literature.

Methods

A systematic literature review was performed in the following databases: Embase, Medline (PubMed), and Cochrane. The analysis was performed according to each "PICO" question (Patient, Intervention, Control, Outcome).

The following English terms were used in the systematic review of the literature: Autoimmune OR Autoimmune Disease OR Autoimmune Diseases OR Systemic OR

* Correspondence: samuel.shinjo@gmail.com
[6]Disciplina de Reumatologia, Faculdade de Medicina FMUSP, Universidade de Sao Paulo, Av. Dr. Arnaldo, 455, 3° andar, sala 3150, Sao Paulo, Cerqueira César CEP: 01246-903, Brazil
Full list of author information is available at the end of the article

Polymyositis OR Idiopathic Polymyositis OR Idiopathic OR Dermatomyositis OR Dermatopolymyositis OR Dermatopolymyositis OR Myositis OR Inflammatory Muscle Diseases OR Inflammatory Myopathy OR Inflammatory Myopathies) AND (Muscular Disease OR Myopathies OR Muscle Disorders OR Muscle Disorders OR Myopathic Conditions OR Myopathic Conditions.

With the application of a random filter, the terms related to each modality of investigation and diagnoses for SAM were included.

The inclusion criteria for the present study were: randomized and controlled trials (RCT) addressing SAM diagnosis and investigation, extension studies derived from RCTs with the criteria mentioned above and systematic reviews with RCT meta-analysis. In some cases, review articles and historical cohort studies were included and, in the absence of RCTs for specific modalities of therapy, open studies or low-quality cohort studies were accepted.

The steps in this systematic review followed the PRISMA guidelines [5]. The selected studies were evaluated, and the quality of the evidence and level of agreement for each question was based on the level of evidence from the studies (Tables 1 and 2) [6–8]. Ten recommendations were developed addressing different aspects of SAM investigation and diagnosis.

Recommendations

What are the classification criteria for SAM?
From 3297 records identified through database searching, 10 studies were selected to answer the present question (Additional file 1).

Literature review and analysis
A series of diagnostic criteria for SAM was developed by Bohan and Peter, Dalakas, Tanimoto, Targoff and the European Neuromuscular Center (ENMC). The classification of Dalakas, with a sensitivity of 77.1% and a specificity of 99.0%, showed better performance, followed by the ENMC criterion, with a sensitivity of 71.4% and a specificity of 82.4% (B) [9–14].

Table 2 Quality of evidence

Quality of evidence	Definition
A	Consistent level 1 studies
B	Consistent level 2 or 3 studies or extrapolations from level 1 studies
C	Level 4 studies or extrapolations of level 2 or 3 studies
D	Level 5 evidence or studies of any level with inconsistency or inconclusiveness

Medical records of adults diagnosed with DM according to the classification of Bohan and Peter were submitted to the European League Against Rheumatism / American College of Rheumatology (EULAR / ACR) criteria due to the inclusion of cutaneous rash (heliotrope rash and Gottron's sign or papules) [15]. DM cutaneous findings were measured by activity using the Severity Index and cutaneous dermatomyositis disease area (CDASI) to show which variables presented more frequently in patients with active DM including classic, amyopathic and hypomyopathic forms (C) [15].

The evaluation of the performance of EULAR / ACR in patients for whom a muscle biopsy was performed resulted in a sensitivity of 93% and specificity of 88%; disregarding the histological criterion indicated a sensitivity of 87% and a specificity of 82% (B) [2, 16]. Of note, the EULAR / ACR classification criteria [2] excluded the necessity of the electroneuromyography exam and aldolase serum dosing.

Similarly, all analyzed criteria showed the relevance of muscle biopsy, whose main objective is to rule out other possible causes of myopathies, in addition to helping to characterize the type of SAM. Biopsy is an important complementary exam in suspected cases of myopathies, especially in patients without characteristic skin involvement.

Overall, among the criteria, those of EULAR / ACR and ENMC performed better in the comparisons evaluated.

Table 1 Categories of evidence in studies

Levels	Evidence
1a	Systematic review and RCT meta-analysis
1b	At least one RCT with narrow confidence interval
2a	Systematic review and meta-analysis of cohort studies
2b	At least one cohort study or low quality RCT
3a	Systematic review and meta-analysis of case-control studies
3b	At least one case control study
4	At least one case series or cohort study and low quality case-control studies
5	Expert opinion without critical evaluation explicit or based on physiology, bench research or "fundamental principles"

RCT randomized clinical trial

Recommendations

SAM classification criteria may help with diagnoses, provided other myopathies have been ruled out. Specifically, the EULAR / ACR criteria deserve special mention, mainly when associated with muscle biopsy (quality of evidence B; level of agreement > 90%).

When should muscle biopsy be indicated in patients with SAM?

From 9275 records identified through database searching, 14 studies were selected to answer the present question (Additional file 1).

Literature review and analysis

In defined DM, perifascicular, perimysial or perivascular infiltrate and perifascicular atrophy are present (D) [17]. In immune-mediated necrotizing myopathy, the biopsy predominantly shows necrotic muscle fibers, sparse inflammatory cells in the perivascular space, and infiltrate of the perimysium (D) [12].

In PM, muscle biopsy shows cytotoxic CD8+ T lymphocyte endomysial inflammatory infiltrate, in necrotic and nonnecrotic fibers expressing major histocompatibility complex (MHC)-I [18–22].

Due to the presence of inflammatory infiltrate and mononuclear cells in muscle biopsy, the diagnostic utility of MHC-I has been studied to differentiate in SAMs from other muscular diseases and may show interference by variations, for example, in antibody type and staining (B) [18–22].

When comparing the histology of PM and DM with muscle biopsies of patients with muscular dystrophy, it was observed that MHC-I was regulated along the membrane of muscle fibers in patients with SAM, which helps in the differentiation from neuromuscular diseases (B) [18, 23, 24].

Therefore, when possible, rheumatologists should obtain muscle biopsy samples from all patients unless they present with unequivocal DM skin lesions (B) [24]. Moreover, immunohistochemistry (i.e., MHC staining) should b also be included in routine muscle biopsy panel analysis whenever possible.

As mentioned in the previous recommendation, all criteria include muscle biopsy to better characterize SAM and to exclude myopathies from another origin.

Recommendations

Muscle biopsy in patients with SAM may aid in the diagnosis of their subtypes and differentiate this disease from noninflammatory myopathies. MHC labeling mainly contributes to differentiating SAM from muscular dystrophies (quality of evidence B, level of agreement > 90%).

When should magnetic resonance imaging of muscles be indicated in patients with SAM?

From 428 records identified through database searching, 5 studies were selected to answer the present question (Additional file 1).

Literature review and analysis

Analysis of the distribution and extension of muscle inflammation through full-body magnetic resonance imaging (MRI) in SAM patients and subsequent biopsy of the muscle guided by these findings are described as a potential aid in the diagnosis of these diseases (B) [25–27].

This technique allows for the early identification of oligosymptomatic myositis, accurately detecting the most severely affected muscle candidates for biopsy, providing a reliable baseline method to monitor disease progression and response to treatment (B) [25–27].

Although imaging diagnostic methods with MRI have not been included in the EULAR / ACR classification criteria [2], the ability to demonstrate possible patterns of tissue alteration shows the possibility of their use as a complementary method in differentiating acquired and hereditary myopathies.

Recommendations

Magnetic resonance images can be used as a guide to muscle biopsy, to identify oligosymptomatic myositis and possible kinds of myopathies, and to monitor disease progression and response to treatment (quality of evidence B, level of agreement > 90%).

When should electroneuromyography be indicated in patients with SAM?

From 2064 records identified through database searching, 14 studies were selected to answer the present question (Additional file 1).

Literature review and analysis

Studies have demonstrated variable accuracy of electroneuromyography in different SAM, at similar rates in DM compared to PM (B) [28], and the evaluation of muscle fiber conduction velocity did not help to discriminate SAM from other myopathies (B) [29, 30].

In European centers, patients with myopathies of different etiologies, and even those with unknown etiologies were evaluated using three different diagnostic consensuses: clinical, electrodiagnostic and final consensus (clinical evaluations and electroneuromyography results). High sensitivity (90.2%) of electroneuromyography was observed in SAM [31–33]. Nevertheless, due to its low specificity, electroneuromyography has been withdrawn from the new EULAR / ACR 2017 [2].

Complementary tests before and after 6 months and 12 months of treatment indicated that increased muscle strength and decreased serum enzyme levels were associated with decreased spontaneous activity and the proportion of high-frequency components in electroneuromyography, except during the initial treatment period, when a temporary increase of high-frequency components was recorded (C) [34].

It was also shown that fiber density was slightly higher in the normal or neurogenic subgroup than in the myogenic subgroup, but without statistical significance (C) [35]. Finally, motor unit potentials and a myopathic interference pattern were present in equal numbers in treated and non-treated DM patients (B) [36]. Therefore, electroneuromyography may have an additional role in the diagnosis of SAM but plays no role in its follow-up (B) [36]. The exam is also important to distinguish eventual muscular weakness secondary to neurogenic affection.

Recommendations
Electroneuromyography in the diagnostic investigation can identify patients with myopathies, but it plays no role in the follow-up (quality of evidence B; level of agreement > 90%).

What are the myositis-specific or myositis-related antibodies that can assist in the diagnosis and/or follow-up of SAM patients in daily practice?
From 2974 records identified through database searching, 36 studies were selected to answer the present question (Additional file 1).

Literature review and analysis
Among the several antibodies identified, we present some antibodies that stand out in SAM.

Eight anti-aminoacyl-tRNA synthetase autoantibodies are described (A) [37]. The most prevalent is anti-Jo-1 (histidyl-tRNA synthetase), which can be identified in more than 20% of adult patients with a diagnosis of SAM (B) [38, 39] (C) [40], and due to its importance, this was included in the new EULAR / ACR 2017 SAM classification criteria [2]. Anti-Jo-1 is usually associated with manifestations that constitute the antisynthetase syndrome characterized by interstitial lung disease (ILD), Raynaud's phenomenon, arthritis and hyperkeratosis of the lateral part of the fingers and palms, a condition known as "mechanic hands." This antibody can also be found in cases of typical antisynthetase syndrome skin rashes. Other antisynthetase autoantibodies such as anti-PL-17 (threonyl-tRNA), anti-PL-12 (alanyl-tRNA), anti-EJ (glycyl-tRNA), anti-Ha (tyrosyl-tRNA), anti-OJ (isoleucyl-tRNA), anti-Zo (phenylalanyl-tRNA) and anti-KS (asparagil-tRNA) are less commonly found in this clinical condition [37–40].

In addition, evidence suggests that some aspects of the disease could vary depending on which antibody is present. Muscle disease, for example, is most frequently present among patients positive for anti-Jo-1, anti-PL-7, and anti-EJ (B) [41]. Arthritis is most associated with anti-Jo-1 and anti-PL-7; on the other hand, positivity of anti-KS, anti-OJ and anti-PL-12 is more associated with ILD (B) [37–42]. In addition, other myositis-specific and myositis-associated autoantibodies may be present, such as anti-melanoma differentiation-associated protein 5 (anti-MDA-5) and anti-PM/Scl, respectively (B) [43]. The presence of anti-MDA-5 is associated with rapidly progressive ILD (A) [44]. It has been used as a marker of response to treatment (B) [43, 45] (C) [46] and of poor prognosis; more than 40% of anti-MDA-5 positive patients die of respiratory failure (B) [47]. On the other hand, patients with anti-Jo-1 autoantibodies have better survival rates (B) [48].

Immune-mediated necrotizing myopathy is an SAM subtype associated with rapid development of muscle weakness and the presence of anti-signal recognition particle (anti-SRP), a specific myositis autoantibody that occurs in the context of acute onset of the disease, with severe myopathy and aggressive disease (C) [49, 50]. Dysphagia and ILD are also found in anti-SRP-positive patients (B) [51]. Anti-3-hydroxy-3-methylglutaryl-coenzyme A reductase (anti-HMGCR) is also associated with this myositis subtype, especially in patients with a previous history of statin use (B) [52] (D) [53]. An observational study designed to evaluate the severity of the disease and response to therapy in patients with myositis associated with the anti-HMGCR autoantibody found that young individuals had a more severe disease and a worse prognosis compared to older individuals (B) [54].

Anti-Mi-2 (directed against the nucleosome deacetylase complex) is associated with the phenotype of cutaneous signs ("shawl" sign, heliotrope rash and photosensitivity), clinically significant weakness, and high levels of muscle enzymes. The prognosis of patients with anti-Mi-2 is a good response to glucocorticoid treatment and a decreased risk of neoplasia and pulmonary disease (B) [55].

Myositis-specific autoantibodies related to a higher risk of malignancy in SAM patients include anti-transcriptional intermediary factors (TIF)-γ and anti-nuclear matrix protein (NXP)-2 (B) [56–58].

Anti-Ku, anti-PM/Scl and anti-nuclear ribonucleoprotein (anti-RNP) antibodies are generally identified in patients with overlapping manifestations of myositis and other autoimmune systemic diseases such as scleroderma, systemic lupus erythematosus and mixed connective tissue disease [59]. These individuals are probably the largest subgroup of patients who are diagnosed with SAM, with a prevalence of up to 50% of all adult individuals (D) [59]. Although these manifestations are nonspecific, they may correlate with some clinical characteristics of SAM (B) [60, 61].

Anti-PM / Scl is most commonly found in the association of systemic sclerosis, conferring an increased risk of interstitial lung disease, arthritis, mechanic's hands and Raynaud's phenomenon, increased CPK, constitutional disease activity, severity of dysphagia, and poor prognosis [61]. Anti-Ku was originally found in a variety of connective tissue disease conditions, being associated with higher rates of arthralgia, Raynaud's phenomenon, musculoskeletal manifestations, and a high frequency of interstitial lung disease [60]. Finally, patients with anti-U1-RNP rarely have myositis at initial presentation and respond favorably to glucocorticoid treatment, suggesting that this is a marker of good prognosis [59].

Myositis-specific autoantibodies are not essential to the treatment but are useful in some cases, especially when it is not possible to obtain a definitive diagnosis with muscle biopsy, being useful to accrue prognostic information and evaluate associated manifestations (B) [60, 61].

Recommendations
Autoantibodies can be found in patients diagnosed with SAM. They are not essential to the treatment but are useful in doubtful cases to accrue prognostic information and associated manifestations (quality of evidence B; level of agreement > 90%).

In the initial and late phases, which types of cancers should be searched for SAM? How often should the screening be done?
From 36,547 records identified through database searching, 18 studies were selected to answer the present question (Additional file 1).

Literature review and analysis
Individuals with DM present a higher risk of malignancy compared to those diagnosed with PM (overall relative risk of 4.6 and 1.7, respectively) (A) [62], Although increased incidence of cancer in these patients can partially be attributed to the investigations requested for these individuals, particularly during the first year after diagnosis in tertiary centers (B) [63], evidence has pointed to a real higher incidence even before the diagnosis is established, thus suggesting a true association between the diagnosis of SAM and cancer (A) [64]. Despite the recognition of this association, the types of cancer remain somewhat controversial, including a broad spectrum of malignancies such as breast, lung colorectal, nasopharynx, body of the uterus, and gastric cancer, which are significantly influenced by gender and ethnicity [62–69].

In particular, a multicenter study of patients with DM found a significantly elevated risk for lung, ovarian, pancreatic, gastric, and colorectal cancer and non-Hodgkin's lymphoma [69]. In patients with PM, an increased risk of non-Hodgkin's lymphoma and lung and bladder cancer was observed (B) [70]. The most common type of

cancer was adenocarcinoma, accounting for 70% of all tumors associated with both diseases (B) [70].

There is a higher risk of neoplasms occurring among older individuals (B) [71, 72]. The evaluation should include prostate and testicular examination in men, breast and pelvic examination in women and rectal examination in all patients. Women with a recent SAM diagnosis should be extensively examined and submitted to mammography and pelvic ultrasonography [71, 72]. Some neoplasms may not yet be identified in a screening program such as lymphoma, ovarian, pancreatic, or lung cancer [71, 72]. Thus, computed tomography examination of the thorax, abdomen, and pelvis may be considered in a subgroup of patients with SAM who have risk factors for specific types of neoplasia, such as a positive family history of ovarian or breast cancer [71, 72]. Gastrointestinal endoscopy and colonoscopy should be utilized on a case-by-case basis [71, 72].

Studies show a lack of uniformity in the definition of the temporal association between neoplasia and the diagnosis of SAM [62–72]. Thus, there has been no consensus until recently regarding how and when this screening should be conducted.

Recommendations
There is no concise information about the screening of neoplasms, and no consensus, regarding how and when this screening should be conducted. However, in our opinion, adults with this diagnosis, highlighting DM, should be screened, requesting specific tests mainly according to gender, age, ethnicity, and familiar history (quality of evidence B; level of agreement > 90%).

Which comorbidities should be (re) evaluated regularly in patients with SAM?
From 36,547 records identified through database searching, 22 studies were selected to answer the present question (Additional file 1).

Literature review and analysis
Virtually all individuals with conditions associated with muscle weakness, such as those found in SAM, are susceptible to the development of low bone mass density (B) [73–75] (A) [76, 77]. Moreover, these individuals are exposed to an additional risk factor since glucocorticoids represent the first-line treatment (B) [78] (D) [79, 80]. Individuals who face significant deterioration of bone mass density and/or bone microarchitecture impairment are at a high risk of fracture (A) [81], making it imperative to periodically investigate using the X-ray dual-density densitometry method (B) [82]. An observational study conducted with the objective of assessing the prevalence of osteoporosis and occurrence of fractures in adults with SAM identified that osteoporosis was

more frequently diagnosed compared to controls with a high prevalence of fractures (B) [82].

Although rarely symptomatic, subclinical cardiac manifestations are usually identified in patients with myopathies, and their prevalence varies widely according to the way the patient is investigated (electrocardiogram, echocardiogram, Holter, cardiac MRI) [83, 84]. The most frequent abnormalities are cardiomyopathy, dilated cardiomyopathy, heart failure, myocarditis, pericarditis, conduction defects and arrhythmias (A) [83] (D) [84]. The occurrence of arterial microvascular disease associated with acute myocardial infarction has also been reported [84, 85]. Nevertheless, patients may demonstrate combinations of more than one type of heart involvement [84, 85]. Clinical evaluation, including detailed anamnesis and physical examination is of paramount importance at the time of diagnosis, and some tests are recommended, such as an electrocardiogram, to check for cardiac involvement with the presence of arrhythmias and conduction abnormalities (C) [85]. Other investigations such as echocardiography, myocardial scintigraphy, and MRI are indicated when clinically relevant at the time of diagnosis and during the follow-up period (C) [86].

The lung is the organ most frequently affected in SAM, which is also the main cause of death in this group of patients [84]. The main types of lung involvement are hypoventilation due to respiratory muscle weakness, interstitial pneumonia, and aspiration (D) [87] (B) [88]. Therefore, patients with myopathies should undergo pulmonary function evaluation at the time of diagnosis. Moreover, patients with a high risk of pulmonary function impairment and/or vital capacity reduction should be monitored more frequently (B) [88–90]. In these cases, assessment of noninvasive oxygenation of patients by oximetry may be indicated. The evaluation of pulmonary function may also include a 6-min walking test, respiratory video fluoroscopy and ergospirometry [88–90].

Dysphagia has been reported in 32–84% of SAM patients, and esophageal involvement assessed by high-resolution manometry is common in patients with SAM, but it correlates poorly with esophageal symptoms. Failed waves and decreased upper esophageal sphincter pressure are more common in PM than in DM patients (B) [91].

Recommendations
The management of patients with myopathies should consider care aimed at limiting the effects of muscle weakness, on joints, bones and other systems. In addition, comorbidities should be screened for and treated when necessary, optimizing the functional capacity and thereby improving quality of life of patients (quality of evidence B; level of agreement > 90%).

What are the main differential diagnoses of SAM?
From 36,547 records identified through database searching, 9 studies were selected to answer the present question (Additional file 1).

Literature review and analysis
The identification of certain extramuscular manifestations may suggest the possibility of mitochondrial myopathy such as the presence of cognitive alterations, hearing and extraocular muscle impairment, convulsions, and neuropathy in patients with mitochondrial encephalomyopathy (D) [92]. Serum CK levels may be normal, and muscle biopsy stained by the Gomori trichrome revealed the presence of fibers with increased reddish granulation [92]. It should be noted, however, that although these findings are indicative of mitochondrial dysfunction, they may be identified in many other disorders and are not specific to the diagnosis of hereditary mitochondrial myopathy (D) [93].

Another important differential diagnosis is metabolic myopathies, characterized by defects in muscle tissue utilization of carbohydrates or fats, resulting in a decrease in energy supply [94, 95]. These myopathies manifest as cramp attacks and muscle weakness, often associated with myoglobinuria [94, 95]. Some metabolic myopathies, such as acid maltase deficiency (Pompe's disease) and glycogen storage disease type V (McArdle's disease) may manifest with episodic proximal muscle weakness [75, 94]. This pattern may eventually lead to confusion with the diagnosis of SAM, especially in the presence of a history of chronicity and nonidentification of myoglobinuria (C) [94, 95].

Endocrine myopathies should also be considered in the differential diagnosis [96]. Myopathy related to hypothyroidism is typically characterized by muscle discomfort associated with mild to moderate proximal muscle weakness [96]. Serum CK levels may be slightly elevated, and there appears to be no association between the degree of muscle weakness and the severity of hypothyroidism (B) [96]. Hyperthyroidism is also associated with myopathy, although it seems to be a less common occurrence than that observed in cases of hypothyroidism [96]. A study identified that approximately 60% of patients with untreated hyperthyroidism showed clinical evidence of proximal muscle weakness; however, only 10% had myopathic changes in electromyography (B) [95]. Hyperparathyroidism may occasionally cause proximal muscle weakness syndrome. Additionally, CK levels that are normal or slightly elevated with muscle biopsy may indicate atrophy without alteration in muscle fiber arrangement [96].

Drug-induced myopathies are also a differential diagnosis [97]. As a classic example, statins may be associated with varying forms of muscle symptoms and toxicity, such as myalgia (1 to 10%), myositis (defined by muscle symptoms and increased CK levels), and rhabdomyolysis (increases in

CK with evidence of injury) (D), most commonly observed in patients with hypothyroidism, in those who are using multiple drugs, and even in those who abuse alcoholic beverages (D) [97].

Some infections may cause chronic myopathy that may resemble PM [98]. These infections are often triggered by acute viral illness, such as the Coxsackie or influenza virus [98]. Human immunodeficiency virus may also be associated with muscle weakness, either as a characteristic of the infection itself or in later stages of the disease [98]. In addition to myopathic changes, there may be evidence of axonal sensory neuropathy [98]. Bacterial infections, except for Lyme disease and syphilis, may present with focal pyomyositis (D) [98].

Finally, muscular dystrophies should also be considered as differential diagnoses, mainly in PM or PM-like conditions, since these conditions may mimic the clinical manifestations of SAM. Some features may suggest the diagnosis of muscular dystrophies, such sa positive family history, prolonged course of muscle weakness, facial weakness, abnormalities of eye movement, distal weakness equal to or greater than proximal weakness, and asymmetrical weakness.

Recommendations
Several conditions may mimic the clinical manifestations of SAM. Moreover, the absence of specific autoantibodies and systemic features related to autoimmunity and refractoriness to immunosuppressive drugs should also raise the suspicion of alternative diagnoses (quality of evidence B; level of agreement > 90%).

Which clinical / laboratory findings result in poor response to drug treatment in SAM?
From 9275 records identified through database searching, 14 studies were selected to answer the present question (Additional file 1).

Literature review and analysis
The International Myositis Assessment & Clinical Studies Group (IMACS) suggested, regarding the status of the disease, some measures as a global evaluation of the disease activity perceived by the patient and physician. Muscle strength assessed by Muscle Manual Testing (MMT); functional capacity measured by the Health Assessment Questionnaire (HAQ); elevated serum levels of at least two muscle enzymes (CK, aldolase, lactate dehydrogenase, aspartate and alanine aminotransferases); and extramuscular manifestations of the disease assessed by the Myositis Disease Activity Assessment Tool (MDAAT) may be used for the purpose of monitoring disease activity and as indicative of poor response to treatment (D) [99]. However, in addition to few measures being fully validated, it is still difficult to differentiate disease activity from accrual damage [99].

Despite the relationship with ILD, antisynthetase antibody positivity is a predictor of clinical response to rituximab in individuals with refractory myositis (B) [100–102]. Reports indicate that patients with ILD-positive anti-OJ present a good prognosis as well as a positive response to glucocorticoid therapy (C) [103]. Anti-exosome (anti-PM/Scl) presence does not appear to be a good prognostic factor and is associated with pulmonary and esophageal involvement (C) [104].

Recommendations
Cytokines and specific or related myositis antibodies aiming to discriminate the disease activity and to predict the prognosis of the treatment. However, it is important to note that the available evidence on the use of laboratory findings for this purpose shows variable results in terms of performance, lacking a standardized approach (quality of evidence B; level of agreement > 90%).

The available evidence on the use of laboratory tests or other standardized tools to evaluate disease activity and/or to predict the response to treatment shows variable results in terms of performance, lacking a standardized approach. At this point, we recommend the use of laboratory markers, such as CPK, and tools, such as physician and patient global evaluation of the disease activity as guides to disease activity, and treatment response (quality of evidence B; level of agreement > 90%).

Which organs and/or systems should be routinely reevaluated in patients with SAM?
From 36,892 records identified through database searching, 20 studies were selected to answer the present question (Additional file 1).

Literature review and analysis
In addition to the considerable heterogeneity in the presentation and prognosis of the SAM, extramuscular involvement is often observed. There may be concurrent involvement of cardiovascular, respiratory, digestive, kidney, endocrine, ocular, dermatological, hematological, and nervous systems (B) [83, 87, 105–109]. The extent and severity of systemic organ involvement also vary substantially in each SAM category (DM, PM, immune-mediated necrotizing myopathy) [83, 87, 105–109].

SAM patients present survival rates estimated between approximately 60 and 70%, with deaths mainly related to cardiac and pulmonary involvement, as well as the occurrence of cancers and infections affecting the respiratory and gastrointestinal tract (B) [88, 110]. The cause of death in individuals depends on the duration of the disease. Death related to pulmonary complications usually occurs in the first year of disease, while cardiovascular complications are the most common cause of death 5 years after diagnosis (B) [111]. Therefore, all individuals should be referred for cardiac and lung function assessment at the time of diagnosis of SAM, and clinical evaluation, including detailed anamnesis and physical examination is essential [108]. Some tests are recommended, such as electrocardiogram and the evaluation of pulmonary function, to verify cardiac involvement with arrhythmias and conduction abnormalities and impairment of pulmonary function as a reduction in vital capacity (B) [90, 112] (C) [85] (D) [113].

Gastrointestinal disorders compromise the oropharynx, esophagus, stomach, liver, small intestine, colon, and rectum, and there is a substantial increase in the risk of occult malignancies, including gastrointestinal cancers, mainly observed in the first year after diagnosis (B) [70, 114, 115]. Thus, extensive anamnesis and physical examination are mandatory in newly diagnosed patients, and a high suspicion of underlying malignancy should be maintained. High-risk characteristics for malignancy include advanced age, myopathy refractory to glucocorticoid treatment, presence of severe cutaneous rash, and being negative for some autoantibodies [anti-histidyl tRNA synthetase (Jo-1), anti-PM/Scl, anti-U1-RNP, anti-U3-RNP and anti-Ku antigen] [116, 117], requiring a more complete evaluation in regard to cancer screening and surveillance.

Recommendations
The manifestation of SAM is heterogeneous. Therefore, cardiovascular, respiratory and gastrointestinal evaluations should be performed when indicated. Care should also be taken to ensure a neoplasm screening and surveillance program (quality of evidence B; level of agreement > 90%).

Conclusions
Among all criteria, the EULAR / ACR 2017 stands out for the diagnosis of SAM. Muscular biopsy is essential, aided by muscular magnetic resonance images and electroneuromyography in complementary research. Analysis of factors related to prognosis with evaluation of extramuscular manifestations, and comorbidities and intense investigation regarding differential diagnoses are mandatory.

Supplementary information

> **Additional file 1.** The studies selection process during the systematic review.

Abbreviations
ACR: American College of Rheumatology; CDASI: Cutaneous dermatomyosis disease area; CPK: Creatine phosphokinase; DM: Dermatomyositis; ENMC: European Neuromuscular Center; EULAR: European League Against Rheumatism; HAQ: Health Assessment Questionnaire; HMGCR: 3-hydroxy-3-methylglutaryl-coenzyme A reductase; IL: Interleukin; ILD: Interstitial lung disease; IMACS: International Myositis Assessment and Clinical Studies Group; IP: Interferon gamma-induced protein; MDA: Melanoma differentiation-associated gene; MDAAT: Myositis Disease Activity Assessment Tool; MMT: Muscle Testing Manual; MRI: Magnetic resonance imaging; NXP: Nuclear Matrix Protein; PICO: Patient, Intervention, Control, Outcome; PM: Polymyositis; RCT: Randomized controlled trials; RNP: Nuclear ribonucleoprotein; SAM: Systemic autoimmune myopathies; SDF: Stromal cell-derived factor; SRP: Signal recognition particle; TIF: Transcriptional intermediary factor; TNF: Tumor necrosis factor

Acknowledgments
Renata Miossi, and Mailze Campos Bezerra who contributed to the elaboration of questions.

Authors' contributions
FHCS contributed to the elaboration of questions. He was a major contributor in writing and reviewing the manuscript. DBA contributed to the elaboration of questions and the manuscript revision. VSS contributed to the elaboration of question and the manuscript revision. RSS contributed to systematic literature review. WMB contributed to systematic literature review. TAF contributed to systematic literature review. BMC contributed to the elaboration of questions and the manuscript revision. SKS contributed to the manuscript organization, elaboration of questions and manuscript revision. All authors read and approved the final manuscript.

Author details
[1]Hospital das Clinicas HCFMUSP, Faculdade de Medicina, Universidade de Sao Paulo, São Paulo, SP, Brazil. [2]Universidade Federal de Pelotas (UFP), Pelotas, RS, Brazil. [3]Universidade do Estado do Rio de Janeiro (UERJ), Rio de Janeiro, RJ, Brazil. [4]Programa Diretrizes da Associação Médica Brasileira (AMB), Brasília, Brazil. [5]Rede Sarah de Hospitais de Reabilitação, Brasília, Brazil. [6]Disciplina de Reumatologia, Faculdade de Medicina FMUSP, Universidade de Sao Paulo, Av. Dr. Arnaldo, 455, 3° andar, sala 3150, Sao Paulo, Cerqueira César CEP: 01246-903, Brazil.

References
1. Feldman BM, Rider LG, Reed AM, Pachman LM. Juvenile dermatomyositis and other idiopathic inflammatory myopathies of childhood. Lancet. 2008;371:201–12.
2. Lundberg IE, Tjamlund A, Bottai M, Pikington C, de Visser M, Alfredson L, et al. 2017 European league against rheumatism / American College of Rheumatology classification criteria for adult and juvenile idiopathic inflammatory myopathies and their major subgroups. Arthritis Rheum. 2017;69:2271–82.
3. Dalakas MC. Inflammatory muscle diseases. N Engl J Med. 2015;372:1734–47.
4. Lundberg IE, Miller FW, Tjärnlund A, Bottai M. Diagnosis and classification of idiopathic inflammatory myopathies. J Intern Med. 2016;280:39–51.
5. Iberati A, Altman DG, Tetzlaff J, Mulrow C, Gøtzsche PC, Ioannidis JP, et al. The PRISMA statement for reporting systematic reviews and meta-analyses of studies that evaluate healthcare interventions: explanation and elaboration. BMJ. 2009;339:b2700.
6. Guyatt GH, Oxman AD, Vist GE, Kunz R, Falck-Ytter Y, Alonso-Coello P, et al. GRADE: an emerging consensus on rating quality of evidence and strength of recommendations. BMJ. 2008;336:924-6.
7. Guyatt GH, Oxman AD, Kunz R, Falck-Ytter Y, Vist GE, Liberati A, et al. GRADE working group. Going from evidence to recommendations. BMJ. 2008;336:1049–51.
8. Guyatt GH, Oxman AD, Vist GE, Kunz R, Falck-Ytter Y, Alonso-Coello P, et al. GRADE working group. GRADE: an emerging consensus on rating quality of evidence and strength of recommendations. BMJ. 2008;336:924–6.
9. Linklater H, Pipitone N, Rose MR, Norwood F, Campbell R, Salvarani C, et al. Classifying idiopathic inflammatory myopathies: comparing the performance of six existing criteria. Clin Exp Rheumatol. 2013;31:767–9.
10. Bohan A, Peter JB. Polymyositis and dermatomyositis (first of two parts). N Engl J Med. 1975;292:344–7.
11. Bohan A, Peter JB. Polymyositis and dermatomyositis (second of two parts). N Engl J Med. 1975;292:403–7.
12. Hoogendijk JE, Amato AA, Lecky BR, Choy EH, Lundberg IE, Rose MR, et al. 119th ENMC international workshop: trial design in adult idiopathic inflammatory myopathies, with the exception of inclusion body myositis, 10-12 October 2003, Naarden, the Netherlands. Neuromuscul Disord. 2004;14:337–45.

13. Tanimoto K, Nakano K, Kano S, Mori S, Ueki H, Nishitani H, et al. Classification criteria for polymyositis and dermato-myositis. J Rheumatol. 1995;22:668–74.

14. Targoff IN, Miller FW, Medsger TA Jr, Oddis CV. Classification criteria for the idiopathic inflammatory myopathies. Curr Opin Rheumatol. 1997;9:527–35.

15. Patel B, Khan N, Werth VP. Applicability of EULAR/ACR classification criteria for dermatomyositis to amyopathic disease. J Am Acad Dermatol. 2018;79:77–83.

16. Hocevar A, Rotar Z, Krosel M, Cucnik S, Tomsic M. Performance of the 2017 European league against rheumatism/American College of Rheumatology classification criteria for adult and juvenile idiopathic inflammatory myopathies in clinical practice. Ann Rheum Dis. 2018;77:e90.

17. Dalakas MC, Hohlfeld R. Polymyositis and dermatomyositis. Lancet. 2003;362:971–82.

18. Nagappa M, Nalini A, Narayanappa G. Major histocompatibility complex and inflammatory cell subtype expression in inflammatory myopathies and muscular dystrophies. Neurol India. 2013;61:614–21.

19. Salaroli R, Baldin E, Papa V, Rinaldi R, Tarantino L, De Giorgi LB, et al. Validity of internal expression of the major histocompatibility complex class I in the diagnosis of inflammatory myopathies. J Clin Pathol. 2012;65:14–9.

20. Rodríguez Cruz PM, Luo YB, Miller J, Junckerstorff RC, Mastaglia FL, Fabian V. An analysis of the sensitivity and specificity of MHC-I and MHC-II immunohistochemical staining in muscle biopsies for the diagnosis of inflammatory myopathies. Neuromuscul Disord. 2014;24:1025–35.

21. Jain A, Sharma MC, Sarkar C, Bhatia R, Singh S, Handa R. Major histocompatibility complex class I and II detection as a diagnostic tool in idiopathic inflammatory myopathies. Arch Pathol Lab Med. 2007;131:1070–6.

22. van der Pas J, Hengstman GJ, ter Laak HJ, Borm GF, van Engelen BG. Diagnostic value of MHC class I staining in idiopathic inflammatory myopathies. J Neurol Neurosurg Psychiatry. 2004;75:136–9.

23. Sallum AM, Kiss MH, Silva CA, Wakamatsu A, Sachetti S, Lotufo S, et al. MHC class I and II expression in juvenile dermatomyositis skeletal muscle. Clin Exp Rheumatol. 2009;27:519–26.

24. Dai TJ, Li W, Zhao QW, Zhao YY, Liu SP, Yan CZ. CD8/MHC-I complex is specific but not sensitive for the diagnosis of polymyositis. J Int Med Res. 2010;38:1049–59.

25. O'Connell MJ, Powell T, Brennan D, Lynch T, McCarthy CJ, Eustace SJ. Whole-body MR imaging in the diagnosis of polymyositis. AJR Am J Roentgenol. 2002;179:967–71.

26. Elessawy SS, Abdelsalam EM, Abdel Razek E, Tharwat S. Whole-body MRI for full assessment and characterization of diffuse inflammatory myopathy. Acta Radiol Open. 2016;5:2058460116668216.

27. Van De Vlekkert J, Maas M, Hoogendijk JE, De Visser M, Van Schaik IN. Combining MRI and muscle biopsy improves diagnostic accuracy in subacute-onset idiopathic inflammatory myopathy. Muscle Nerve. 2015;51:253–8.

28. Lyu RK, Cornblath DR, Chaudhry V. Incidence of irritable electromyography in inflammatory myopathy. J Clin Neuromuscul Dis. 1999;1:64–7.

29. Blijham PJ, Hengstman GJ, Ter Laak HJ, Van Engelen BG, Zwarts MJ. Muscle-fiber conduction velocity and electromyography as diagnostic tools in patients with suspected inflammatory myopathy: a prospective study. Muscle Nerve. 2004;29:46–50.

30. Yang F, Jing F, Chen Z, Ling L, Wang R, Wang X, et al. Electrophysiological and clinical examination of polymyositis: a retrospective analysis. Am J Med Sci. 2014;348:162–6.

31. Pugdahl K, Johnsen B, Tankisi H, Camdessanch JP, de Carvalho M, Fawcett PR, et al. Added value of electromyography in the diagnosis of myopathy: a consensus exercise. Clin Neurophysiol. 2017;128:697–701.

32. Kim NR, Nam EJ, Kang JW, Song HS, Im CH, Kang YM. Complex repetitive discharge on electromyography as a risk factor for malignancy in idiopathic inflammatory myopathy. Korean J Intern Med. 2014;29:814–21.

33. Mechler F. Changing electromyographic findings during the chronic course of polymyositis. J Neurol Sci. 1974;23:237–42.

34. Sandstedt PE, Henriksson KG, Larrsson LE. Quantitative electromyography in polymyositis and dermatomyositis. Acta Neurol Scand. 1982;65:110–21.

35. Jian F, Cui LY, Li BH, Du H. Changes of single fiber electromyography in patients with inflammatory myopathies. Chin Med Sci J. 2005;20:1–4.

36. Blijham PJ, Hengstman GJ, Hama-Amin AD, van Engelen BG, Zwarts MJ. Needle electromyographic findings in 98 patients with myositis. Eur Neurol. 2006;55:183–8.

37. Lega JC, Fabien N, Reynaud Q, Durieu I, Durupt S, Dutertre M, et al. The clinical phenotype associated with myositis-specific and associated autoantibodies: a meta-analysis revisiting the so-called antisynthetase syndrome. Autoimmun Rev. 2014;13:883–91.

38. Hengstman GJ, Brouwer R, Egberts WT, Seelig HP, Jongen PJ, van Venrooij WJ, et al. Clinical and serological characteristics of 125 Dutch myositis

39. Zampeli E, Venetsanopoulou A, Argyropoulou OD, Mavragani CP, Tektonidou MG, Vlachoyiannopoulos PG, et al. Myositis autoantibody profiles and their clinical associations in Greek patients with inflammatory myopathies. Clin Rheumatol. 2018;38(1):125.

40. Nishikai M, Reichlin M. Heterogeneity of precipitating antibodies in polymyositis and dermatomyositis. Characterization of the Jo-1 antibody system. Arthritis Rheum. 1980;23:881–8.

41. Hamaguchi Y, Fujimoto M, Matsushita T, Kaji K, Komura K, Hasegawa M, et al. Common and distinct clinical features in adult patients with anti-aminoacyl-tRNA synthetase antibodies: heterogeneity within the syndrome. PLoS One. 2013;8:e60442.

42. Klein M, Mann H, Pleštilová L, Betteridge Z, McHugh N, Remáková M, et al. Arthritis in idiopathic inflammatory myopathy: clinical features and autoantibody associations. J Rheumatol. 2014;41:1133–9.

43. Koga T, Fujikawa K, Horai Y, Okada A, Kawashiri SY, Iwamoto N, et al. The diagnostic utility of anti-melanoma differentiation-associated gene 5 antibody testing for predicting the prognosis of Japanese patients with DM. Rheumatology (Oxford). 2012;51:1278–84.

44. Chen Z, Cao M, Plana MN, Liang J, Cai H, Kuwana M, et al. Utility of anti-melanoma differentiation-associated gene 5 antibody measurement in identifying patients with dermatomyositis and a high risk for developing rapidly progressive interstitial lung disease: a review of the literature and a meta-analysis. Arthritis Care Res. 2013;65:1316–24.

45. Gono T, Sato S, Kawaguchi Y, Kuwana M, Hanaoka M, Katsumata Y, et al. Anti-MDA5 antibody, ferritin and IL-18 are useful for the evaluation of response to treatment in interstitial lung disease with anti-MDA5 antibody-positive dermatomyositis. Rheumatology (Oxford). 2012;51:1563–70.

46. Endo Y, Koga T, Suzuki T, Hara K, Ishida M, Fujita Y, et al. Successful treatment of plasma exchange for rapidly progressive interstitial lung disease with anti-MDA5 antibody-positive dermatomyositis: a case report. Medicine (Baltimore). 2018;97:e0436.

47. Moghadam-Kia S, Oddis CV, Sato S, Kuwana M, Aggarwal R. Anti-melanoma differentiation-associated gene 5 is associated with rapidly progressive lung disease and poor survival in us patients with amyopathic and myopathic dermatomyositis. Arthritis Care Res. 2016;68:689–94.

48. Aggarwal R, Cassidy E, Fertig N, Koontz DC, Lucas M, Ascherman DP, et al. Patients with non-Jo-1 anti-tRNA-synthetase autoantibodies have worse survival than Jo-1 positive patients. Ann Rheum Dis. 2014;73:227–32.

49. Suzuki S, Hayashi YK, Kuwana M, Tsuburaya R, Suzuki N, Nishino I. Myopathy associated with antibodies to signal recognition particle: disease progression and neurological outcome. Arch Neurol. 2012;69:728–32.

50. Wang L, Liu L, Hao H, Gao F, Liu X, Wang Z, et al. Myopathy with anti-signal recognition particle antibodies: clinical and histopathological features in Chinese patients. Neuromuscul Disord. 2014;24:335–41.

51. Kao AH, Lacomis D, Lucas M, Fertig N, Oddis CV. Anti-signal recognition particle autoantibody in patients with and patients without idiopathic inflammatory myopathy. Arthritis Rheum. 2004;50:209–15.

52. Allenbach Y, Drouot L, Rigolet A, Charuel JL, Jouen F, Romero NB, et al. French myositis network. Anti-HMGCR autoantibodies in European patients with autoimmune necrotizing myopathies: inconstant exposure to statin. Medicine (Baltimore). 2014;93:150–7.

53. Mohassel P, Mammen AL. Anti-HMGCR myopathy. J Neuromuscul Dis. 2018;5:11–20.

54. Tiniakou E, Pinal-Fernandez I, Lloyd TE, Albayda J, Paik J, Werner JL, Parks CA, et al. More severe disease and slower recovery in younger patients with anti-3-hydroxy-3-methylglutaryl-coenzyme a reductase-associated autoimmune myopathy. Rheumatology (Oxford). 2017;56:787–94.

55. Targoff IN, Reichlin M. The association between anti-Mi2 antibodies and dermatomyositis. Arthritis Rheum. 1985;28:796–803.

56. Kaji K, Fujimoto M, Hasegawa M, Kondo M, Saito Y, Komura K, et al. Identification of a novel autoantibody reactive with p155 and 140 kDa nuclear proteins in patients with dermatomyositis: an association with malignancy. Rheumatology (Oxford). 2007;46:25–8.

57. Targoff IN, Mamyrova G, Trieu EP, Perurena O, Koneru B, O'Hanlon TP, et al. A novel autoantibody to a 155-kd protein is associated with dermatomyositis. Arthritis Rheum. 2006;54:3682–9.

58. Albayda J, Pinal-Fernandez I, Huang Y, Parks C, Casciola-Rosen L, Danoff SK, et al. Antinuclear matrix protein 2 autoantibodies and edema, muscle disease and malignancy risk in dermatomyositis patients. Arthritis Care Res. 2017;69:1771–6.

59. Fredi M, Cavazzana I, Franceschini F. The clinic-serological spectrum of overlap myositis. Curr Opin Rheumatol. 2018;30:637–43.

60. Rigolet A, Musset L, Dubourg O, Maisonobe T, Grenier P, Charuel JL, et al. Inflammatory myopathies with anti-Ku antibodies: a prognosis dependent on associated lung disease. Medicine (Baltimore). 2012;91:95–102.

61. Muro Y, Hosono Y, Sugiura K, Ogawa Y, Mimori T, Akiyama M. Anti-PM/Scl antibodies are found in Japanese patients with various systemic autoimmune conditions besides myositis and scleroderma. Arthritis Res Ther. 2015;17:57.

62. Qiang JK, Kim WB, Baibergenova A, Alhusayen R. Risk of malignancy in dermatomyositis and polymyositis. J Cutan Med Surg. 2017;21:131–6.

63. Zhang Y, Felson D. The overall and temporal association of cancer with polymyositis and dermatomyositis. J Rheumatol. 1994;21:1855–9.

64. Yang Z, Lin F, Qin B, Liang Y, Zhong R. Polymyositis/dermatomyositis and malignancy risk: a meta-analysis study. J Rheumatol. 2015;42:282–91.

65. Chen YJ, Wu CY, Huang YL, Wang CB, Shen JL, Chang YT. Cancer risks of dermatomyositis and polymyositis: a nationwide cohort study in Taiwan. Arthritis Res Ther. 2010;12:R70.

66. Azuma K, Yamada H, Ohkubo M, Yamasaki Y, Yamasaki M, Mizushima M, al e. Incidence and predictive factors for malignancies in 136 Japanese patients with dermatomyositis, polymyositis and clinically amyopathic dermatomyositis. Mod Rheumatol. 2011;21:178–83.

67. Wakata N, Kurihara T, Saito E, Kinoshita M. Polymyositis and dermatomyositis associated with malignancy: a 30-year retrospective study. Int J Dermatol. 2002;41:729–34.

68. Toumi S, Ghnaya H, Braham A, Harrabi I, Laouani-Kechrid C. Groupe tunisien d'étude des myosites inflammatoires. [polymyositis and dermatomyositis in adults. Tunisian multicentre study]. Rev Med Interne. 2009;30:747–53.

69. Diallo M, Fall AK, Diallo I, Diédhiou I, Ba PS, Diagne M, et al. Dermatomyositis and polymyositis: 21 cases in Senegal. Med Trop (Mars). 2010;70:166–8.

70. Hill CL, Zhang Y, Sigurgeirsson B, Pukkala E, Mellemkjaer L, Airio A, et al. Frequency of specific cancer types in dermatomyositis and polymyositis: a population-based study. Lancet. 2001;357:96–100.

71. Chow WH, Gridley G, Mellemkjaer L, McLaughlin JK, Olsen JH, Fraumeni JF Jr. Cancer risk following polymyositis and dermatomyositis: a nationwide cohort study in Denmark. Cancer Causes Control. 1995;6:9–13.

72. Airio A, Pukkala E, Isomäki H. Elevated cancer incidence in patients with dermatomyositis: a population based study. J Rheumatol. 1995;22:1300–3.

73. Heinonen A, Kannus P, Sievänen H, Pasanen M, Oja P, Vuori I. Good maintenance of high-impact activity-induced bone gain by voluntary, unsupervised exercises: an 8-month follow-up of a randomized controlled trial. J Bone Miner Res. 1999;14:125–8.

74. Kalluru R, Hart H, Corkill M, Ng KP. Long-term follow-up of patients with idiopathic inflammatory myopathy at Waitemata District health board. N Z Med J. 2016;129:50–6.

75. So H, Yip ML, Wong AK. Prevalence and associated factors of reduced bone mineral density in patients with idiopathic inflammatory myopathies. Int J Rheum Dis. 2016;19:521–8.

76. Martyn-St James M, Carroll S. Effects of different impact exercise modalities on bone mineral density in premenopausal women: a meta-analysis. J Bone Miner Metab. 2010;28:251–67.

77. Marques EA, Mota J, Carvalho J. Exercise effects on bone mineral density in older adults: a meta-analysis of randomized controlled trials. Age (Dordr). 2012;34:1493–515.

78. van de Vlekkert J, Hoogendijk JE, de Haan RJ, Algra A, van der Tweel I, van der Pol WL. Et al; Dexa myositis trial. Oral dexamethasone pulse therapy versus daily prednisolone in sub-acute onset myositis, a randomized clinical trial. Neuromuscul Disord. 2010;20:382–9.

79. Compston J. Glucocorticoid-induced osteoporosis: an update. Endocrine. 2018;61:7–16.

80. Sato AY, Peacock M, Bellido T. Glucocorticoid excess in bone and muscle. Clin Rev Bone Miner Metab. 2018;16:33–47.

81. Health Quality Ontario. Utilization of DXA bone mineral densitometry in Ontario: an evidence-based analysis. Ont Health Technol Assess Ser. 2006;6:1–180.

82. de Andrade DC, de Magalhães Souza SC, de Carvalho JF, Takayama L, Borges CT, Aldrighi JM, et al. High frequency of osteoporosis and fractures in women with dermatomyositis/polymyositis. Rheumatol Int. 2012;32:1549–53.

83. Zhang L, Wang GC, Ma L, Zu N. Cardiac involvement in adult polymyositis or dermatomyositis: a systematic review. Clin Cardiol. 2012;35:686–91.

84. Lundberg IE. The heart in dermatomyositis and polymyositis. Rheumatology (Oxford). 2006;45:iv18–21.

85. Stern R, Godbold JH, Chess Q, Kagen LJ. ECG abnormalities in polymyositis. Arch Intern Med. 1984;144:2185–9.

86. Allanore Y, Vignaux O, Arnaud L, Puéchal X, Pavy S, Duboc D, et al. Effects of corticosteroids and immunosuppressors on idiopathic inflammatory myopathy related myocarditis evaluated by magnetic resonance imaging. Ann Rheum Dis. 2006;65:249–52.

87. Fathi M, Lundberg IE, Tornling G. Pulmonary complications of polymyositis and dermatomyositis. Semin Respir Crit Care Med. 2007;28:451–8.

88. Obert J, Freynet O, Nunes H, Brillet PY, Miyara M, Dhote R, et al. Outcome and prognostic factors in a French cohort of patients with myositis-associated interstitial lung disease. Rheumatol Int. 2016;36:1727–35.

89. Fujisawa T, Hozumi H, Kono M, Enomoto N, Hashimoto D, Nakamura Y, et al. Prognostic factors for myositis-associated interstitial lung disease. PLoS One. 2014;9:e98824.

90. Fujisawa T, Hozumi H, Kono M, Enomoto N, Nakamura Y, Inui N, et al. Predictive factors for long-term outcome in polymyositis/dermatomyositis-associated interstitial lung diseases. Respir Investig. 2017;55:130–7.

91. Casal-Dominguez M, Pinal-Fernandez I, Mego M, Accarino A, Jubany L, Azpiroz F, et al. High-resolution manometry in patients with idiopathic inflammatory myopathy: elevated prevalence of esophageal involvement and differences according to autoantibody status and clinical subset. Muscle Nerve. 2017;56:386–92.

92. Magner M, Kolarova H, Honzik T, Svandová I, Zeman J. Clinical manifestation of mitochondrial diseases. Dev Period Med. 2015;19:441–9.

93. Milone M, Wong LJ. Diagnosis of mitochondrial myopathies. Mol Genet Metab. 2013;110:35–41.

94. Hagemans ML, Winkel LP, Van Doorn PA, Hop WJ, Loonen MC, Reuser AJ, et al. Clinical manifestation and natural course of late-onset Pompe's disease in 54 Dutch patients. Brain. 2005;128:671–7.

95. Lucia A, Ruiz JR, Santalla A, Nogales-Gadea G, Rubio JC, García-Consuegra I, et al. Genotypic and phenotypic features of McArdle disease: insights from the Spanish national registry. J Neurol Neurosurg Psychiatry. 2012;83:322–8.

96. Duyff RF, Van den Bosch J, Laman DM, van Loon BJ, Linssen WH. Neuromuscular findings in thyroid dysfunction: a prospective clinical and electrodiagnostic study. J Neurol Neurosurg Psychiatry. 2000;68:750–5.

97. Ramkumar S, Raghunath A, Raghunath S. Statin therapy: review of safety and potential side effects. Acta Cardiol Sin. 2016;32:631–9.

98. Crum-Cianflone NF. Bacterial, fungal, parasitic, and viral myositis. Clin Microbiol Rev. 2008;21:473–94.

99. Rider LG, Giannini EH, Harris-Love M, Joe G, Isenberg D, Pilkington C, et al. International myositis Assesment and clinical studies group. Defining clinical improvement in adult and juvenile myositis. J Rheumatol. 2003;30:603–17.

100. Aggarwal R, Bandos A, Reed AM, Ascherman DP, Barohn RJ, Feldman BM, et al. Predictors of clinical improvement in rituximab-treated refractory adult and juvenile dermatomyositis and adult polymyositis. Arthritis Rheum. 2014;66:740–9.

101. Joffe MM, Love LA, Leff RL, Fraser DD, Targoff IN, Hicks JE, et al. Drug therapy of the idiopathic inflammatory myopathies: predictors of response to prednisone, azathioprine, and methotrexate and a comparison of their efficacy. Am J Med. 1993;94:379–87.

102. Koreeda Y, Higashimoto I, Yamamoto M, Takahashi M, Kaji K, Fujimoto M, et al. Clinical and pathological findings of interstitial lung disease patients with anti-aminoacyl-tRNA synthetase autoantibodies. Intern Med. 2010;49:361–9.

103. Kunimasa K, Arita M, Nakazawa T, Tanaka M, Tsubouchi K, Konishi S, et al. The clinical characteristics of two anti-OJ (anti-isoleucyl-tRNA synthetase) autoantibody-positive interstitial lung disease patients with polymyositis/dermatomyositis. Intern Med. 2012;51:3405–10.

104. Marie I, Lahaxe L, Benveniste O, Delavigne K, Adoue D, Mouthon L, et al. Long-term outcome of patients with polymyositis / dermatomyositis and anti-PM-Scl antibody. Br J Dermatol. 2010;162:337–44.

105. Ng KP, Ramos F, Sultan SM, Isenberg DA. Concomitant diseases in a cohort of patients with idiopathic myositis during long-term follow-up. Clin Rheumatol. 2009;28:947–53.

106. Sultan SM, Ioannou Y, Moss K, Isenberg DA. Outcome in patients with idiopathic inflammatory myositis: morbidity and mortality. Rheumatology (Oxford). 2002;41:22–6.

107. Ríos G. Retrospective review of the clinical manifestations and outcomes in Puerto Ricans with idiopathic inflammatory myopathies. J Clin Rheumatol. 2005;11:153–6.

108. Torres C, Belmonte R, Carmona L, Gómez-Reino FJ, Galindo M, Ramos B, et al. Survival, mortality and causes of death in inflammatory myopathies. Autoimmunity. 2006;39:205–15.

109. Diederichsen LP. Cardiovascular involvement in myositis. Curr Opin Rheumatol. 2017;29:598–603.

110. Nuño-Nuño L, Joven BE, Carreira PE, Maldonado-Romero V, Larena-Grijalba C, Cubas IL, et al. Mortality and prognostic factors in idiopathic inflammatory myositis: a retrospective analysis of a large multicenter cohort of Spain. Rheumatol Int. 2017;37:1853–61.

111. Amaral Silva M, Cogollo E, Isenberg DA. Why do patients with myositis die? A retrospective analysis of a single-Centre cohort. Clin Exp Rheumatol. 2016;34:820–6.

112. Deveza LM, Miossi R, de Souza FH, Shimabuco AY, Favarato MH, Grindler J, et al. Electrocardiographic changes in dermatomyositis and polymyositis. Rev Bras Reumatol. 2016;56:95–100.

113. Chen F, Peng Y, Chen M. Diagnostic approach to cardiac involvement in idiopathic inflammatory myopathies. Int Heart J. 2018;59:256–62.

114. Buchbinder R, Forbes A, Hall S, Dennett X, Giles G. Incidence of malignant disease in biopsy-proven inflammatory myopathy. A population-based cohort study. Ann Intern Med. 2001;134:1087–95.

115. András C, Ponyi A, Constantin T, Csiki Z, Szekanecz E, Szodoray P, et al. Dermatomyositis and polymyositis associated with malignancy: a 21-year retrospective study. J Rheumatol. 2008;35:438–44.

116. Ceribelli A, Isailovic N, De Santis M, Generali E, Fredi M, Cavazzana I, et al. Myositis-specific autoantibodies and their association with malignancy in Italian patients with polymyositis and dermatomyositis. Clin Rheumatol. 2017;36:469–75.

117. Chinoy H, Fertig N, Oddis CV, Ollier WE, Cooper RG. The diagnostic utility of myositis autoantibody testing for predicting the risk of cancer-associated myositis. Ann Rheum Dis. 2007;66:1345–9.

12

Gait in children and adolescents with idiopathic musculoskeletal pain

Maria da Conceição Costa[1], Jamil Natour[2], Hilda A. V. Oliveira[2], Maria Teresa Terreri[1] and Claudio A. Len[1*] (iD)

Abstract

Introduction: Musculoskeletal pain is a constant complaint in pediatric practice. The pain may be related to a number of organic diseases and / or be part of the *amplified* musculoskeletal *pain syndromes*. Idiopathic musculoskeletal pain (IMSP) is defined as the presence of intermittent pain in three or more body regions for at least three months, excluding organic diseases that could explain the symptoms.

Objective: To study the gait of children and adolescents with IMSP by dynamic baropodometry.

Methodology: Thirty-two patients with IMSP and 32 healthy controls, matched by age, sex, social class, and body mass index (BMI) were enrolled. All were evaluated for pain intensity through the visual analogue scale (VAS) and gait evaluation using dynamic baropodometry.

Results: The mean age of the IMSP group was 13.6 years (SD = 2.1, range 9.8–16.9) and of the control group was 13.5 years (SD = 2.0, range 9.6–16.5). The mean pain scale was 5.4 cm in the IMSP group and 0 cm in the control group ($p < 0.001$). In gait, the mean right foot velocity of the IMSP group was significantly lower ($p = 0.034$), the time of the step of the IMSP group was significantly higher ($p = 0.003$) and the pace of the IMSP group was significantly lower ($p = 0.001$).

Conclusion: In our study we observed differences between the gait of children with IMSP and healthy controls according to the dynamic baropodometry. This finding indicates the need for individualized attention to the gait of children with musculoskeletal pain.

Keywords: Musculoskeletal pain, Children, Adolescents, Gait, Baropodometry

Introduction

Musculoskeletal pain is a constant complaint in pediatric practice, being a frequent reason for outpatient and emergency appointments [1]. Pain may be related to a number of organic diseases and / or may be part of *amplified* musculoskeletal *pain syndromes,*.

The main condition related to diffuse pain is the idiopathic musculoskeletal pain (IMSP), defined as the presence of intermittent pain in three or more body regions for at least three months, excluding organic diseases that could explain the symptoms, such as inflammatory, neoplastic and infectious diseases, among others [2].

The etiopathogenesis of *amplified* musculoskeletal *pain syndromes* is multifactorial and includes physical factors such as lower central pain threshold, increased nociceptive receptor sensitivity, autonomic nervous system disorders [3], emotional factors such as increased stress and anxiety and environmental aspects [4]. In some patients, there may be other clinical findings related to pain, such as joint hypermobility and obesity, among others [5–8]. Some points of the etiopathogenesis of IMSP are still unknown, among them, gait disorders.

Gait can be evaluated by subjective or objective methods. Muro-de-la-Herran et al. [9] carried out a review of the methods used in the recognition and analysis of human gait from three different approaches: image processing, floor sensors and body sensors.

* Correspondence: claudiolen@gmail.com
[1]Rheumatology Unit of Pediatrics Department of Escola Paulista de Medicina (EPM), Universidade Federal de São Paulo (UNIFESP), Rua Borges Lagoa, 802, São Paulo, SP 04038.001, Brazil
Full list of author information is available at the end of the article

In a study using body sensors of adults with fibromyalgia and controls (Locomotrix, Centaure Metrix, France), Auvinet et al. observed that gait may be slowed and the number of strides may be decreased in patients with pain [10]. These aspects should be taken into account in the daily clinical approach, since aerobic physical activities are part of the therapeutic arsenal [11]. However, according to our knowledge, there are no published studies on possible gait changes in children with IMSP.

Dynamic baropodometry is an objective method of gait evaluation and allows the identification of a series of abnormalities, since it automatically recognizes the right and left feet, records all steps, and stipulates the closest average step. It also allows you to view all recorded steps and force curves overlapping. Its use is not associated with any discomfort for patients. Although used for the evaluation of the gait of patients with musculoskeletal disorders, such as rheumatoid arthritis [12] and plantar fasciitis [13], this method has not yet been used for gait evaluation in patients with *amplified* musculoskeletal *pain syndromes*, whether adults or children.

Therefore, our proposal was to carry out a study on the characteristics of the gait of children and adolescents with IMSP, through dynamic baropodometry, a modern method capable of providing information still unknown up to this date.

Material and methods
Study design
Cross-sectional and observational study.

Patients
The sample consisted of patients with diffuse IMSP between the ages of 10 and 16, of both genders, consecutively selected in the outpatient clinic of musculoskeletal pain, of which 164 patients with IMSP were followed regularly. Inclusion criteria were: 1) diagnosis of IMSP according to the Malleson criteria [2], which include the presence of three or more episodes of musculoskeletal pain in a period of three months; and 2) outpatient follow-up time of at least six months. The exclusion criterion was: 1) presence of scoliosis or organic disease in which pain could be a symptom.

The control group consisted of apparently healthy children and adolescents, with no complaint of musculoskeletal pain. Controls were family members and / or friends of patients, or those enrolled in a recreation center for children and adolescents, matched by age, gender, nutritional status, socioeconomic level [14] and school level with patients. The controls were invited through direct or telephone contact with their parents / legal guardians.

This study was approved by the Research Ethics Committee of the local institution. All subjects or parents signed an informed consent form.

Study procedures
All subjects underwent a three-step process: clinical evaluation, performed by a qualified pediatric rheumatologist, to verify the inclusion and exclusion criteria, questionnaire completion, and gait evaluation.

Demographics
We collected demographic data from individuals who were weighed and measured, without shoes and with the least amount of clothing.

Pain measurement
To measure pain, a Visual Analogue Scale (VAS) was used, ranging from 0 (no pain) to 10 cm (maximum intensity pain), according to the last 30 days before the evaluation.

Evaluation of gait by dynamic baropodometry
The FootWork Pro, AM cube®, Gargas, France marching track, with four platforms (A, B, C, and D), was used for a 196 cm path by 49 cm of active dimension, with a thickness of 4 mm / 5 mm of rubber, polycarbonate coated, weighing 18 kg. This track has two sensors per 2 cm^2, totaling approximately 16,384 sensors automatically calibrated. The device contains a Footwork Pro software (IST Informatique - Intelligence Service et Technique, France), which automatically recognizes the right and left feet, records all steps and stipulates the closest step to the average. It allows to visualize all the registered steps and the overlap of force curves. This assessment was performed within 30 days after a medical appointment.

In the test, patients and controls walked once for six minutes on the equipment's digital mat.

Statistical analysis
The SPSS software version 22.0 was used to perform the statistical analysis of the data. Descriptive statistics (mean, standard deviation, 95% confidence interval) was used to characterize patients and controls. The continuous variables of the two groups were compared by the Student's t-test for variables with normal distribution, and the Mann-Whitney test for variables with a distribution not considered normal. Categorical variables were assessed using the chi-square test.

The level of statistical significance adopted was 5%.

Results
Thirty-four patients with diffuse IMSP were initially recruited. Two patients refused to participate in the study and were excluded. In the control group 33 individuals were initially recruited included, but one individual was

excluded for complaint of musculoskeletal pain. There-fore, 32 IMSP and 32 controls were enrolled in the study. Demographic and clinical data are presented in Table 1. It was observed that the sample is homogeneous with respect to age, gender, and body mass index (BMI). The mean age in the IMSP group was 13.6 (SD = 2.1) and in the control group was 13.5 (SD = 2.0) (p = 0.880). There was a prevalence of the female gender (84.4%).

Statistically significant dynamic baropodometry results are shown in Figs. 1, 2 and 3.

There was a statistically significant difference in the following baropodometry parameters: 1) mean right foot velocity with the IMSP group p values lower than those in the control group (p = 0.034), 2) step time with IMSP values higher than those of the control group (p = 0.003), 3) pace with IMSP values lower than those of the control group (p = 0.001). No differences were observed in the following variables: mean left foot velocity(mm/s), mean static right foot pressure (kpa), mean static left foot pressure (kpa), body strength surface on right foot (cm^2), body strength surface on left foot (cm^2), right forefoot load distribution (%); left forefoot load distribution (%); load distribution in the right hindfoot (%); load distribution in the left hindfoot (%); center of force on the left foot (cm^2); center of force on the right foot (cm^2), and center of force of the body (cm^2) (Table 2).

Discussion

Our data show that the gait of children and adolescents with IMSP, evaluated by dynamic baropodometry, is different when compared to healthy children in relation to the mean velocity of the right foot, time of the step, and pace. These results were achieved based on a technology in which sensors are located on a platform that records several aspects of the gait. Since IMSP has a multifactorial etiology, we believe that these changes are part of a complex gear whose final result is a decrease in the patients' quality of life [4].

The methods used in human gait recognition and analysis are based on image processing and can be classified according to two different approaches: 1) non-portable

Table 1 Demographic and clinical data

	Study		Control		
	(n = 32)		(n = 32)		p Value
Age (years) (Mean and SD)	13.6	2.1	13.5	2.0	0.880[a]
Female Gender (n and %)	27	84.4	27	84.4	1.000[b]
Weight (kg) (Mean and SD)	49.9	10.8	51.2	14.4	0.689[a]
Height (cm) (Mean and SD)	156.0	8.9	155.3	10.8	0.772[a]
BMI (kg/m^2) (Mean and SD)	20.43	3.82	21.05	4.72	0.568[a]
Pain (cm) (Mean and SD)	5.42	2.60	–	–	–

[a]– Student's t-test; [b] – chi-square test

sensors (NWS) and 2) portable sensors (WS) [10]. NWS systems require the use of controlled research facilities and rely on sensors that pick up gait data while the patient walks on a catwalk. In contrast, in WS systems, data analysis is performed outside the laboratory, capturing information about human gait during the individual's daily activities. In this specific case, the sensors are coupled in various locations of the locomotor apparatus. There is also a third group of hybrid systems that uses a combination of both methods.

Children and adolescents with gait disorders may experience musculoskeletal pain [12]. However, it is not possible to know if alterations in walking lead to pain or if the presence of pain alters gait.

Wassmer et al. [13] evaluated 103 children with gait disorders; in eight there was no apparent cause for this disorder. In these cases, pain was significant, as there was functional impairment and school absenteeism. Thus, it is known that in a considerable number of children without apparent locomotor disorders, they present impairment in quality of life. In our non-inflammatory musculoskeletal pain outpatient clinic, we observed that many patients present changes in posture and sedentary lifestyle. We know that walking may be altered in these cases, but there are no studies specifically conducted in children with IMSP.

Dynamic baropodometry, NWS system, allows precise identification of a series of gait abnormalities. For this reason, it has been used in the evaluation of patients with varied diseases, such as neurological, orthopedic, rheumatic, and even physiological, as in the case of longevity [9, 15–21]. However, some authors have evaluated the gait of individuals with musculoskeletal pain with other reliable methods, especially fibromyalgia patients. In these evaluations, the gait was altered [21], which justifies its detailed study in the *amplified* musculoskeletal *pain syndromes*. Dynamic baropodometry is an useful tool for the physiotherapist, since it helps in the diagnosis and treatment of gait disorders.

Auvinet et al. [5] analyzed the gait of 14 adult females with fibromyalgia and 14 healthy controls by means of equipment specially developed to measure walking speed, size, laterality, and regularity of the step (LocometrixTM Centaure Metrix, France). The gait of patients with fibromyalgia was altered, with a decrease in gait velocity in relation to the decrease in step size and pace. In other words, gait was irregular in patients when compared to controls regardless of age. In our study, although we used the technology of dynamic baropodometry to evaluate gait, we observed similar results, for example, gait slowing in patients with pain.

Sil et al. [22] evaluated gait biomechanics in juvenile fibromyalgia using a 10-camera 3D analysis device (Raptor-E, Motion Analysis Corp, Santa Rosa, CA). In this

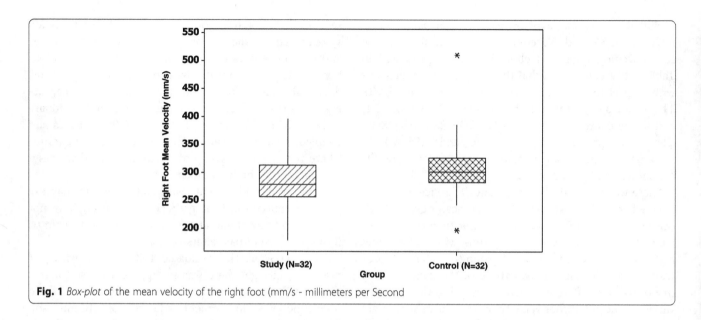

Fig. 1 *Box-plot* of the mean velocity of the right foot (mm/s - millimeters per Second

study, functional gait deficits were observed in 17 female adolescents with juvenile fibromyalgia when compared to 14 healthy controls. In addition, these authors measured isometric strength in lower limbs (Biodex System II equipment, Shirley, NY). Differently from our results, they observed no difference in gait velocity between patients and controls. On the other hand, they observed that the strides were significantly lower in the patient group. The isometric strength in the lower limbs was lower in the patient group, especially in knee flexion and extension and hip adduction. In our study, we did not assess muscle strength. We believe that a specific strength assessment would complement our findings.

Since the prescription of regular physical exercises and aerobic physical activities is part of the treatment of children and adolescents with IMSP [6], a deeper understanding of gait is necessary so that these guidelines are more accurate and appropriate to the characteristics of each patient.

Pain often leads to inertia and slower movement. The antalgic postures are common, with muscular compensations and with the inadequate use of the joints in the movement, generating tiredness and fatigue. These compensations manifest themselves as abnormal gait patterns and are invariably less efficient and more expensive in energy expenditure than normal mechanisms [23].

However, the prescription of physical activities for patients with musculoskeletal pain is consecrated in current literature [6, 24]. In our daily practice, we follow these guidelines and we also encourage patients.

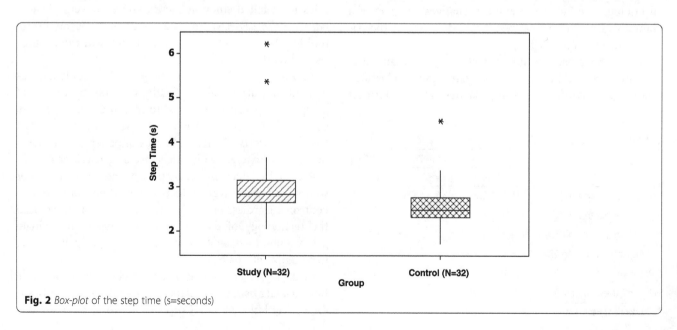

Fig. 2 *Box-plot* of the step time (s=seconds)

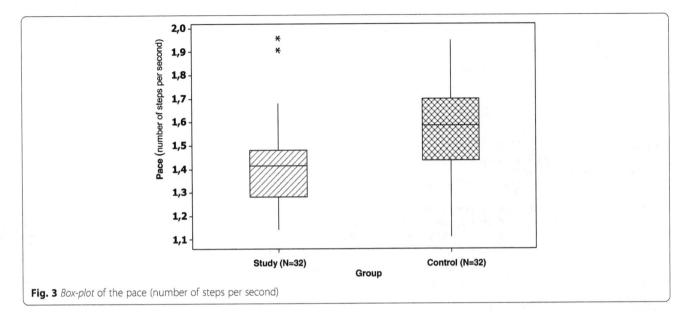

Fig. 3 *Box-plot* of the pace (number of steps per second)

Table 2 Mean baropodometry parameters of patients with idiopathic musculoskeletal pain and healthy controls

Variables	Study (n = 32)		Control (n = 32)		P value
Mean velocity of the right foot (# mm/s)	284.40	54.1	311.10	54.5	**0.034***
Mean velocity of the left foot (# mm/s)	286.10	44.8	309.50	53.3	0.063
Step time (# s)	3.00	0.83	2.56	0.51	**0.003***
Pace (# steps/second)	1.41	0.19	1.56	0.2	**0.001***
Right static mean pressure (# kpa)	37.30	12.4	35.30	12.1	0.517
Left static mean pressure (# kpa)	40.10	8.1	38.60	10.5	0.519
Right body strength surface (# cm²)	81.50	17.5	87.40	13.9	0.135
Left body strength surface (# cm²)	84.20	16.4	87.10	16.7	0.478
Right forefoot load distribution (%)	19.20	5.1	20.20	5.2	0.432
Left forefoot load distribution (%)	21.80	5.1	20.30	4.9	0.250
Load distribution in the right hindfoot (%)	27.30	5.9	27.30	7.8	0.999
Load distribution in the left hindfoot (%)	31.70	7.8	32.10	7.2	0.826
Center of force of the right foot (# cm²)	2.03	2.89	3.61	5.09	0.888
Center of force of the left foot (# cm²)	1.52	2.04	3.09	5.44	0.417
Mean center of force of the body (# cm²)	4.68	4.04	5.99	6.57	0.727

mm/s millimeters per second, *s* seconds, *Kpa* kilopascoal, *cm²* square centimeter
Mann-Whitney test, #
* *p* < 0.05

However, before prescribing physical activity, we firstly have as a therapeutic exercise the subjective evaluation of gait, followed by a training, motivating the adequacy and distribution of body weight on the lower limbs, in addition to the proper positioning of the head, so that the body is sustained against the action of gravity, thus seeking balance.

To the best of our knowledge, this is the first study to study the gait in children and adolescentes with musculoskeletal pain. The main limitation of our study was the reduced number of patients. To minimize this problem, we selected healthy controls matched by age, gender, nutritional status, school level, and socioeconomic level.

Conclusions

In our study we observed differences between the gait of children with IMSP and healthy controls according to the dynamic baropodometry. This finding indicates the need for individualized attention to the gait of children with musculoskeletal pain.

Acknowledgements
Not applicable.

Authors' contributions
MCC: design of the project, main responsible by ethics approval and data collection. MCC also participated in the data interpretation and writing of the manuscript. JN: design of the project. JN also participated in the data interpretation and writing of the manuscript. HAVO: was co-responsible by data collection and participated in the writing of the manuscript. MTT participated in the data interpretation and writing of the manuscript. CAL participated in the study design, data interpretation, writing of the manuscript and paper submission. All authors read and approved the final manuscript.

Author details

[1]Rheumatology Unit of Pediatrics Department of Escola Paulista de Medicina (EPM), Universidade Federal de São Paulo (UNIFESP), Rua Borges Lagoa, 802, São Paulo, SP 04038.001, Brazil. [2]Rheumatology Division, Medicine Department of Escola Paulista de Medicina (EPM), Universidade Federal de São Paulo (UNIFESP), São Paulo, Brazil.

References

1.   Goodman JE, McGrath PJ. The epidemiology of pain in children and adolescents: a review. Pain. 1991;46(3):247–64.
2.   Malleson PN, Matar M, Petty RE. Idiopathic musculoskeletal pain syndromes in children. J Rheumatol. 1992;19(11):1786–9.
3.   Maia MM, Gualano B, Sá-Pinto AL, Sallum AM, Pereira RM, Len CA, et al. Juvenile fibromyalgia syndrome: blunted heart rate response and cardiac autonomic dysfunction at diagnosis. Semin Arthritis Rheum. 2016;46(3):338–43.
4.   Adib N, Davies K, Grahame R, Woo P, Murray KJ. Joint hypermobility syndrome in childhood. A not so benign multisystem disorder? Rheumatology (Oxford). 2005;44(6):744–50.
5.   Houghton KM. Review for the generalist: evaluation of pediatric hip pain. Pediatr Rheumatol Online J. 2009;7:10.
6.   Zapata A, Moraes AJ, Leone C, Doria-Filho U, Silva CA. Pain and musculoskeletal pain syndromes in adolescents. J Adolesc Health. 2006; 38(6):769–71.
7.   Al Z, Moraes AJ, Leone C, Doria-Filho U, Silva CA. Pain and musculoskeletal pain syndromes related to computer and video game use in adolescents. Eur J Pediatr. 2006;165(6):408–14.
8.   Jannini SN, Dória-Filho U, Damiani D, Silva CAA. Musculoskeletal pain in obese adolescents. JPediatr (Rio J). 2011;87(4)329-35.
9.   Muro-de-la-Herran A, Garcia-Zapirain B, Mendez-Zorrilla A. Gait analysis methods: an overview of wearable and non-wearable systems, highlighting clinical applications. Sensors (Basel). 2014;14(2):3362–94.
10. Auvinet B, Bileckot R, Alix AS, Chaleil D, Barrey E. Gait disorders in patients with fibromyalgia. Joint Bone Spine. 2006;73(5):543–6.
11. MacPhee RS, McFall K, Perry SD, Tiidus PM. Metabolic cost and mechanics of walking in women with fibromyalgia syndrome. BMC Res Notes. 2013;6:420.
12. Houghton KM. Review for the generalist: evaluation of pediatric hip pain. Pediatric Rheumatology Online J. 2009;7:10.
13. Oliveira HA, Jones A, Moreira E, Jennings F, Natour J. Effectiveness of total contact insoles in patients with plantar fasciitis. J Rheumatol. 2015;42(5):870–8.
14. ABEP. Associação Nacional de Empresas de Pesquisa. Critério de Classificação Econômica Brasil (2015, April). Retreived from www.abep.org.
15. Wassmer E, Wright E, Rideout S, Whitehouse WP. Idiopathic gait disorder among in patients with acquired gait disorder admitted to a children's hospital. Pediatr Rehabil. 2002;5(1):21–8.
16. Mummolo C, Mangialardi L, Kim JH. Quantifying dynamic characteristics of human walking for comprehensive gait cycle. J Biomech Eng. 2013;135(9):91006.
17. Kerrigan DC, Todd MK, Della Croce U, Lipsitz LA, Collins JJ. Biomechanical gait alterations independent of speed in the healthy elderly: evidence for specific limiting impairments. Arch Phys Med Rehabil. 1998;79(3):317–22.
18. Stolze H, Klebe S, Petersen G, Raethjen J, Wenzelburger R, Witt K. Typical features of cerebellar ataxic gait. J Neurol Neurosurg Psychiatry. 2002;73(3):310–2.
19. Gehlsen G, Beekman K, Assmann N, Winant D, Seidle M, Carter A. Gait characteristics in multiple sclerosis: progressive changes and effects of exercise on parameters. Arch Phys Med Rehabil. 1986;67(8):536–9.
20. Waters DL, Hale L, Grant AM, Herbison P, Goulding A. Osteoporosis and gait and balance disturbances in older sarcopenic obese. New Zealanders. Osteoporos Int. 2010;21(2):351–7.
21. Arana-Arri E, Gutiérrez-Ibarluzea I, Ecenarro Mugaguren A, Asua Batarrita J. Prevalence of certain osteoporosis-determining habits among post menopausal women in the Basque Country, Spain, in 2003. Rev Esp Salud Publica. 2007;81(6):647–56 Spanish.
22. Sil S, Thomas S, DiCesare C, Strotman D, Ting TV, Myer G, et al. Preliminary evidence of altered biomechanics in adolescents with juvenile fibromyalgia. Arthritis Care Res (Hoboken). 2015;67(1):102–11.
23. Smith LK, Weiss EL, Lehmkuhl LD. Cinesiologia Clínica de Brunnstrom. 5ª ed. São Paulo: Manole; 1997. p. 472–4.
24. Odell S, Logan DE. Pediatric pain management: the multidisciplinary approach. J Pain Res. 2013;6:785–90.

13

Mycophenolate mofetil in patients with refractory systemic autoimmune myopathies

Pablo Arturo Olivo Pallo, Fernando Henrique Carlos de Souza, Renata Miossi and Samuel Katsuyuki Shinjo[*]

Abstract

Background: Currently, there are only few studies (mostly case reports or case series) on mycophenolate mofetil (MMF) in patients with systemic autoimmune myopathies (SAM). Therefore, the goal of the present study was to evaluate the safety and efficacy of MMF (monotherapy or coadjuvant drug) in a specific sample of patients with refractory SAM: dermatomyositis, polymyositis, anti-synthetase syndrome or clinically amyopathic dermatomyositis.

Methods: A case series including 20 consecutive adult patients with refractory SAM from 2010 to 2016 was conducted. After the introduction of MMF, associated or not with other drugs, the patients were followed for 6 consecutive months.

Results: In 17 out of 20 patients MMF was introduced without any intolerance. The clinical symptoms evaluated in these patients were muscular, cutaneous and/or pulmonary activity. During the 6-month follow-up, 11 out of 17 patients had clinical and laboratory activities response with MMF, allowing significant tapering of the prednisone median dose (15 *vs.* 5 mg/day, *P*=0.005). On the other hand, in three out of 20 patients; MMF was discontinued in less than two months, because of gastrointestinal intolerance. There were no cases of serious infection or death.

Conclusions: MMF was relatively well-tolerated, safe and effective in patients with refractory SAM. Further studies are needed to confirm the data found.

Keywords: Dermatomyositis, Drugs, Immunomodulator, Immunosuppressive, Myositis, Polymyositis

Background

Systemic autoimmune myopathies (SAM) are a heterogeneous group of rare systemic autoimmune diseases that result in progressive skeletal muscle weakness and disability [1–3]. Depending on the demographic, clinical, laboratory, histological and disease evaluation, SAM can be classified into dermatomyositis (DM), polymyositis (PM), inclusion body myositis, or immune-mediated necrotizing myopathy, among others [2–4].

There are no randomized controlled clinical trials and glucocorticoid has been used as the first-line drug in SAM [5, 6]. Various immunosuppressive or immunomodulatory drugs have been recommended as glucocorticoid-sparing agents, including methotrexate, azathioprine, cyclosporine, cyclophosphamide, tacrolimus and intravenous human immunoglobulin [5–7]. Moreover, the rituximab, an anti-CD20 immunobiological drug, has been administered in refractory SAM cases [7, 8].

Mycophenolate mofetil (MMF) is an agent that inhibits the mitosis and proliferation of T and B lymphocytes and has been successfully used to treat different autoimmune systemic diseases [9]. However, only a few studies in the literature have investigated the use of MMF in adult patients with SAM [10–20]. Furthermore, as limitations, the majority of these studies are case reports or case series [10, 12, 13, 15–18, 20] and analyzed only SAM patients with pulmonary disease activity [15, 19, 20]. Those who used rituximab [10–17, 19, 20] or anti-synthetase syndrome (ASS) patients [10–20] have not been studied.

The aim of the present case series was to evaluate the safety and efficacy of MMF (monotherapy or coadjuvant drug) in refractory SAM (DM, PM, ASS or clinically

* Correspondence: samuel.shinjo@gmail.com
Division of Rheumatology, Faculdade de Medicina FMUSP, Universidade de Sao Paulo, Av. Dr. Arnaldo, 455, 3 andar, sala 3150 - Cerqueira César, CEP 01246-903 Sao Paulo, Brazil

amyopathic DM) as monotherapy or in combination of immunosuppressants.

Methods

This retrospective, case series included 21 consecutive adult patients with refractory SAM: classical DM or PM, according to Bohan and Peter's criteria [21, 22], clinically amyopathic DM, according to Gerami et al. [23], and ASS which was defined as myositis, arthritis, pulmonary disease, positive anti-synthetase antibody, with or without mechanic's hands, fever and/or Raynaud's phenomenon [24].

Refractoriness was defined as primarily cutaneous (worsing heliotrope rash and/or Gottron's sign, new cutaneous lesions attributed to MAS), muscular (objective and progressive limb weakness), articular (arthritis) and/or pulmonary activity (progressive dyspnea), hampering glucocorticoid tapering and/or inadequate response to at least two immunosuppressive or immunomodulatory drugs at full-dose for a minimum period of three months, given sequentially or concomitantly [25].

To improve the homogeneity of the sample under study, only patients followed up at our outpatient clinic between 2010 and 2016 were included.

MMF treatment was defined as effective when the drug promoted over 50% improvement in the initial: cutaneous (evaluated clinically by the rheumatologists from Outgoing clinic); muscular (clinical muscle strength graded according to the Medical Research Council [26]) and/or laboratory parameters (serum creatine phosphokinase level - reference range: 24 - 173 IU/L - assayed by automated kinetic methods)]; articular (arthritis) or pulmonary (subjective dyspnea associated simultaneously with confirmed "ground-glass" on high-resolution chest computed tomography) activity. Comparisons of creatine phosphokinase level values at initial and after 6 months of MMF were considered as expected when variations ranged up to 20%. Moreover, glucocorticoid tapering of over 50% of initial dose was also considered evidence of efficacy of MMF.

All patients were followed for 6 consecutive months after MMF introduction and were examined at baseline and after 6 months by the same examiner.

Myositis overlap syndromes, neoplasia associated myositis, necrotizing myopathies, muscular dystrophy, inclusion body myositis, metabolic myopathies, irregular or doubt treatment adhesions were excluded.

Data were obtained from the ongoing electronic database protocol applied all patients with SAM at 1 - 6 month intervals entailing extensive clinical and laboratory evaluations, including the assessment relevant to this study.

Statistical analysis. The Kolmogorov-Smirnov test was used to evaluate the distribution of each parameter. The demographic and clinical features are expressed as the means ± standard deviations for the continuous variables or as frequencies and percentages for the categorical variables. The medians (25th - 75th percentiles) were calculated for the continuous variables that were not normally distributed. Comparisons between the patients at initial and after 6 months of MMF were performed using Student's t-test or Wilcoxon test for continuous variables, and $P < 0.05$ was considered significant. All of the analyses were performed with the SPSS 15.0 statistics software (Chicago, USA).

Results

Twenty consecutive patients with refractory SAM treated with MMF were initially analyzed. In 7 patients, previous immunosuppressive drugs were exchanged for MMF (monotherapy), whereas in 13, MMF was associated with previous immunosuppressant (Table 1).

Patients #11 used rituximab 12 months before switch to MMF.

As an internal service protocol, the patients were not using antimalarials, except for one patient (#5).

In 17 out of 20 refractory MAS patients (11 DM, three PM, two ASS, one clinically amyopathic DM) (Table 1), MMF was introduced with good tolerance and with 100% of adhesion. The median dose of MMF was 2 g/day. This group comprised patients that were predominantly women, with a mean age of 46.2 ± 12.6 years and median disease duration of 2.0 years. All 17 patients used glucocorticoids (methylprednisolone or prednisone) and received previously a median of three immunosuppressive drugs (Table 1).

Of this group, 8 had muscle activity, three muscular and skin activities, three cutaneous activities, two pulmonary activities, one cutaneous and pulmonary activity and one had muscular, cutaneous and pulmonary activity. No cases had articular activity.

During the 6-month follow-up, prednisone median dose was significant tapering from 15.0 to 5.0 mg/day ($P = 0.005$). Moreover, the prednisone tapering was achieved in 14 out of 17 patients. However, glucocorticoid tapering of more than half occurred in 11 patients, all of whom had good clinical activity response using MMF.

As an additional analysis, the MAS patients with MMF as monotherapy ($n = 6$) were compare to those with MMF in combination therapy ($n = 11$). All clinical, laboratory, therapeutic and outcome parameters were comparable between both groups ($P > 0.05$).

In three out of 20 refractory female patients (one DM, one PM and one ASS) with cutaneous, articular and/or muscular activity, MMF was suspended in less than two month, because of gastrointestinal intolerance. The maximum dose of MMF in these patients was 1.5 g/day.

There were no cases of death or infection during the follow-up of the patients analyzed.

Table 1 General features of 17 refractory idiopathic systemic autoimmune myopathies

No	Disease	Disease (years)	Treatment			Activity		CPK (U/L)		Prednisone (mg/day)*	
			Previous	Immediately Before MMF	Current	Initial	6 months after MMF treatment	Initial	6 months after MMF treatment	Inicial	6 months after MMF treatment
1	PM	2	MP,Pred,Aza,CYC	CP	CP, MMF	P	P	95	130	5.0	20.0
2	DM	2	Pred,Aza,MTX,CYC	AZA	MMF	P	Remission	48	66	15.0	5.0
3	ASS	1	MP,Pred,IVIg,Aza,MTX,CYC	CYC	MMF	Mu,C,P	Mu	242	139	20.0	10.0
4	ASS	2	Pred,Aza,MTX,CYC	MTX	MTX, MMF	Mu,C	Remission	167	200	10.0	5.0
5	DM	8	Pred,AM,Aza,CP,RTX,Tac	AM,Tac	AM, Tac, MMF	Mu,C	C	141	53	15.0	20.0
6	DM	3	Pred,Aza,MTX	AZA	AZA, MMF	Mu,C	Mu	268	148	15.0	7.5
7	DM	2	MP,Pred,Aza,MTX	MTX	MMF	Mu	Mu	40	20	50.0	30.0
8	DM	6	MP,Pred,Aza,MTX,CP	MTX,CP	CP, MMF	Mu	Mu	249	2120	10.0	15.0
9	PM	6	MP,Pred,Aza,MTX	AZA	AZA, MMF	Mu	Mu	1534	3517	5.0	0
10	DM	1	MP,Pred,Aza,CYC,RTX	RTX	RTX, MMF	Mu	Mu	215	255	15.0	2.5
11	PM	1	Pred,Aza,MTX	-	MMF	Mu	Mu	118	205	60.0	5.0
12	DM	1	MP,AM,AZA,MTX	AZA	MMF	Mu	Mu	35	30	40.0	5.0
13	DM	1	MP,Pred,AZA,MTX	MTX	MTX, MMF	Mu	Remission	245	257	10.0	0
14	DM	5	MP,AM,AZA,MTX,CP	AZA,CP	AZA, MMF	Mu	Mu	858	268	10.0	0
15	DM	1	Pred,AZA,CYC	-	MMF	C,P	C	114	138	15.0	5.0
16	DM	1	MP,Pred,MTX	MTX	MTX, MMF	C	Remission	100	80	12.5	5.0
17	CADM	3	Pred,AZA,MTX,LFN,CYC	AZA,LFN	AZA, MMF	C	C	79	95	60.0	2.5
		2.0 (1.0-4.0)								15.0 (10.0-30.0)	5.0 (2.5-12.5)

AM antimalarials, ASS anti-synthetase syndrome, AZA azathioprine, CPK creatine phosphokinase, CP cyclosporine, C cutaneous, CADM clinically amyopathic dermatomyositis, CYC cyclophosphamide, DM dermatomyositis, F female, IVIg intravenous human immunoglobulin, LFN leflunomide, M male, MP methylprednisolone pulse therapy, MTX methotrexate, Mu muscular, PM polymyositis, P pulmonary, Pred prednisone, RTX rituximab, Tac tacrolymus
*Pred: current vs. 6 months: P = 0.005

Discussion

This case series showed that MMF, as a monotherapy or coadjunt drug, is relatively safe and effective in patients with refractory SAM.

A strict exclusion in rare diseases criteria was employed in this study, however a sample of 20 consecutive patients with refractory SAM was analyzed based on previously standardized and parameterized data. The protocol was performed at the same service adopting the same standardization of reports, thereby reducing inter-examiner variability. Only patients with refractoriness were included.

MMF has been used in several systemic autoimmune diseases, such as systemic sclerosis, rheumatoid arthritis, Sjögre's syndrome, systemic lupus erythematosus [16, 27–29]. However, there are few studies in the literature investigating the use of MMF in adult patients with SAM [10–20].

Most studies are case reports or case series and MMF was found to promote significant clinical and laboratory improvement in patients with SAM [10, 12–16, 19, 20].

According to the study by Majithia and Harisdangkul [10], 6 out of 7 refractory SAM had marked improvement, with good tolerance, in active myositis using MMF. This response rate was higher than ours, however

in a group with less severity and in previous use of a smaller number of immunosuppressive drugs.

In another study [13], MMF was effective for controlling cutaneous activity in all four patients with SAM analyzed, also resulting in glucocorticoid tapering. In 10 out of 12 patients with recalcitrant DM, Edge et al. [14] observed an improvement in muscular and cutaneous activity after four weeks of treatment with MMF.

Probably we found a smaller rate of success because of all patients of our sample had refractory and severe disease.

The heterogeneity of response evaluation in myopathies in the literature is present. Better criteria have been established [30–33], but in relation to DM, for example, there is still a difficulty in assessing improvement, especially in those with little muscle involvement. The response assessment parameter of the present study was based mainly on the clinical criteria.

Previous study showed that antimalarial could predispose patients with DM/PM to developing herpes zoster, particularly women and DM patients [29]. Therefore, as an internal service protocol, our patients were not using antimalarials (except for one patient) at the time of this study.

Facing the previous refractoriness, in two thirds of the patients, the MMF was introduced as a coadjuvant in the present study. However, during follow-up, there was no difference between this group and those who used MMF as monotherapy for the response parameters analyzed.

In the present study, most frequent side effects of MMF were associated with the gastrointestinal tract (nausea, vomiting, abdominal pain and/or diarrhea). Intolerance was observed in three out of the 20 patients in the present analysis, comparable to findings of other studies [12–14].

Akin to the present study, some investigations have also shown that MMF is safe in patients with SAM [10, 14, 16]. There were no cases of infection or death events in our sample. By contrast, Rowin et al. [11] reported that three out of their 10 DM patients developed opportunistic infections with MMF (pulmonary infections: Blastomycosis, *Mycobacterium xenopi*, legionella).

Limitations of this study include the short follow-up of 6 months. In addition, possible inclusion of more severe cases of the disease due to the characteristics of our tertiary care centre should also be considered. Finally, as this is a review of retrospective cases, tools such as Manual Muscle Testing (MMT)-8 [31], 2016 European League Against Rheumatism / American College of Rheumatology (EULAR/ACR) response criteria [34] were not used and pulmonary involvement was not analyzed with pulmonary function test (at baseline and 6 months of MMF) and high-resolution chest computed tomography (6 months of MMF).

Conclusions
MMF was relatively well-tolerated, safe and effective in patients with refractory SAM, at least in the short follow-up of 6 consecutive months. Further studies are needed to confirm the data found in the present study.

Abbreviations
AM: Antimalarials; ASS: Anti-synthetase syndrome; AZA: Azathioprine; C: Cutaneous; CADM: Clinically amyopathic dermatomyositis; CP: Cyclosporine; CPK: Creatine phosphokinase; CYC: Cyclophosphamide; DM: Dermatomyositis; EULAR/ACR: European League Against Rheumatism / American College of Rheumatology; F: Female; IVIg: Intravenous human immunoglobulin; LFN: Leflunomide; M: Male; MMF: Mycophenolate mofetil; MMT: Manual Muscle Testing; MP: Methylprednisolone pulse therapy; Mu: Muscular; P: Pulmonary; PM: Polymyositis; Pred: Prednisone; RTX: Rituximab; SAM: Systemic autoimmune myopathies; Tac: Tacrolymus

Authors' contributions
All authors contributed equally to write and review the manuscript. All authors read and approved the final manuscript.

References
1. Dalakas MC. Inflammatory muscle diseases. N Engl J Med. 2015;372:1734–47.
2. Dalakas MC. Pathogenesis and therapies of immune-mediated myopathies. Autoimmun Rev. 2012;11:203–6.
3. Nava A, Orozco-barocio G. Approach to the differential diagnosis of inflammatory myopathies. Rheumatol Clin. 2009;5:32–4.
4. Irazoque-Palazuelos F, Barragán-Navarro Y. Inflammatory myopathies: epidemiology, etiology and classification. Rheumatol Clin. 2009;5:2–5.
5. Aggarwal R, Oddis CV. Therapeutic advances in myositis. Curr Opin Rheumatol. 2012;24:635–41.
6. Distad BJ, Amato AA, Weiss MD. Inflammatory myopathies. Curr Treat Options Neurol. 2011;13:19–30.
7. Ernste FC, Reed AM. Idiopathic inflammatory myopathies: current trends in pathogenesis, clinical features, and up-to-date treatment recommendations. Mayo Clin Proc. 2013;88:83–105.
8. Ytterberg SR. Treatment of refractory polymyositis and dermatomyositis. Curr Rheumatol Rep. 2006;8:167–73.
9. Bandelier C, Guerne PA, Genevay S, Finckh A, Gabay C. Clinical experience with mycophenolate mofetil in systemic autoimmune conditions refractory to common immunosuppressant therapies. Swiss Med Wkly. 2009;139:41–6.
10. Majithia V, Harisdangkul V. Mycophenolate mofetil (CellCept): an alternative therapy for autoimmune inflammatory myopathy. Rheumatology. 2005;44:386–9.
11. Rowin J, Amato AA, Deisher N, Cursio J, Meriggioli MN. Mycophenolate mofetil in dermatomyositis: is it safe? Neurology. 2006;66:1245–7.
12. Tausche AK, Meurer M. Mycophenolate mofetil for dermatomyositis. Dermatology. 2001;202:341–3.
13. Gelber AC, Nousari HC, Wigley FM. Mycophenolate mofetil in the treatment of severe skin manifestations of dermatomyositis: a series of 4 cases. J Rheumatol. 2000;27:1542–5.
14. Edge JC, Outland JD, Dempsey JR, Callen JP. Mycophenolate mofetil as an effective corticosteroid-sparing therapy for recalcitrant dermatomyositis. Arch Dermatol. 2006;142:65–9.
15. Morganroth PA, Kreider ME, Werth VP. Mycophenolate mofetil for interstitial lung disease in dermatomyositis. Arthritis Care Res. 2010;62:1496–501.
16. Saketkoo LA, Espinoza LR. Experience of mycophenolate mofetil in 10 patients with autoimmune-related interstitial lung disease demonstrates promising effects. Am j Med Sci. 2009;337:329–35.
17. Danieli MG, Calcabrini L, Calabrese V, Marchetti A, Loqullo F, Gabrielli A. Intravenous immunoglobulin as add on treatment with mycophenolate mofetil in severe myositis. Autoimmun Rev. 2009;9:124–9.
18. Parziale N, Kovacs SC, Thomas CB, Srinivasan J. Rituximab and mycophenolate combination therapy in refractory dermatomyositis with multiple autoimmune disorders. J Clin Neuromuscul Dis. 2011;13:63–7.
19. Mira-Avendano IC, Parambil JG, Yadav R, Arrossi V, Xu M, Chapman JT, et al. A retrospective review of clinical features and treatment outcomes in steroid-resistant interstitial lung disease from polymyositis / dermatomyositis. Respir Med. 2013;107:890–6.
20. Tsuchiya H, Tsuno H, Inoue M, Takahashi Y, Yamashita H, Kaneko H, et al. Mycophenolate mofetil therapy for rapidly progressive interstitial lung disease in a patient with clinically amyopathic dermatomyositis. Mod Rheumatol. 2014;24:694–6.
21. Bohan A, Peter JB. Polymyositis and dermatomyositis (first of two parts). N Engl J Med. 1975;292:344–7.
22. Bohan A, Peter JB. Polymyositis and dermatomyositis (second of two parts). N Engl J Med. 1975;292:403–7.
23. Gerami P, Schope JM, McDonald L, Alling HW, Sontheimer RD. A systematic review of adult-onset clinically amyopathic dermatomyositis (dermatomyositis sine myositis): a missing link within the spectrum of the idiopathic inflammatory myopathies. J Am Acad Dermatol. 2006;54:597–613.
24. Mahler M, Miller FW, Fritzler MJ. Idiopathic inflammatory myopathies and the anti-synthetase syndrome: a comprehensive review. Autoimmun Rev. 2014;13:367–71.
25. Brandão M, Marinho A. Idiopathic inflammatory myopathies: Definition and management of refractory disease. Autoimmun Rev. 2011;10:720–4.
26. Medical Research Council: Aids to the investigation of peripheral nerve injuries. War Memorandun. No 7, 2. Ed. London: Her Majesty's Stationery Office, 1943.
27. Appel GB, Gerald B, Radhakrishnan J, Ginzler EM. Use of mycophenolate mofetil in autoimmune and renal diseases. Transplantation. 2005;80:S265–71.
28. Iaccarino L, Rampudda M, Canova M, Libera SD, Sarzi-Puttinic P, Doria A. Mycophenolate mofetil: what is its place in the treatment of autoimmune rheumatic diseases? Autoimmun Rev. 2007;6:190–5.
29. Cunha GF, Souza FH, Levy-Neto M, Shinjo SK. Chloroquine diphosphate: a risk factor for herpes zoster in patients with dermatomyositis / polymyositis. Clinics. 2013;68:621–7.
30. Bruce B, Fries JF. The Stanford Health Assessment Questionnaire: dimensions and practical applications. Health Qual Life Outcomes. 2003;1:20.

31. Rider LG, Koziol D, Giannini EH, Jain MS, Smith MR, Whitney-Mahoney K, et al. Validation of manual muscle testing and a subset of eight muscles for adult and juvenile idiopathic inflammatory myopathies. Arthritis Care Research (Hoboken). 2010;62:465–72.
32. Rider LG, Feldman BM, Perez MD, Rennebohm RM, Lindsley CB, Zemel LS, et al. Development of validated disease activity and damage indices for the juvenile idiopathic inflammatory myopathies: I. Physician, parent, and patient global assessments. Juvenile Dermatomyositis Disease Activity Collaborative Study Group. Arthritis Rheum. 1997;40:1976–83.
33. Sultan SM, Allen E, Oddis CV, Kiely P, Cooper RG, Lundberg IE, et al. Reliability and validity of the myositis disease activity assessment tool. Arthritis Rheum. 2008;58:3593–9.
34. Rider LG, Ruperto N, Pistorio A, Erman B, Bayat N, Lachenbruch PA, et al. International Myositis Assessment and Clinical Studies Group and the Paediatric Rheumatology International Trials Organisation. 2016 ACR-EULAR adult dermatomyositis and polymyositis and juvenile dermatomyositis response criteria-methodological aspects. Rheumatology (Oxford). 2017;56:1884–93.

14

Physical exercise among patients with systemic autoimmune myopathies

Diego Sales de Oliveira[1], Rafael Giovani Misse[1], Fernanda Rodrigues Lima[2] and Samuel Katsuyuki Shinjo[1*]

Abstract

Systemic autoimmune myopathies (SAMs) are a heterogeneous group of rare systemic autoimmune diseases that primarily affect skeletal muscles. Patients with SAMs show progressive skeletal muscle weakness and consequent functional disabilities, low health quality, and sedentary lifestyles. In this context, exercise training emerges as a non-pharmacological therapy to improve muscle strength and function as well as the clinical aspects of these diseases. Because many have feared that physical exercise exacerbates inflammation and consequently worsens the clinical manifestations of SAMs, it is necessary to evaluate the possible benefits and safety of exercise training among these patients. The present study systematically reviews the evidence associated with physical training among patients with SAMs.

Keywords: Dermatomyositis, Physical exercise, Myositis, Polymyositis

Background

Systemic autoimmune myopathies (SAMs) are a heterogeneous group of rare autoimmune systemic diseases that primarily affect skeletal muscles [1, 2]. Depending on demographic, clinical, laboratory, histopathological, and evolutionary data, SAMs can be subdivided into dermatomyositis (DM), polymyositis (PM), inclusion body myositis (IBM), and others [3].

Patients with SAMs share a common clinical presentation characterized by skeletal muscle weakness, which ultimately leads to functional disability and increased morbidity and mortality [4].

Until the 1960s, absolute rest was recommended for patients with autoimmune rheumatic diseases to help treat the disease [5]. However, this recommendation has changed because sedentary behavior is now known to be associated with increases in triglyceride levels, blood pressure, insulin resistance, and cardiovascular risk [6, 7]. In this context, exercise training emerged as a non-pharmacological therapy for patients with SAMs, thereby contributing to the restoration of the muscle strength and functional capacity of these individuals and improving their clinical condition. Because exercise training among these patients was prohibited for many years, it is necessary to understand the mechanisms through which physical exercise acts to improve these parameters, as well as the safety of recommending exercise training to treat these diseases. Thus, the purpose of this review was to describe the safety of exercise training among patients, particularly those with SAMs.

Methods

For the present study, a bibliographic search was performed using the electronic databases Medline and PubMed.

The descriptors were selected in January 2017 and were defined based on the following keywords (in English): dermatomyositis, inclusion body myositis, polymyositis, idiopathic inflammatory myopathies, aerobic capacity, muscle strength, functional capacity, physical activity, exercise training, resistance training, vascular occlusion training, and resistance training with vascular occlusion. These keywords were combined using the Boolean operators "AND" and "OR" and adapted to each database as needed. In addition, the reference lists of all retrieved articles were manually reviewed.

The following inclusion criteria were adopted: no time limit; published in English; original articles, case reports, case series, controlled clinical trials, or longitudinal experimental studies (with experimental and control groups); exercise/physical training interventions were conducted for

* Correspondence: samuel.shinjo@gmail.com
[1]Division of Rheumatology, Faculdade de Medicina FMUSP, Universidade de Sao Paulo, Av. Dr. Arnaldo, 455, 3° andar, sala 3150 - Cerqueira César, Sao Paulo 01246-903, Brazil
Full list of author information is available at the end of the article

individuals with SAMs; details of the intervention, such as duration, frequency, types of exercise and intensity, were listed; and muscle strength and/or functionality were evaluated and presented as primary or secondary outcomes through physical performance tests.

Abstracts of congresses, monographs, theses and dissertations, articles about other myopathies (e.g., muscular dystrophy, metabolic myopathy, and neuromuscular disease), and letters to the editor that were purely commentary were excluded from this review.

The search identified 26 articles. The concepts used in this study are explained in Table 1.

Literature review

The first studies that evaluated the effect of physical exercise on patients with SAMs were performed in the 1990s by Hicks et al. [8] (Table 2) and Escalante et al. [9] (Table 3). Hicks et al. [8] demonstrated that a 4-week quadriceps and biceps isometric strengthening program for patients with PM effectively increased isometric strength without increasing muscle enzyme serum levels. Escalante et al. [9] were the first to suggest that patients with active SAMs can participate in rehabilitation programs involving strength training. Furthermore, these programs were associated with a clinical improvement in strength without increasing muscle enzyme serum levels.

Wiesinger et al. [10] was the first to conduct a prospective, controlled, and randomized study evaluating the effects of physical training on patients with SAMs. In that study, 14 patients with DM/PM (seven undergoing physical training and seven controls) were prospectively evaluated over a 6-week period. Patients undergoing physical training demonstrated significant improvements in aerobic capacity, isometric muscle strength, activities of

daily living, and quality of life compared with the control group. In addition, patients undergoing physical training showed an elevation in the inflammatory markers of the disease, suggesting that physical training is safe for these patients. Several additional studies have built on those preliminary studies to better understand the effects of physical training among patients with SAMs.

Physical exercise among patients with DM/PM

Patients with DM/PM have decreased aerobic capacity, with a lower peak oxygen consumption (VO_2 peak) [11, 12]. In addition, this decrease in aerobic capacity is positively correlated with a decrease in isometric strength, suggesting that the decrease in muscle strength among these patients impairs aerobic capacity [11].

The impairment in the aerobic capacity of these patients might also be related to elevated levels of blood lactate and the low proportion of type 1 muscle fibers, suggesting that patients with DM/PM show an impaired skeletal muscle oxidative capacity [13, 14]. Because one of the causes of mortality among patients with SAMs is cardiopulmonary diseases [15, 16] and decreases in aerobic capacity are associated with an increased risk of these diseases [17, 18], it is essential to employ strategies that can improve these parameters among these patients.

Based on this assumption, Wiesinger et al. [19] studied eight patients with DM/PM in remission who engaged in a physical training program. These authors observed a 28% improvement in aerobic capacity after 6 months of training, which was considered clinically significant. The same authors [10] demonstrated a significant improvement in aerobic capacity after 6 weeks of physical training among 14 patients with DM/PM (7 in the training group and 7 controls) in a randomized study. Munters

Table 1 Concepts used in physical training

Term	Concept
Aerobic capacity	Maximum capacity of the individual to capture oxygen from the environment, transport it through the bloodstream, and use it in cellular respiration. It can be estimated using peak oxygen consumption (peak VO_2) via ergospirometry
Aerobic training	Training characterized by low and moderate intensity efforts with a prolonged duration (over 150 s). This training predominantly uses oxygen (O_2)-dependent bioenergetic pathways to meet the energy demand required by the activity
1RM	Test used to determine the maximum muscle strength of the individual, determined as the maximum amount of weight lifted in only one repetition during a standardized exercise
MVC	Test used to determine the maximum number of repetitions/contractions that the participant can perform with a preset load
Strength training	Training that uses exercises requiring a level of strength above that used in everyday tasks to increase muscle function. When prescribing this training, the 1RM and/or MVC test is necessary, and the training is based on the percentage of each participant's 1RM (usually between 50 and 80% of 1RM/MVC)
Isometric exercise	During this exercise, the production of muscle tension equals the external load imposed on the muscle. Moreover, this exercise is characterized by the absence of joint movement during its execution
Dynamic exercise	This exercise involves the displacement of the body in time and space, and it is characterized by alternations between eccentric and concentric contractions

1RM 1-repetition maximum test, *MVC* maximum voluntary contraction test

Table 2 Physical exercise in patients with chronic stable dermatomyositis, polymyositis, or both

Author	Patients (n)	Protocol (Exercises)	Time (week)	Evaluated Components	Inflammatory markers	Results
Hicks et al. [8]	1	Isometric strength	4	Isometric strength 3 MVC	↔ CPK	↑ Isometric strength
Wiesinger et al. [10]	14	Aerobic	6	VO₂ peak Isometric strength Activities of daily living	↔ CPK	↑ VO₂ peak ↑ Isometric strength ↑ Activities of daily living
Wiesinger et al. [19]	13	Aerobic	24	VO₂ peak Isometric strength Activities of daily living	↔ CPK	↑ VO₂ peak ↑ Isometric strength ↑ Activities of daily living
Alexanderson et al. [23]	10	Strength Dynamic	12	Muscle function Walking distance Quality of life	↔ CPK ↔ Immune / inflammatory markers	↑ Muscle function ↑ Walking distance ↑ Quality of life
[a]Heikkilä et al. [44]	22	Strength Dynamic	3	Functional capacity Pain	↔ CPK	↑ Muscle function ↔ Pain
[b]Varvu et al. [45]	19	Strength Dynamic	3	Respiratory function (Spirometry) Muscle strength	↔ CPK	↑ Respiratory function ↑ Muscle function
Harris-Love et al. [46]	1	Strength Eccentric	12	Isometric strength	↔ Muscle enzymes	↑ Isometric strength ↑ Concentric strength
Alexanderson et al. [23]	8	Strength Dynamic	7	10–15 MVC Functional capacity	↔ CPK	↑ 10–15 MVC ↔ Disease activity ↔ Functional capacity
Dastmalchi et al. [14]	9	Aerobic Strength	12	Type of muscle fiber Quality of life Functional capacity	Not reported	↑ Type I Fiber ↑ Functional Capacity ↑ Quality of Life
Chung et al. [47]	37	Strength Dynamic Creatine supplementation	20	Functional capacity Muscle strength Quality of life Pain and fatigue Anxiety and depression	↔ CPK	↑ Functional capacity ↑ Muscle strength ↔ Quality of life ↔ Anxiety and depression ↔ Pain and fatigue
Nader et al. [21]	8	Strength Dynamic	7	Genes related to inflammation and fibrosis	↓ CPK	↓ Genes related to inflammation and fibrosis ↓ Tissue fibrosis
Munters et al. [12]	9	Aerobic	12	Aerobic capacity Activity of mitochondrial enzymes	↔ CPK	↑ Aerobic capacity ↑ Activity of mitochondrial enzymes
Munters et al. [20]	11	Aerobic	12	Aerobic capacity Disability Disease activity Quality of life 5 MVC	↔ CPK	↓ Disease activity ↑ Muscle strength ↑ Quality of life ↑ Aerobic capacity ↑ Quality of life
Mattar et al. [25]	13	Strength Dynamic Vascular occlusion	12	Muscle strength Functional capacity Quality of life	↔ CPK ↔ Aldolase	↑ Muscle strength ↑ Functional capacity ↑ Quality of life
Munters et al. [22]	15	Aerobic	12	Aerobic capacity Proteomic analysis Molecular profile	↔ CPK	↑ Aerobic capacity ↑ Genes related to capillary growth, mitochondrial biogenesis, protein synthesis, cytoskeletal remodeling and muscular hypertrophy ↑ Genes related to the immune and inflammatory response and sarcoplasmic reticulum stress

CPK creatine phosphokinase, *DM* dermatomyositis, *PM* polymyositis, *MVC* maximum voluntary contraction, *VO₂ peak* oxygen consumption, ↑: increase, ↔: no change, ↓: decrease
[a] included patients with inclusion body myositis
[b] included patients with active disease

Table 3 Physical exercise among patients with dermatomyositis, newly diagnosed polymyositis, clinically active disease, or some combination therein

Author	Patients (n)	Disease activity	Protocol (Exercises)	Time (week)	Evaluated components	Inflammatory markers	Results
Escalante et al. [9]	5	Active	Strength Dynamic	8	Isometric strength	↔ CPK	↑ Isometric strength
Alexanderson et al. [24]	11	Active	Strength Dynamic	12	Muscle function Quality of life	↔ CPK	↑ Muscle function ↑ Quality of life
[a]Varvu et al. [45]	19	Chronic/Active	Strength Dynamic	3	Respiratory function (Spirometry) Muscle strength	↔ CPK	↑ Respiratory function ↑ Muscle function
Mattar et al. [29]	3	Active	Strength Aerobic	12	Muscle strength Functional capacity Quality of life	↔ CPK↔ Aldolase	↑ Muscle strength ↑ Functional capacity ↑ Quality of life

CPK creatine phosphokinase, DM dermatomyositis, PM polymyositis, ↑: increase, ↔: no change
[a] Active disease but with chronic evolution

et al. [12] corroborated these findings by demonstrating that aerobic training over a 12-week period effectively improved the aerobic capacity of patients with DM/PM and increased the activity of the mitochondrial enzymes in their skeletal muscles. Aerobic training also led to a change in muscle fiber type (increased type I fibers) in these patients as well as an increase in the cross-sectional area of the muscle, which contributed to improvements in aerobic capacity and decreases in muscle fatigue [14]. In addition, Munters et al. [20] demonstrated that aerobic training improves the overall health of patients with DM/PM in a multicenter study; furthermore, improved aerobic capacity through training was associated with reduced disease activity.

Although aerobic training has important benefits for patients with DM/PM, the molecular effects of physical exercise on the skeletal muscles of these patients are unknown. Physical exercise might positively modulate the genetic profile of patients with DM/PM. Nader et al. [21] evaluated the genes related to inflammation and fibrosis in eight patients with DM/PM undergoing strength training. After 7 weeks of training, the expression levels of genes related to skeletal muscle inflammation and fibrosis were reduced, and these changes were accompanied by a reduction in tissue fibrosis among these patients. Similarly, Munters et al. [22] evaluated the effect of a 12-week aerobic training program on the molecular profile of the skeletal muscles of seven patients with DM/PM compared with eight controls. After 12 weeks, the patients undergoing training showed increased expression levels of genes related to capillary growth, mitochondrial biogenesis, protein synthesis, cytoskeletal remodeling, and muscle hypertrophy as well as decreased expression of genes related to inflammation, immune response, and endoplasmic reticulum stress [22]. These data suggest that the training activates an aerobic phenotype and promotes muscle growth as

well as suppresses the inflammatory response in the muscles of these patients.

As with aerobic capacity, patients with DM/PM show a significant decrease in muscle strength, primarily in the proximal muscles, which in turn leads to functional impairment [1, 2]. Several studies have demonstrated that physical training plays an important role in reversing the losses in muscle strength and function in patients with DM/PM [19, 23–25]. Escalante et al. [9] was the first to demonstrate an increase in muscle strength among three patients with DM/PM who engaged in physical training for 2 weeks. Based on these preliminary data, Wiesinger et al. [25] studied eight patients with DM/PM who participated in a physical training program for 6 months and observed increases in isometric strength, which led to improvements in activities of daily living (e.g., sitting down, standing up, and walking) in these patients. Alexanderson et al. [23] corroborated these data when they demonstrated that an intensive 7-week physical training program led to increases in muscle strength, helping to improve the impairments and limitations in daily activities without increasing inflammatory markers.

Strength training with intensities ranging from 70 to 80% of one-repetition maximum (1RM) has been recommended to increase muscle strength and mass [26]. As an alternative to this type of exercise, the practice of low-intensity strength training (20 to 30% of 1RM) combined with partial blood flow restriction likely induces similar improvements in muscle strength and hypertrophy in both healthy individuals and patients with chronic diseases [25–27]. Because patients with SAMs are generally unable to exercise at high intensities, this type of training is an alternative to conventional strength training. Mattar et al. [25] were the first to demonstrate that low-intensity strength training combined with partial blood flow restriction was a safe and effective method of increasing muscle strength, function, and mass and that it could lead to significant improvements in the quality of life of patients with DM/PM. These results suggest that this type of training act as a new non-pharmacological therapy to reverse the clinical manifestations associated with these diseases.

Physical exercise among patients with DM/PM during clinical disease activity

The data presented above lead us to believe that physical exercise is a powerful aid in improving the impaired physical abilities of patients with DM/PM. In addition, because inflammatory markers were not exacerbated in the studies presented, exercise training might be safe for these patients.

However, newly diagnosed patients and those with clinical disease activity are often fearful regarding the use of exercise training. Because patients present with a high degree of inflammation, fear remains about exercising during these periods.

Alexanderson et al. [28] evaluated the effect of intensive physical training performed at home five times per week over a 12-week period on the clinical disease activity of patients with DM/PM. After 12 weeks, significant increases were observed in muscle strength and function, which in turn led to an improvement in the quality of life of these patients. These authors suggested that this physical exercise program was safe because the inflammatory markers did not increase; therefore, exercise training was recommended for the rehabilitation of these patients. Similarly, Mattar et al. [29] conducted a case series study of three patients with clinical DM/PM activity and assessed the safety and effect of aerobic training combined with supervised strength training over a 12-week period. After this period, physical training was well tolerated and safe (i.e., increases in creatine phosphokinase (CPK) and aldolase levels were not found). In addition, specific parameters of aerobic capacity, muscle function, and quality of life improved, suggesting that supervised physical training positively affects these parameters during clinical disease activity.

Alexanderson et al. [24] were the first to demonstrate that physical exercise is safe during this period for patients newly diagnosed with DM/PM. A total of 19 patients newly diagnosed with DM/PM receiving high doses of prednisone were selected. The patients were randomized into a training group ($n = 10$) and a control group ($n = 9$). The patients in the training group were instructed to perform an intensive physical training program (five times per week for 12 weeks); the patients were then evaluated at the 24th, 52nd, 78th and 104th weeks. No significant differences were found between the training and control groups with regard to the parameters evaluated; however, intensive physical training was found to be safe for these patients because it did not exacerbate inflammation during the evaluated period, suggesting that exercise training is safe even for newly diagnosed patients.

Physical exercise in patients with IBM

Although the effects of physical training on patients with DM/PM have been well described in the literature, few studies have evaluated the effect of physical training on patients with IBM.

Studies comparing the aerobic capacity of these patients with healthy controls are scarce. Because patients with IBM also present with significant impairments in their mitochondrial oxidative capacity [30, 31], studies are necessary to determine whether these patients have impaired aerobic capacity. To date, only one study has evaluated the effect of 12 weeks of stationary bicycle training combined with strength training on the aerobic capacity of seven patients with IBM (Table 4). After 12 weeks of physical training, a 38% increase in aerobic capacity was observed among these patients [32].

Like those with DM/PM, patients with IBM present with an important impairment in muscle strength as a characteristic of the disease [33, 34]. Spector et al. [35] examined five patients with IBM who completed a 12-week progressive strength-training program. These authors did not observe an increase in the cross-sectional area of the muscle; however, a significant increase in muscle strength was shown without the exacerbation of inflammatory markers. Low-intensity strength training combined with partial blood flow restriction is also an important aid when reversing the losses in strength and muscular function as well as stimulating the increase of muscle mass in these patients. Gualano et al. [36] were the first authors to demonstrate that strength training combined with partial blood flow restriction for 12 weeks effectively and safely increased muscle strength (through the 1RM test), balance, and function as well as lead to 15.9, 60, and 4.7% increases in the cross-sectional area of muscle in a case study of a patient with IBM resistant to all types of treatment. In addition, there was an improvement in quality of life, varying from 18 to 600%. In addition to these effects, the same research group [37] demonstrated that strength training combined with the partial restriction of blood flow for 12 weeks decreased the expression of the myostatin gene and increased the expression of endogenous myostatin inhibitors. These data might partially explain the increase in muscle mass observed in the aforementioned case study [36]. Corroborating the previous findings, Jorgensen et al. [38] examined a 74-year-old man with who participated in strength training combined with partial blood flow restriction over a 12-week period. These authors observed substantial increases in mechanical muscle strength and gait speed, suggesting that this type of training reverses the losses in strength and functional capacity associated with these patients.

Table 4 Physical exercise in patients with chronic inclusion body myositis

Author	Patients (n)	Protocol (Exercises)	Time (week)	Evaluated Components	Inflammatory markers	Results
Spector et al. [35]	5	Strength Dynamic	12	Isometric strength 3 MVC	↔ CPK ↔ Immune / inflammatory markers	↑ Isometric strength ↑ 3 MVC ↔ Increased cross-sectional area
Arnardottir et al. [39]	7	Strength Dynamic	12	Isometric strength	↔ CPK ↔ Cytokines ↔ Adhesion molecules	↑ Isometric strength
Johnson et al. [32]	7	Aerobic	12	VO$_2$ peak Functional Capacity	↔ CPK	↑ VO$_2$ peak ↔ Functional capacity
	7	Strength Dynamic	16	Muscle strength Functional capacity	↔ CPK	↑ Muscle strength ↑ Functional capacity
Gualano et al. [36]	1	Strength Dynamic With vascular occlusion	12	Muscle strength Balance Quality of life Cross-sectional area	↔ CPK	↑ Muscle strength ↑ Balance ↑ Quality of life ↑ Cross-sectional area
Santos et al. [37]	1	Strength Dynamic With vascular occlusion	12	Myostatin gene Myostatin inhibitor genes	↔ CPK	↓ Myostatin gene ↑ Myostatin inhibitor genes
Jorgensen et al. [38]	1	Strength Dynamic With vascular occlusion	12	Isometric strength Functional capacity Gait speed	↔ CPK	↑ Isometric strength ↑ Functional capacity ↑ Gait speed

CPK creatine phosphokinase, MVC maximum voluntary contraction, VO$_2$ peak oxygen consumption, ↑: increase, ↔: no change

Physical exercise performed at home is also an important therapy for patients with IBM. Intensive home training (5 days per week for 12 weeks) was also found to be safe (no increase in creatine phosphokinase levels) and effective at increasing the muscle strength and function of these patients [39], suggesting that this practice effectively rehabilitates patients with IBM.

Future prospects and final considerations

SAMs are characterized by periods of clinical activity and remission. During clinical disease activity, patients present with a significant decrease in skeletal muscle strength, which remains lower throughout the lifespan. This decrease in strength leads to functional impairment and consequent decreases in daily activities, resulting in marked sedentary lifestyles among these patients.

The data presented in this review suggest that physical training is an important non-pharmacological tool for increasing muscle strength, improving functional impairment, and improving the quality of life of patients with SAMs. In addition, physical training likely improves the impaired aerobic capacity of patients with SAMs. This effect is likely associated with the ability of physical training to improve the molecular profile (thereby increasing the expression of the genes related to mitochondrial neoangiogenesis and biogenesis) and leading to increases in the activities of mitochondrial enzymes and the type I fibers in the skeletal muscle [12, 21, 22].

Additional studies are needed to better understand how physical exercise acts in the pathogenesis of SAMs. The causes of these diseases are not yet known; however, immune and nonimmune mechanisms are most likely involved [40–43]. Studies that demonstrate how physical exercise affects these parameters might help to understand how exercise training acts toward the clinical improvement of these diseases.

Clinical, controlled, and randomized studies of patients with IBM are necessary to show the real effects of physical exercise among this population. Physical training likely stimulates increases in muscle strength and improves the aerobic capacities of these patients; however, without an increase in the cross-sectional area of the muscle [32, 35, 39]. Strength training with vascular occlusion appears to efficiently increase strength, function, balance, and the cross-sectional area of muscle in these patients [36, 37]. Thus, this type of training is an alternative to conventional training that is capable of stimulating increases in the muscle mass of patients with IBM. Because these patients are generally resistant to drug therapy, the use of strength training with vascular occlusion is an important aid to minimize the clinical manifestations of this disease.

Studies have yet to evaluate the effect of physical exercise among patients with immune-mediated necrotizing myopathy; therefore, future trials should explore this area.

Conclusions

The data presented in this review suggest that physical training is an important cal tool for increasing muscle strength, improving functional impairment, and improving the quality of life of patients with SAMs. In addition, physical training likely improves the impaired aerobic capacity of patients with SAMs.

Abbreviations

CPK: Creatine phosphokinase; DM: Dermatomyositis; IBM: Inclusion body myositis; PM: Polymyositis; RM: repetition maximum; SAMs: Systemic

Authors' contributions

All authors contributed equally to write and review the manuscript. All authors read and approved the final manuscript.

Author details

[1]Division of Rheumatology, Faculdade de Medicina FMUSP, Universidade de Sao Paulo, Av. Dr. Arnaldo, 455, 3° andar, sala 3150 - Cerqueira César, Sao Paulo 01246-903, Brazil. [2]Division of Rheumatology, Hospital das Clinicas HCFMUSP, Faculdade de Medicina, Universidade de Sao Paulo, Sao Paulo, Brazil.

References

1. Feldman BM, Rider LG, Reed AM, Pachman LM. Juvenile dermatomyositis and other idiopathic inflammatory myopathies of childhood. Lancet. 2008; 371:2201–12.
2. Greenberg SA. Inflammatory myopathies: evaluation and management. Semin Neurol. 2008;28:241–9.
3. Dalakas MC. Review: an update on inflammatory and autoimmune myopathies. Neuropathol Appl Neurobiol. 2011;37:226–42.
4. Dimanckhie MM, Barohn R, Amato AA. Idiopathic inflammatory myopathies. Neurol Clin. 2014;32:595–628.
5. Partridge RE, Duthie JJ. Controlled trial of the effect of complete immobilization of the joints in rheumatoid arthritis. Ann Rheum Dis. 1963;22:91–9.
6. Lim MS, Park B, Kong IG, Sim S, Kim SY, Kim JH, et al. Leisure sedentary time is differentially associated with hypertension, diabetes mellitus, and hyperlipidemia depending on occupation. BMC Public Health. 2017;17:278–87.
7. Garelnabi M, Veledar E, Abramson J, White-Welkley J, Santanam N, Weintraub W, et al. Physical inactivity and cardiovascular risk: baseline observations from men and premenopausal women. J Clin Lab Anal. 2010;24:100–5.
8. Hicks JE, Miller F, Plotz P, Chen TH, Gerber L. Isometric exercise increases strength and does not produce sustained creatinine phosphokinase increases in a patients with polymyositis. J Rheumatol. 1993;20:1399–401.
9. Escalante A, Miller L, Beardmore TD. Resistive exercise in the rehabilitation of polymyositis/dermatomyositis. J Rheumatol. 1993;41:1124–32.
10. Wiesinger GF, Quittan M, Aringer M, Seeber A, Volc-platzer B, Smolen J, et al. Improvement of physical fitness and muscle strength in polymyositis/dermatomyositis patients by a training programme. Br J Rheumatol. 1998;37:196–200.
11. Wiesinger GF, Quittan M, Nuhr M, Volc-Platzer B, Ebenbichler G, Zehetgruber M, et al. Aerobic capacity in adult dermatomyositis/polymyositis patients and healthy controls. Arch Phys Med Rehabil. 2000;81:1–5.
12. Alemo Munters L, Dastmalchi M, Katz A, Esbjörnsson M, Loell I, Hanna B, et al. Improved exercise performance and increased aerobic capacity after endurance training of patients with stable polymyositis and dermatomyositis. Arthritis Res Ther. 2013;15:83–96.
13. Bertolucci F, Neri R, Dalise S, Venturi M, Rossi B, Chisari C. Abnormal lactate levels in patients with polymyositis and dermatomyositis: the benefits of a specific rehabilitative program. Eur J Phys Rehabil Med. 2014;50:161–9.
14. Dastmalchi M, Alexanderson H, Loell I, Stahlberg M, Borg K, Lundberg IE, et al. Effect of physical training on the proportion of slow-twitch type I muscle fibers, a novel nonimmune-mediated mechanism for muscle impairment in polymyositis or dermatomyositis. Arthritis Rheum. 2007;57:1303–10.
15. Moraes MT, De Souza FH, De Barros TB, Shinjo SK. An analysis of metabolic syndrome in adult dermatomyositis with a focus on cardiovascular disease. Arthritis Care Res. 2013;65:793–9.
16. Limaye V, Hakendorf P, Woodman RJ, Blumbergs P, Roberts-Thomson P. Mortality and its predominant causes in a large cohort of patients with biopsy-determined inflammatory myositis. Intern Med J. 2012;42:191–8.
17. Ladenvall P, Persson CU, Mandalenakis Z, Wilhelmsen L, Grimby G, Svärdsudd K, et al. Low aerobic capacity in middle-aged men associated with increased mortality rates during 45 years of follow-up. Eur J Prev Cardiol. 2016;23:1557–64.
18. Sui X, LaMonte MJ, Laditka JN, Hardin JW, Chase N, Hooker SP, et al. Cardiorespiratory fitness and adiposity as mortality predictors in older adults. JAMA. 2007;298:2507–16.
19. Wiesinger GF, Quittan M, Graninger M, Seeber A, Ebenbichler G, Sturm B, Kerschan K, Smolen J, Graninger W. Benefit of 6 months long-term physical training in polymyositis/dermatomyositis patients. Br J Rheumatol. 1998;37:1338–42.
20. Alemo Munters L, Dastmalchi M, Andgren V, Emilson C, Bergegård J, Regardt M, et al. Improvement in health and possible reduction in disease activity using endurance exercise in patients with established polymyositis and dermatomyositis: a multicenter randomized controlled trial with a 1-year open extension followup. Arthritis Care Res (Hoboken). 2013;65:1959–68.
21. Nader GA, Dastmalchi M, Alexanderson H, Grundtman C, Gernapudi R, Esbjörnsson M, et al. A longitudinal, integrated, clinical, histological and mRNA profiling study of resistance exercise in myositis. Mol Med. 2010;16:455–64.
22. Munters LA, Loell I, Ossipova E, Raouf J, Dastmalchi M, Lindroos E, et al. Endurance exercise improves molecular pathways of aerobic metabolism in patients with myositis. Arthritis Rheumatol. 2016;68:1738–50.
23. Alexanderson H, Dastmalchi M, Esbjornsson-Liljedahl M, Opava CH, Lundberg IE. Benefits of intensive resistance training in patients with chronic polymyositis or dermatomyositis. Arthritis Rheum. 2007;57:768–77.
24. Alexanderson H, Stenström CH, Jenner G, Lundberg I. The safety of a resistive home exercise program in patients with recent onset active polymyositis or dermatomyositis. Scand J Rheumatol. 2000;29:295–301.
25. Mattar MA, Gualano B, Perandini LA, Shinjo SK, Lima FR, Sá-Pinto LA, et al. Safety and possible effects of low-intensity resistance training associated with partial blood flow restriction in polymyositis and dermatomyositis. Arthritis Res Ther. 2014;16:473.
26. Scott BR, Loenneke JP, Slattery KM, Dascombe BJ. Exercise with blood flow restriction: an updated evidence-based approach for enhanced muscular development. Sports Med. 2015;45(3):313–25.
27. Scott BR, Loenneke JP, Slattery KM, Dascombe BJ. Blood flow restricted exercise for athletes: a review of available evidence. J Sci Med Sport. 2016;19:360–7.
28. Alexanderson H, Stenström CH, Lundberg I. Safety of a home exercise programme in patients with polymyositis and dermatomyositis: a pilot study. Rheumatology (Oxford). 1999;38:608–11.
29. Mattar MA, Gualano B, Roschel H, Perandini LA, Dassouki T, Lima FR, Shinjo SK, de Sá Pinto AL. Exercise as an adjuvant treatment in persistent active polymyositis. J Clin Rheumatol. 2014;20:11–5.
30. Lindgren U, Roos S, Hedberg Oldfors C, Moslemi AR, Lindberg C, et al. Mitochondrial pathology in inclusion body myositis. Neuromuscul Disord. 2015;25:281–8.
31. Joshi PR, Vetterke M, Hauburger A, Tacik P, Stoltenburg G, Hanisch F. Functional relevance of mitochondrial abnormalities in sporadic inclusion body myositis. J Clin Neurosci. 2014;21:1959–63.
32. Johnson LG, Collier KE, Edwards DJ, Philippe DL, Eastwood PR, Walters SE, et al. Improvement in aerobic capacity after an exercise program in sporadic inclusion body myositis. J Clin Neuromuscul Dis. 2009;10:178–84.
33. Gallay L, Petiot P. Sporadic inclusion-body myositis: recent advances and the state of the art in 2016. Rev Neurol (Paris). 2016;172:581–6.
34. Needham M, Mastaglia FL. Sporadic inclusion body myositis: a review of recent clinical advances and current approaches to diagnosis and treatment. Clin Neurophysiol. 2016;127:1764–73.
35. Spector SA, Lemmer JT, Koffman BM, Fleisher TA, Feuerstein IM, Hurley BF, et al. Safety and efficacy of strength training in patients with sporadic inclusion body myositis. Muscle Nerve. 1997;20:1242–8.
36. Gualano B, Neves M Jr, Lima FR, Pinto AL, Laurentino G, Borges C, et al. Resistance training with vascular occlusion in inclusion body myositis: a case study. Med Sci Sports Exerc. 2010;42:250–4.
37. Santos AR, Neves MT Jr, Gualano B, Laurentino GC, Lancha AH Jr, Ugrinowitsch C, et al. Blood flow restricted resistance training attenuates myostatin gene expression in a patient with inclusion body myositis. Biol Sport. 2014;31:121–4.

38. Jørgensen AN, Aagaard P, Nielsen JL, Frandsen U, Diederichsen LP. Effects of blood-flow-restricted resistance training on muscle function in a 74-year-old male with sporadic inclusion body myositis: a case report. Clin Physiol Funct Imaging. 2016;36:504–9.

39. Arnardottir S, Alexanderson H, Lundberg IE, Borg K. Sporadic inclusion body myositis: pilot study on the effects of a home exercise program on muscle function, histopathology and inflammatory reaction. J Rehabil Med. 2003;35:31–5.

40. Grundtman C, Malmström V, Lundberg IE. Immune mechanisms in the pathogenesis of idiopathic inflammatory myopathies. Arthritis Res Ther. 2007;9:208–20.

41. Rayavarapu S, Coley W, Kinder TB, Nagaraju K. Idiopathic inflammatory myopathies: pathogenic mechanisms of muscle weakness. Skelet Muscle. 2013;3:13–26.

42. Lightfoot AP, Nagaraju K, McArdle A, Cooper RG. Understanding the origin of non-immune cell-mediated weakness in the idiopathic inflammatory myopathies - potential role of ER stress pathways. Curr Opin Rheumatol. 2015;27:580–5.

43. Ceribelli A, De Santis M, Isailovic N, Gershwin ME, Selmi C. The immune response and the pathogenesis of idiopathic inflammatory myositis: a critical review. Clin Rev Allergy Immunol. 2017;52:58–70.

44. Heikkila S, Viitanen JV, Kautiainen H, et al. Rehabilitation in myositis. Physiother. 2001;87:301–9.

45. Varjú C, Pethö E, Kutas R, Czirják L. The effect of physical exercise following acute disease exacerbation in patients with dermato/polymyositis. Clin Rehabil. 2003;17:83–7.

46. Harris-Love MO. Safety and efficacy of submaximal eccentric strength training for a subject with polymyositis. Arthritis Rheum. 2005;53:471–4.

47. Chung YL, Alexanderson H, Pipitone N, Morrison C, Dastmalchi M, Ståhl-Hallengren C, et al. Creatine supplements in patients with idiopathic inflammatory myopathies who are clinically weak after conventional pharmacologic treatment: six-month, double-blind, randomized, placebo-controlled trial. Arthritis Rheum. 2007;57:694–702.

15

Revisiting hydroxychloroquine and chloroquine for patients with chronic immunity-mediated inflammatory rheumatic diseases

Edgard Torres dos Reis Neto[1], Adriana Maria Kakehasi[2]* (iD), Marcelo de Medeiros Pinheiro[1], Gilda Aparecida Ferreira[2], Cláudia Diniz Lopes Marques[3], Licia Maria Henrique da Mota[4], Eduardo dos Santos Paiva[5], Gecilmara Cristina Salviato Pileggi[6], Emília Inoue Sato[1], Ana Paula Monteiro Gomides Reis[4], Ricardo Machado Xavier[7] and José Roberto Provenza[8]

Abstract

Hydroxychloroquine and chloroquine, also known as antimalarial drugs, are widely used in the treatment of rheumatic diseases and have recently become the focus of attention because of the ongoing COVID-19 pandemic. Rheumatologists have been using antimalarials to manage patients with chronic immune-mediated inflammatory rheumatic diseases for decades. It is an appropriate time to review their immunomodulatory and anti-inflammatory mechanisms impact on disease activity and survival of systemic lupus erythematosus patient, including antiplatelet effect, metabolic and lipid benefits. We also discuss possible adverse effects, adding a practical and comprehensive approach to monitoring rheumatic patients during treatment with these drugs.

Keywords: Hydroxychloroquine, Chloroquine, Antimalarials, Chronic immune-mediated inflammatory rheumatic diseases

Background

Hydroxychloroquine (HCQ) and chloroquine (CQ), known as antimalarial (AM) drugs, are widely used in the treatment of rheumatic disorders, especially in immune-mediated such as systemic lupus erythematosus (SLE), cutaneous lupus [1–4] and rheumatoid arthritis (RA) [5, 6]. Besides that, both the Brazilian Society of Rheumatology (SBR) and the European League Against Rheumatism (EULAR) recommend, in specific circumstances, the use of HCQ for primary Sjögren syndrome (pSS) [7, 8] and antiphospholipid syndrome (APS) [9]. HCQ is currently preferred over chloroquine as it has a better safety profile [10], especially regarding the risk of retinopathy [11].

In this narrative review, the mechanism of action of these medications, as well as their main clinical, biological and safety effects in patients with chronic immune-mediated inflammatory rheumatic diseases (CIMID) will be discussed. Therefore, studies of these drugs related to COVID-19 will not be addressed in this review.

Methods

The new scenario of COVID-19 pandemic brought many medical challenges to physicians and health care systems. In view of this situation, The Brazilian Society of Rheumatology established a team of specialists from its commissions to respond to the demands related to the topic, especially those come from the Brazilian

---

* Correspondence: amkakehasi@gmail.com
[2]Serviço de Reumatologia do Hospital das Clínicas da Universidade Federal de Minas Gerais, Belo Horizonte, Brazil
Full list of author information is available at the end of the article

Ministry of Health. The discussion about the possible use of AM in SARS-cov2 infection showed the opportunity to revisit the topic by rheumatologists. A writing committee started gathering published research and analyzed it carefully. After discussion and debate, the committee members agreed on what would be the most useful knowledge to be highlighted about AM for rheumatologists, and prepared this manuscript. In a time of rapid response to a public health emergency, this type of document needed to be produced quickly and was evidence-informed, but not supported by complete evidence reviews.

Pharmacological characteristics

CQ is a 4-aminoquinoline known since 1934, discovered in the first half of the twentieth century as an effective substitute for quinine. Currently, CQ is the drug of choice for the treatment of malaria [12]. Hydroxychloroquine is a hydroxylated analogue of CQ that has both antimalarial and antiinflammatory activities (Fig. 1). These two molecules enter cells as non-protonated forms and become protonated, inversely proportional to pH, according to Henderson-Hasselbach's law. Therefore, these drugs are concentrated in acidic organelles, including endosomes, lysosomes and Golgi vesicles, increasing the pH [13].

Both drugs are weak bases and have a large volume of distribution with a half-life of about 50 days. These drugs interfere with lysosomal activity and autophagy, interact with membrane stability and may alter signaling pathways and transcriptional activity, resulting in inhibition of cytokine production and modulation of certain co-stimulatory molecules. At the cellular level, they inhibit

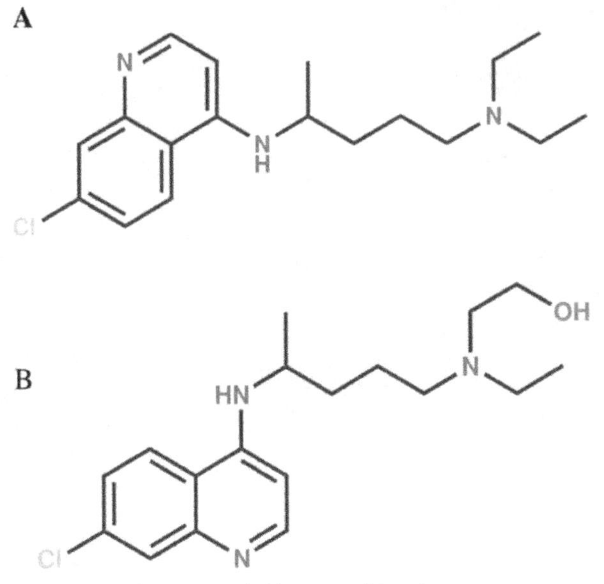

Fig. 1 Chemical structure of chloroquine (**a**) and hydroxychloroquine (**b**)

the Toll-like receptors signaling and reduce the CD154 molecule expression in T cells. Effects on plasmacytoid dendritic cells (pDCs), B cells and other antigen presenting cells have also been described [13].

HCQ is administered as a sulfate while chloroquine is administered as a phosphate salt. The differences between the pharmacokinetic properties of CQ and HCQ are presented in Table 1.

Mechanisms of action

The exact mechanism of action of HCQ and CQ in the treatment of CIMID is not yet fully understood, but there is strong evidence that they have an immunomodulatory and antithrombotic effect [13, 14]. The proposed mechanisms to explain these effects are (Fig. 2):

- Alkalinization of lysosomes and other intracellular acid compartments with interference in phagocytosis. The increase of intracellular pH causes a selective change in the presentation of proper antigens;
- Blockage of T-cell response and reduction of pro-inflammatory cytokine production, including INF-γ, TNF, IL-1 and IL-6;
- Blockage of Toll-like receptors 7 and 9, especially in plasmacytoid dendritic cell with inhibition of INF-α, which plays an important role in the pathophysiology of SLE;
- cGAS-STING signaling inhibition;
- Inhibition of phospholipase A2 activity;
- Stimulation of nitric oxide production by endothelial cells with antiproliferative effect;
- Antithrombotic effect through the inhibition of platelet aggregation in a dose-dependent manner, decreased production of arachidonic acid by activated platelets and action on antiphospholipid antibodies.
- Action on glucose metabolism and lipid profile as a non-immunomodulatory mechanism

Benefits in SLE

This class of medication has been used in the treatment of SLE for more than 50 years. It is a chronic autoimmune inflammatory disease that can affect several organs and systems and has a variable incidence, with 8.7 cases/100,000 inhabitants in Brazil [15]. It mainly affects young women aged from 15 to 45 years-old with heterogeneous and pleomorphic clinical manifestations [16, 17].

In 1976, Urowitz et al. described a bimodal mortality pattern in lupus patients, with premature deaths related to disease activity or infection, while late rate was more associated with atherosclerotic disease [18]. Considering the improvements in diagnosis and treatment, as well as

Table 1 Pharmacokinetic properties of chloroquine and hydroxychloroquine

	Chloroquine	Hydroxychloroquine
Oral absorption	Upper gastrointestinal tract	Upper gastrointestinal tract
Distribution volume	Blood 65,000 L Plasma 15,000 L	Blood 47,257 L Plasma 5500 L
Hepatic metabolism	Desethylchloroquine 39%	Desethylchloroquine 18% Desethyl-hydroxychloroquine 16%
Renal clearance	51%	21%
Unmetabolized excretion	58%	62%
Terminal half-life	41 ± 11 days	45 ± 15 days

Adapted from: Schrezenmeier E et al. [13]

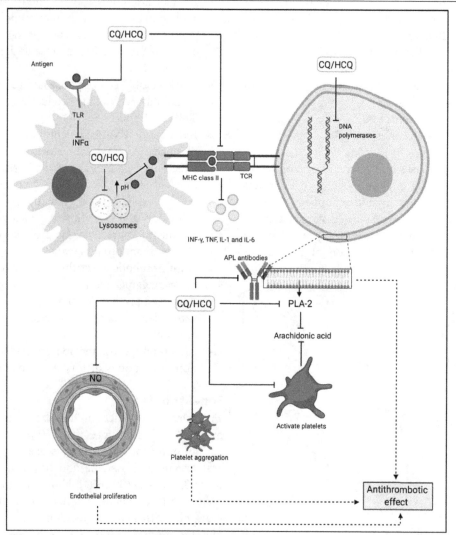

*APL: antiphospholipids; CQ: chloroquine; HCQ: hydroxychloroquine; IL-1: interleukin 1; IL-6: interleukin-6;
INF-α: interferon alpha; INF-γ: interferon gama; PLA-2: phospholipase A-2; TCR: T cell receptor; TLR: toll
like receptor; TNF: tumor necrose factor*

Fig. 2 Proposed mechanisms of action of antimalarials (chloroquine and hydroxychloroquine). APL: antiphospholipids; CQ: chloroquine; HCQ: hydroxychloroquine; IL-1: interleukin 1; IL-6: interleukin-6; INF-α: interferon alpha; INF-γ: interferon gama; PLA-2: phospholipase A-2; TCR: T cell receptor; TLR: toll like receptor; TNF: tumor necrose factor

the reduction of complications related to disease itself or its own treatment, the survival rate has increased in the two last decades [19].

The treatment of SLE patients may be individualized and targeted, according to the disease activity and severity. Additionally, patient education about the disease, sun exposure protection, regular physical exercise, diet, treatment of comorbidities (hypertension, diabetes, dyslipidemia, osteoporosis), avoiding smoking and performing adequate contraception and vaccines are important approaches and should be stimulated for all patients. The main goals of treatment in SLE are to increase long-term survival, to induce and maintain remission, to prevent damage and to improve quality of life [10].

CQ or preferably HCQ should be always recommended for lupus patients, regardless other immunosuppressive medications and severity or type of clinical manifestations, except if some contraindication or previous toxicity [10, 11]. Both of them promote multiple benefits, including direct or indirect effects [20], such as reducing disease activity and new flares [21]; improvement of skin lesions and joint symptoms [22, 23]; prevention of accrual damage [24, 25]; possible mortality risk reduction [26, 27]; as well as some benefits on glucose and lipid metabolism and reduction of thrombotic phenomena [14].

Disease activity

AMs are widely used and recommended for the treatment of SLE, since they promote an immunomodulatory effect of the immune response and better control of disease activity [2].

Tsakonas et al. demonstrated 57%-risk reduction of severe activity in quiescent lupus patients after HCQ, suggesting some prevention benefit on disease activity (RR = 0.43; 95% CI 0.17–1.12) [21]. The Canadian Hydroxychloroquine Study Group randomized 47 lupus patients, who were with stable dose of HCQ, to maintain on (n = 25) or to switch to placebo (n = 22). After 6-month HCQ withdrawal, there was significant 2.5-increase of SLE activity (95% CI 1.08–5.58; p = 0.02). Interestingly, there was a non-significant higher risk for severe activity, including vasculitis, transverse myelitis and nephritis, in those that had stopped the medication (RR = 6.1; 95% CI 0.72–52.54) [28]. Additionaly, some other studies have shown clinical worsening after drug discontinuation [29].

Regarding lupus nephritis, Petri et al. have demonstrated higher remission rate in 450 patients using HCQ when compared to non-users after 1-year follow-up (64% vs. 22%; p = 0.036) [30]. Also, the HCQ was a stronger predictor of complete renal remission in lupus patients when combined to mycophenolate than mycophenolate in monotherapy [31]. Thus, the SBR, the

ACR, and the EULAR consensus and recommendations for treating lupus patients have recommended the HCQ as an adjunctive treatment [1–4].

Damage accrual

Several studies have found relevant damage accrual in SLE patients [24, 32–35]. Accordingly to the LUMINA study, HCQ users had lower risk of developing new damage in patients with less than 5 years of disease (HR = 0.73; CI 95% 0.52–1.00; p = 0.05), especially in patients with no damage at baseline (HR = 0.55; CI 95% 0.34–0.87; p = 0.011) [24]. Another LUMINA analysis in 203 patients with lupus nephritis without renal damage found that HCQ delayed the onset of kidney failure (HR = 0.12; CI 95% 0.02–0.97; p = 0.046). The accumulated kidney damage was higher in HCQ non-users in class IV lupus nephritis [35]. Petri et al. evaluated 2054 patients and found that age, hypertension and use of corticosteroids were main predictors of damage, while HCQ had a protective effect (p = 0.06) [34].

Thrombotic events

HCQ reduces platelet aggregation and its antithrombotic effect can be explained by the reduction of the formation of antiphospholipid-β2-glycoprotein complexes on monocytes surfaces [36] with protective effect in patients with SLE [26, 37–40] (OR = 0.17; CI 95% 0.07–0.44; p < 0.0001) [38] and HR = 0.28; CI95% 0.08–0.90) [26]. Jung et al. compared 54 patients with SLE and prior thrombosis with 108 lupus patients with no thrombosis and demonstrated that AM were associated with lower risk of thrombotic events, both arterial and venous (OR = 0.31; CI 95% 0.13–0.71) [41].

Glucose metabolism and lipid profile

In vitro and experimental models demonstrated that HCQ improves insulin secretion and peripheral insulin sensitivity [14]. Penn et al. found HCQ was associated with lower fasting glycemia and Homeostatic Model Assessment (HOMA) index in patients with SLE [42].

Moreover, AM in monotherapy or associated with glucocorticoids (GC) have also improved the lipid profile in lupus patients because they provide hepatic cholesterol synthesis reduction with inhibition of lysosomal function, as well as lysosomal cholesterol transport and metabolism blockage. Other explanations are related to lower LDL receptor activity and bile steroid precursors and HMG-CoA reductase function gain [14]. Besides that, chloroquine diphosphate increases low-density lipoprotein removal from plasma in SLE patients [43].

Petri et al. found that HCQ was associated with lower total cholesterol serum levels, regardless dosage (200 mg or 400 mg/day), and it was able to mitigate the deleterious prednisone effect (10 mg/day) on total cholesterol

[44]. Rahman et al. reported 4.1%-reduction of total cholesterol serum levels after starting AM in 3 months ($p = 0.02$). In 181 patients using GC and AM, the mean total cholesterol was 11% lower than in 201 patients receiving comparable dosage of GC (p = 0.002) [45]. Cairoli et al. demonstrated a significant decrease in total cholesterol (198 ± 33.7 vs. 183 ± 30.3 mg/dL; $p = 0.023$) and LDL levels (117 ± 31.3 vs. 101 ± 26.2 mg/dL; $p = 0.023$) after the 3 months of HCQ therapy in SLE patients which determined a significant decrease in the frequency of dyslipidemia (26% vs. 12.5%; $p = 0.013$) [46].

A recent systematic review and meta-analysis involving data from nine studies and 823 participants has stated that HCQ significantly reduced mean total cholesterol plasmatic levels (26.8 mg/dL; 95% CI 8.3–45.3), as well as mean LDL serum levels (24.3 mg/dL; CI95% 8.9–39.8). However, it is important to note that other studies had an extensive heterogeneity among them, including lack of information about statin use [47]. Similarly, there are controversial data regarding HDL status [14].

Survival
Ruiz-Irastorza et al. evaluated a cohort with 232 lupus patients (64% on AMs). Among 23 patients who died, 19 (83%) had never received AMs. The cumulative 15-year survival rate was higher in those using AM drugs (0.98 vs. 0.15; $p < 0.001$) [26]. Shinjo et al., analyzing 1480 patients from the GLADEL (Grupo Latino Americano para Estudo do Lupus) found lower mortality rate in AMs users for at least six consecutive months (4.4% vs. 11.5%; $p < 0.001$). In addition, the protective effect on mortality rate increased according to longer exposition time to AMs [6 to 11 months: 3.85 (95%CI 1.41 to 8.37); 12 to 24 months: 2.7 (95%CI 1.41 to 4.76); and more than 24 months: 0.54 (95%CI 0.37 to 0.77)]. After adjustment to potential confounders, AMs were associated with a 38% reduction in mortality (HR = 0.62; 95%CI 0.39–0.99) [27].

Pregnancy and lactation
The use of CQ and HCQ is not only allowed but is recommended during pregnancy and lactation in SLE patients [14]. A HCQ placebo-controlled study suggested beneficial effect on disease activity [48] and the interruption of HCQ was related to higher risk of flares during pregnancy. In other words, AMs are recommended during the preconception period, pregnancy and lactation [49].

The presence of anti-Ro/SSA and anti-La/SSB antibodies are associated with 1 to 2% risk of congenital total atrioventricular block. When there is a maternal history of an affected fetus or child, the recurrence rate can increase 13 to 18%. HCQ is associated with lower

occurrence of neonatal cardiac lupus, especially if recurrent [50, 51].

More recently, a systematic review and meta-analysis involving 6 studies and 870 pregnancies have found no difference concerning prematurity and restricted intrauterine growth in lupus patients exposed (n = 308) or not exposed (n = 562) to HCQ. It is important to emphasize that these results should be addressed with caution due to huge heterogeneity among the studies [52].

Benefits in RA
AMs are important as adjunctive therapy to treatment with disease-modifying drugs (DMARDs) in RA, including recommendations for treatment of SBR [5] and ACR [6]. HCQ has been shown to improve clinical and laboratory findings in RA, particularly in early and mild disease, although there was no protective effect on radiographic progression [53]. Because of its good safety profile, it currently being studied for the prevention of future onset of rheumatoid arthritis (RA) in individuals who have elevations of anti-cyclic citrullinated peptide (anti-CCP3) antibodies [54].

Similarly to data from lupus patients, most of effects are also seen in RA, including improvement in lipid profile and insulin resistance [55, 56]. In a multicenter study with 4905 RA patients, Wasko et al. demonstrated that HCQ was associated with lower risk of diabetes mellitus (HR = 0.62; 95% CI 0.42–0.92) [56] and could be used for controlling traditional cardiovascular risk factors [57].

Benefits in other immune-mediated diseases
Antimalarial drugs may be used to treat sarcoidosis, including cutaneous sarcoidosis, pulmonary sarcoidosis, neurosarcoidosis, and arthritis [58]. Although less effective than in patients with SLE, AM can be useful in for cutaneous manifestations in dermatomyositis [59].

Safety
AMs are usually effective, safe, and well tolerated. According to the SBR, the Brazilian Society of Dermatology and The Study Group on Inflammatory Bowel Diseases, patients with CIMID on AMs are considered as non-immunosuppressant medications [60]. There is no increased risk of infections or even neoplasms in the short- and long-term [61]. More frequently the adverse events are related to gastrointestinal complaints, such as abdominal pain, nausea, vomiting and diarrhea. To decrease these adverse effects, the HCQ can be taken once or twice daily with a meal [62].

Patients with psoriasis, porphyria and alcoholism may be more susceptible to adverse skin events, usually without severity. In rare cases, hemolysis may occur in patients with glucose-6-phosphate dehydrogenase deficiency [63]. Besides G6PD deficiency, the concomitant use of HCQ with dapsone may enhance the risk of hemolytic reactions [64].

There is no current recommendation to reduce the dose of HCQ in patients with chronic kidney disease [13]. Some experts recommend reducing the dose of chloroquine phosphate by 50% if the glomerular filtration rate is less than 10 mL/minute, and in hemodialysis or peritoneal dialysis patients [65]. Neither safety nor efficacy of HCQ has been established for chronic use in children for juvenile idiopathic arthritis or for juvenile SLE.

The main adverse events related to the use of AM are summarized in Fig. 3.

Ocular toxicity

Both CQ and HCQ can cause ocular deposition, an effect more associated with CQ. Retinal changes are related to lysosomal degradation of the external photoreceptor with lipofuscin accumulation in retinal pigment epithelium [66].

Once symptomatic, the retinopathy associated with AM is characterized by abnormalities of the retinal pigment epithelium, which are detectable clinically, and may later develop into the classic appearance of 'bull's eye maculopathy' with retinal pigment epithelial loss. At this stage the visual loss is severe and irreversible and may be complicated by secondary cystoid macular oedema, epiretinal membrane and other sequalae [67].

Although rare, the retinopathy is one of main adverse events related to AMs [14]. Considering the recommended dosages, the 5-year, 10-year and 20-year toxicity risk is lesser than 1%, below 2 and 20%, respectively. After 20 years of use, the risk increases 4% each year for those no previous toxicity [11].

More recently, the hydroxychloroquinemia has been reported as a risk factor for retinopathy in 537 lupus patients (total prevalence = 4.3%) [68]. Other risk factors associated with retinopathy were age, duration of use and high body mass index (BMI).

In 2016, the American Society of Ophthalmology updated its recommendations for retinopathy screening in CQ or HCQ users. According to them, the maximum daily dosage of HCQ should be ≤5 mg/kg. The main risk factors for ocular toxicity are daily dose above the recommended, duration of use, renal failure, previous maculopathy or retinopathy and concomitant use of tamoxifen. Other risk factors include advanced age, liver failure and genetic factors related to abnormalities of the ABCA4 gene or cytochrome P450. It is recommended that patients initiating the drug undergo eye examination within the first year of treatment. Although visual field examination and spectral-domain optical coherence tomography (SD OCT) are very useful, they are not mandatory at the beginning of treatment, unless the

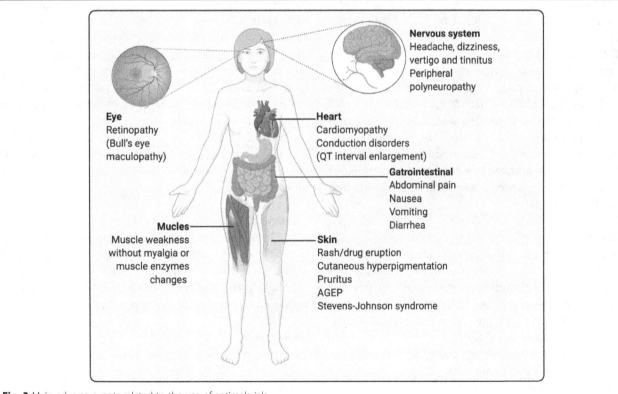

Fig. 3 Main adverse events related to the use of antimalarials

patient has risk factors or other diseases that may affect the initial screening tests. In the absence of major risk factors, screening tests may be performed annually after 5 years of baseline assessment. If risk factors are present, screening tests should be performed annually or at shorter intervals soon after beginning AMs, and automated visual field assessment and OCT-SD are recommended. Additional tests in some situations may be indicated, such as the multifocal electroretinogram (mfERG), which provides objective information of visual field, especially in Asian patients [11].

Adverse dermatologic events

The use of antimalarials may provoke adverse dermatologic effects of varying severity, being drug eruptions or rashes the most common [69]. Both CQ and HCQ bound to melanin and can deposit on the skin, with the possibility of cutaneous hyperpigmentation (grayish color) in long-term, especially with CQ [66].

A study that compared acitretin with HCQ for the treatment of cutaneous lupus found around 27% of patients with dry skin complaints; itching and burning sensation on the skin in 17%; dermatitis in 3% and desquamation in 3% of those using HCQ [70]. Also, grayish pigmentation of the skin and oral mucosa has been associated with longer use, higher levels of hydroxychloroquinemia, as well as the use of acetyl salicylic acid and oral anticoagulants, sometimes with reports of microtrauma and local ecchymosis preceding hyperpigmentation [71, 72]. Cases of worsening psoriasis are also described with the use of medication [73]. Acute generalized exanthematous pustulosis is rare and described in 1/5,000,000 inhabitants [74].

A recent systematic review including ninety-four articles, comprising a total of 689 adverse dermatologic side effects, has shown that drug eruption or rash (358 cases) were the most frequent, followed by cutaneous hyperpigmentation (116 cases), pruritis (62 cases), acute generalized exanthematous pustulosis (27cases), Stevens-Johnson syndrome or toxic epidermal necrolysis (26 cases), hair loss (12 cases), and stomatitis (11 cases) [69].

Cardiotoxicity

Although rare, it can be a serious adverse event [75]. Both cardiomyopathy and conduction disorders (for example, QT prolongation) are described. A possible mechanism involves a lysosomal pathway dysfunction with metabolite products (glycogen and phospholipids) intracellular accumulation [76].

A systematic review about CQ and HCQ cardiotoxicity found 86 articles, comprising only 127 patients in case reports or small case series, most of them were SLE (n = 49) or RA patients (n = 28). Most patients (58.3%) were treated with CQ with a median time of use of 7 years (3 days to 35 years) and median cumulative dose of 803 g (1235 g for HCQ). Heart rhythm problems were the main reported side effects, affecting 85% of patients. Other non-specific cardiac events included ventricular hypertrophy, hypokinesia, valve dysfunction and pulmonary arterial hypertension. It is worth mentioning that 38 cases were classified as probably related to adverse drug events, 69 as possibly associated and in 20 cases it was not possible to indicate this association. It was not possible to classify this association as definitive for any case, using the Naranjo Scale. The authors could not definitively exclude the possibility that some cardiac complications were due to the disease itself or to differential diagnoses (Fabry disease, for example). Determination of the risk for cardiac complications attributed to the medications was not possible because of the lack of randomized controlled trials [75].

Other studies suggest that older age, duration of medication use, dosage above that recommended by weight, use of CQ instead of HCQ, pre-existing heart disease and renal failure may be risk factors for medication cardiotoxicity. In addition, the risk may be greater in those who use other medications that also lead to prolongation of the QT interval or that increase the serum level of QC [77–79]. A study suggested that SLE patients using AM drugs with persistently elevated creatine phosphokinase (CPK) should be monitored periodically and specific biomarkers, such as troponin and brain natriuretic peptide (BNP), may be useful as a screening tool for cardiotoxicity diagnosis by AMs. The electrocardiogram, echocardiogram and magnetic resonance imaging can provide more information in suspicious cases, as well as endomyocardial biopsy, if necessary [80]. At the moment, there are no consensus and guidelines which are the best methods and interval to monitor cardiotoxicity with chronic use of AM.

On the other hand, it is important to highlight HCQ and CQ have a protective effect on cardiovascular risk, anti-thrombotic mechanisms and on survival rate in lupus patients.

Myotoxicity

It has been described in a few cases, especially associated to CQ. Patients with myopathy have proximal muscle weakness without myalgia or muscle enzymes changes (or slightly elevated more rarely). Patients can improve with medication discontinuation [63].

Neurotoxicity

Central nervous system toxicity includes headache, dizziness, vertigo and tinnitus. There are rare case reports of seizures related to reduction of seizure threshold and psychosis, especially when combined to GC.

Neuromyopathy and peripheral polyneuropathy are also rare, occurring in patients with worsening renal function and using CQ [62, 63].

Drug interactions

HCQ and CQ are substrates for cytochrome P450 enzymes, responsible for the metabolism of multiple drugs. Cytochrome P450 enzymes dealkylate AMs to their active metabolites. Thus, the concomitant use of AMs can lead to increased levels of digoxin, cyclosporine and metoprolol [62]. HCQ can reduce gastrointestinal absorption of methotrexate, since it alters the local pH and it can explain lower toxicity of methotrexate when combined. Antacids may decrease oral bioavailability of CQ [13].

Special attention should be given to other concomitant drugs, such as macrolides, quinolones, some antivirals and antipsychotics, because they can also lead to QT interval enlargement (Fig. 4) [13, 81].

Recommendations

Since this is a narrative review, it is not possible to make formal recommendations, but suggestions for monitoring and proposal of key messages are valuable, and provide information about AM use for health-care providers, especially rheumatologists. These key messages are depicted in Table 2.

Table 2 Key messages regarding safety of treatment with antimalarial drugs

- Daily dose not greater than 5 mg/Kg
- Regular screening for retinal toxicity according to risk factors
- Monitoring of complete blood count at the beginning and during prolonged therapy
- Physical examination with attention to muscle strength and reflexes
- Monitoring of QT interval prolongation in at-risk patients
- Caution in hepatic and renal impairment, use of other medications that lead to prolongation of the QT interval or that increase the serum level of antimalarials, alcoholism, concurrent antidiabetic agents, porphyria, psoriasis.

Conclusions

Given its multiple benefits, the use of AMs, preferably HCQ, should be encouraged to SLE patients, unless there is any contraindication. In other diseases like RA, pSS, APS, dermatomyositis and sarcoidosis some studies also show positive data, especially under specific circumstances. The majority of the side effects occur after a wide range of cumulative dosages.

It is a low-cost and widely available medication, whose safety profile is well known and acceptable. In addition, considering its pharmacokinetic properties (long half-life), it is possible to measure its serum concentration as a marker of treatment adherence and potential long-term toxicity, when necessary and available.

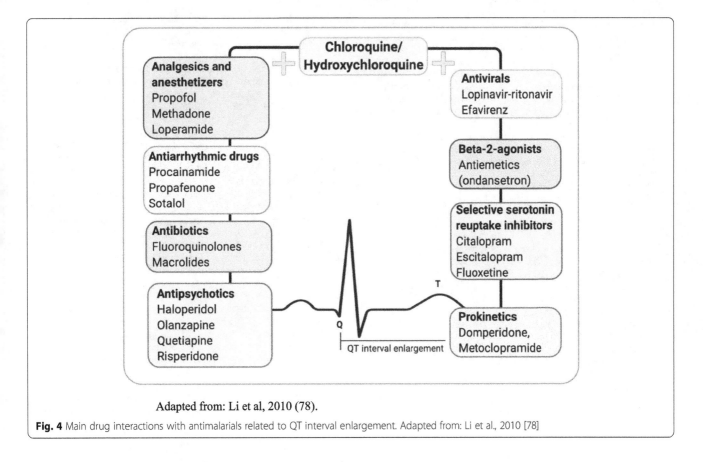

Adapted from: Li et al, 2010 (78).

Fig. 4 Main drug interactions with antimalarials related to QT interval enlargement. Adapted from: Li et al., 2010 [78]

Abbreviations
ACR: American College of Rheumatology; APS: Antiphospholipid syndrome; AM: Antimalarials; CQ: Chloroquine; CIMID: Chronic immune-mediated inflammatory rheumatic diseases; DMARD: Disease-modifying antirheumatic drugs; EULAR: European League Against Rheumatism; GLADEL: Grupo Latino Americano para Estudo do Lupus; HCQ: Hydroxychloroquine; HOMA: Homeostatic Model Assessment; pSS: Primary Sjögren syndrome; SLE: Systemic lupus erythematosus; RA: Rheumatoid arthritis; SBR: Brazilian Society of Rheumatology

Acknowledgements
Not applicable.

Authors' contributions
All of the authors provided critical review, relevant edits, and feedback to direct content during multiple rounds of review. In addition, all authors have read and approved the final version of this manuscript.

Author details
[1]Disciplina de Reumatologia, Escola Paulista de Medicina, Universidade Federal de São Paulo, São Paulo, Brazil. [2]Serviço de Reumatologia do Hospital das Clínicas da Universidade Federal de Minas Gerais, Belo Horizonte, Brazil. [3]Serviço de Reumatologia do Hospital das Clínicas da Universidade Federal de Pernambuco, Recife, Brazil. [4]Hospital Universitário - UnB/EBSERH, Brasília, Brazil. [5]Serviço de Reumatologia do Hospital das Clínicas da Universidade Federal do Paraná, Curitiba, Brazil. [6]Instituto de Ensino e Pesquisa (IEP), Hospital Amor, Barretos, Brazil. [7]Serviço de Reumatologia do Hospital de Clínicas de Porto Alegre da Universidade Federal do Rio Grande do Sul, Porto Alegre, Brazil. [8]Pontifícia Universidade Católica de Campinas, Campinas, Brazil.

References
1. Klumb EM, Silva CA, Lanna CC, Sato EI, Borba EF, Brenol JC, et al. Consensus of the Brazilian Society of Rheumatology for the diagnosis, management and treatment of lupus nephritis. Rev Bras Reumatol. 2015;55:1–21.
2. Fanouriakis A, Kostopoulou M, Alunno A, Aringer M, Bajema I, Boletis JN, et al. 2019 update of the EULAR recommendations for the management of systemic lupus erythematosus. Ann Rheum Dis. 2019;78:736–45.
3. Fanouriakis A, Kostopoulou M, Cheema K, Anders HJ, Aringer M, Bajema I, et al. 2019 update of the joint European league against rheumatism and European renal association-European Dialysis and transplant association (EULAR/ERA-EDTA) recommendations for the management of lupus nephritis. Ann Rheum Dis. 2020. https://doi.org/10.1136/annrheumdis-2020-216924.
4. Hahn BH, McMahon MA, Wilkinson A, Wallace WD, Daikh DI, Fitzgerald JD, et al. American College of Rheumatology guidelines for screening, treatment, and management of lupus nephritis. Arthritis Care Res (Hoboken). 2012;64:797–808.
5. Mota L, Kakehasi AM, Gomides APM, Duarte A, Cruz BA, Brenol CV, et al. 2017 recommendations of the Brazilian Society of Rheumatology for the pharmacological treatment of rheumatoid arthritis. Adv Rheumatol. 2018;58:2.
6. Singh JA, Saag KG, Bridges SL Jr, Akl EA, Bannuru RR, Sullivan MC, et al. 2015 American College of Rheumatology Guideline for the treatment of rheumatoid arthritis. Arthritis Care Res (Hoboken). 2016;68:1–25.
7. Ramos-Casals M, Brito-Zeron P, Bombardieri S, Bootsma H, De Vita S, Dorner T, et al. EULAR recommendations for the management of Sjogren's syndrome with topical and systemic therapies. Ann Rheum Dis. 2020;79:3–18.
8. Valim V, Trevisani VF, Pasoto SG, Serrano EV, Ribeiro SL, Fidelix TS, et al. Recommendations for the treatment of Sjogren's syndrome. Rev Bras Reumatol. 2015;55:446–57.
9. Tektonidou MG, Andreoli L, Limper M, Amoura Z, Cervera R, Costedoat-Chalumeau N, et al. EULAR recommendations for the management of antiphospholipid syndrome in adults. Ann Rheum Dis. 2019;78:1296–304.
10. van Vollenhoven RF, Mosca M, Bertsias G, Isenberg D, Kuhn A, Lerstrom K, et al. Treat-to-target in systemic lupus erythematosus: recommendations from an international task force. Ann Rheum Dis. 2014;73:958–67.
11. Marmor MF, Kellner U, Lai TY, Melles RB, Mieler WF. Recommendations on screening for Chloroquine and Hydroxychloroquine retinopathy (2016 revision). Ophthalmology. 2016;123:1386–94.
12. Rolain JM, Colson P, Raoult D. Recycling of chloroquine and its hydroxyl analogue to face bacterial, fungal and viral infections in the 21st century. Int J Antimicrob Agents. 2007;30:297–308.
13. Schrezenmeier E, Dorner T. Mechanisms of action of hydroxychloroquine and chloroquine: implications for rheumatology. Nat Rev Rheumatol. 2020; 16:155–66.
14. Costedoat-Chalumeau N, Dunogue B, Morel N, Le Guern V, Guettrot-Imbert G. Hydroxychloroquine: a multifaceted treatment in lupus. Presse Med. 2014;43(6 Pt 2):e167–80.
15. Vilar MJ, Sato EI. Estimating the incidence of systemic lupus erythematosus in a tropical region (Natal, Brazil). Lupus. 2002;11:528–32.
16. Amador-Patarroyo MJ, Rodriguez-Rodriguez A, Montoya-Ortiz G. How does age at onset influence the outcome of autoimmune diseases? Autoimmune Dis. 2012;2012:251730.
17. Arnaud L, Mathian A, Boddaert J, Amoura Z. Late-onset systemic lupus erythematosus: epidemiology, diagnosis and treatment. Drugs Aging. 2012; 29:181–9.
18. Urowitz MB, Bookman AA, Koehler BE, Gordon DA, Smythe HA, Ogryzlo MA. The bimodal mortality pattern of systemic lupus erythematosus. Am J Med. 1976;60:221–5.
19. Souza DC, Santo AH, Sato EI. Trends in systemic lupus erythematosus mortality rates in the state of Sao Paulo, Brazil from 1985 to 2004. Clin Exp Rheumatol. 2010;28:519–24.
20. Ruiz-Irastorza G, Ramos-Casals M, Brito-Zeron P, Khamashta MA. Clinical efficacy and side effects of antimalarials in systemic lupus erythematosus: a systematic review. Ann Rheum Dis. 2010;69:20–8.
21. Tsakonas E, Joseph L, Esdaile JM, Choquette D, Senecal JL, Cividino A, et al. A long-term study of hydroxychloroquine withdrawal on exacerbations in systemic lupus erythematosus. Canadian Hydroxychloroquine Study Group. Lupus. 1998;7:80–5.
22. Cavazzana I, Sala R, Bazzani C, Ceribelli A, Zane C, Cattaneo R, et al. Treatment of lupus skin involvement with quinacrine and hydroxychloroquine. Lupus. 2009;18:735–9.
23. Bezerra EL, Vilar MJ, da Trindade Neto PB, Sato EI. Double-blind, randomized, controlled clinical trial of clofazimine compared with chloroquine in patients with systemic lupus erythematosus. Arthritis Rheum. 2005;52:3073–8.
24. Fessler BJ, Alarcon GS, McGwin G Jr, Roseman J, Bastian HM, Friedman AW, et al. Systemic lupus erythematosus in three ethnic groups: XVI. Association of hydroxychloroquine use with reduced risk of damage accrual. Arthritis Rheum. 2005;52:1473–80.
25. Ibanez D, Gladman DD, Urowitz MB. Adjusted mean systemic lupus Erythematosus disease activity index-2K is a predictor of outcome in SLE. J Rheumatol. 2005;32(5):824–7.
26. Ruiz-Irastorza G, Egurbide MV, Pijoan JI, Garmendia M, Villar I, Martinez-Berriotxoa A, et al. Effect of antimalarials on thrombosis and survival in patients with systemic lupus erythematosus. Lupus. 2006;15:577–83.
27. Shinjo SK, Bonfa E, Wojdyla D, Borba EF, Ramirez LA, Scherbarth HR, et al. Antimalarial treatment may have a time-dependent effect on lupus survival: data from a multinational Latin American inception cohort. Arthritis Rheum. 2010;62:855–62.
28. A randomized study of the effect of withdrawing hydroxychloroquine sulfate in systemic lupus erythematosus. N Engl J Med. 1991;324:150–4.
29. Aouhab Z, Hong H, Felicelli C, Tarplin S, Ostrowski RA. Outcomes of systemic lupus Erythematosus in patients who discontinue Hydroxychloroquine. ACR Open Rheumatol. 2019;1:593–9.
30. Petri M, Alarcon GS, Kimberly RP, Reveille JD. Predictors of renal insufficiency in systemic lupus erythematosus (abstract); 2005.
31. Kasitanon N, Fine DM, Haas M, Magder LS, Petri M. Hydroxychloroquine use predicts complete renal remission within 12 months among patients treated with mycophenolate mofetil therapy for membranous lupus nephritis. Lupus. 2006;15:366–70.
32. Molad Y, Gorshtein A, Wysenbeek AJ, Guedj D, Majadla R, Weinberger A, et al. Protective effect of hydroxychloroquine in systemic lupus erythematosus. Prospective long-term study of an Israeli cohort. Lupus. 2002;11:356–61.
33. Akhavan PS, Su J, Lou W, Gladman DD, Urowitz MB, Fortin PR. The early protective effect of hydroxychloroquine on the risk of cumulative damage in patients with systemic lupus erythematosus. J Rheumatol. 2013;40:831–41.

34. Petri M, Purvey S, Fang H, Magder LS. Predictors of organ damage in systemic lupus erythematosus: the Hopkins lupus cohort. Arthritis Rheum. 2012;64:4021–8.

35. Pons-Estel GJ, Alarcon GS, McGwin G Jr, Danila MI, Zhang J, Bastian HM, et al. Protective effect of hydroxychloroquine on renal damage in patients with lupus nephritis: LXV, data from a multiethnic US cohort. Arthritis Rheum. 2009;61:830–9.

36. Rand JH, Wu XX, Quinn AS, Chen PP, Hathcock JJ, Taatjes DJ. Hydroxychloroquine directly reduces the binding of antiphospholipid antibody-beta2-glycoprotein I complexes to phospholipid bilayers. Blood. 2008;112:1687–95.

37. Petri M. Thrombosis and systemic lupus erythematosus: the Hopkins lupus cohort perspective. Scand J Rheumatol. 1996;25:191–3.

38. Mok MY, Chan EY, Fong DY, Leung KF, Wong WS, Lau CS. Antiphospholipid antibody profiles and their clinical associations in Chinese patients with systemic lupus erythematosus. J Rheumatol. 2005;32:622–8.

39. Tektonidou MG, Laskari K, Panagiotakos DB, Moutsopoulos HM. Risk factors for thrombosis and primary thrombosis prevention in patients with systemic lupus erythematosus with or without antiphospholipid antibodies. Arthritis Rheum. 2009;61:29–36.

40. Kaiser R, Cleveland CM, Criswell LA. Risk and protective factors for thrombosis in systemic lupus erythematosus: results from a large, multi-ethnic cohort. Ann Rheum Dis. 2009;68:238–41.

41. Jung H, Bobba R, Su J, Shariati-Sarabi Z, Gladman DD, Urowitz M, et al. The protective effect of antimalarial drugs on thrombovascular events in systemic lupus erythematosus. Arthritis Rheum. 2010;62:863–8.

42. Penn SK, Kao AH, Schott LL, Elliott JR, Toledo FG, Kuller L, et al. Hydroxychloroquine and glycemia in women with rheumatoid arthritis and systemic lupus erythematosus. J Rheumatol. 2010;37:1136–42.

43. Sachet JC, Borba EF, Bonfa E, Vinagre CG, Silva VM, Maranhao RC. Chloroquine increases low-density lipoprotein removal from plasma in systemic lupus patients. Lupus. 2007;16:273–8.

44. Petri M, Lakatta C, Magder L, Goldman D. Effect of prednisone and hydroxychloroquine on coronary artery disease risk factors in systemic lupus erythematosus: a longitudinal data analysis. Am J Med. 1994;96:254–9.

45. Rahman P, Gladman DD, Urowitz MB, Yuen K, Hallett D, Bruce IN. The cholesterol lowering effect of antimalarial drugs is enhanced in patients with lupus taking corticosteroid drugs. J Rheumatol. 1999;26:325–30.

46. Cairoli E, Rebella M, Danese N, Garra V, Borba EF. Hydroxychloroquine reduces low-density lipoprotein cholesterol levels in systemic lupus erythematosus: a longitudinal evaluation of the lipid-lowering effect. Lupus. 2012;21:1178–82.

47. Babary H, Liu X, Ayatollahi Y, Chen XP, Doo L, Uppaluru LK, et al. Favorable effects of hydroxychloroquine on serum low density lipid in patients with systemic lupus erythematosus: a systematic review and meta-analysis. Int J Rheum Dis. 2018;21:84–92.

48. Levy RA, Vilela VS, Cataldo MJ, Ramos RC, Duarte JL, Tura BR, et al. Hydroxychloroquine (HCQ) in lupus pregnancy: double-blind and placebo-controlled study. Lupus. 2001;10:401–4.

49. Andreoli L, Bertsias GK, Agmon-Levin N, Brown S, Cervera R, Costedoat-Chalumeau N, et al. EULAR recommendations for women's health and the management of family planning, assisted reproduction, pregnancy and menopause in patients with systemic lupus erythematosus and/or antiphospholipid syndrome. Ann Rheum Dis. 2017;76:476–85.

50. Izmirly PM, Costedoat-Chalumeau N, Pisoni CN, Khamashta MA, Kim MY, Saxena A, et al. Maternal use of hydroxychloroquine is associated with a reduced risk of recurrent anti-SSA/Ro-antibody-associated cardiac manifestations of neonatal lupus. Circulation. 2012;126:76–82.

51. Tunks RD, Clowse ME, Miller SG, Brancazio LR, Barker PC. Maternal autoantibody levels in congenital heart block and potential prophylaxis with antiinflammatory agents. Am J Obstet Gynecol. 2013;208:64.e1–7.

52. Vivien G, Alice B, Thomas B, Christophe R, Marie-Elise T, Julien S, et al. Hydroxychloroquine for the prevention of fetal growth restriction and prematurity in lupus pregnancy: a systematic review and meta-analysis. Joint Bone Spine. 2018;85:663–8.

53. HERA Study Group. A randomized trial of hydroxychloroquine in early rheumatoid arthritis: the HERA study. Am J Med. 1995;98:156–68.

54. Strategy to Prevent the Onset of Clinically-Apparent Rheumatoid Arthritis - Full Text View - ClinicalTrials.gov 2020. Available from: https://clinicaltrials.gov/ct2/show/NCT02603146]. Acessed 22 Apr 2020.

55. Rempenault C, Combe B, Barnetche T, Gaujoux-Viala C, Lukas C, Morel J, et al. Metabolic and cardiovascular benefits of hydroxychloroquine in patients with rheumatoid arthritis: a systematic review and meta-analysis. Ann Rheum Dis. 2018;77:98–103.

56. Wasko MC, Hubert HB, Lingala VB, Elliott JR, Luggen ME, Fries JF, et al. Hydroxychloroquine and risk of diabetes in patients with rheumatoid arthritis. Jama. 2007;298:187–93.

57. Avina-Zubieta JA, Choi HK, Sadatsafavi M, Etminan M, Esdaile JM, Lacaille D. Risk of cardiovascular mortality in patients with rheumatoid arthritis: a meta-analysis of observational studies. Arthritis Rheum. 2008;59:1690–7.

58. Beegle SH, Barba K, Gobunsuy R, Judson MA. Current and emerging pharmacological treatments for sarcoidosis: a review. Drug Des Devel Ther. 2013;7:325–38.

59. Sontheimer RD. Aminoquinoline antimalarial therapy in dermatomyositis-are we missing opportunities with respect to comorbidities and modulation of extracutaneous disease activity? Ann Transl Med. 2018;6:154.

60. Pileggi GS, Da Mota LMH, Kakehasi AM, De Souza AW, Rocha A, de Melo AKG, et al. Brazilian recommendations on the safety and effectiveness of the yellow fever vaccination in patients with chronic immune-mediated inflammatory diseases. Adv Rheumatol. 2019;59:17.

61. Ruiz-Irastorza G, Olivares N, Ruiz-Arruza I, Martinez-Berriotxoa A, Egurbide MV, Aguirre C. Predictors of major infections in systemic lupus erythematosus. Arthritis Res Ther. 2009;11:R109.

62. Ponticelli C, Moroni G. Hydroxychloroquine in systemic lupus erythematosus (SLE). Expert Opin Drug Saf. 2017;16:411–9.

63. Fiehn C, Ness T, Weseloh C, Specker C, Hadjiski D, Detert J, et al. Safety management in treatment with antimalarials in rheumatology Interdisciplinary recommendations on the basis of a systematic literature review. Z Rheumatol. 2020. https://doi.org/10.1007/s00393-020-00785-4.

64. Haar D, Solvkjaer M, Unger B, Rasmussen KJ, Christensen L, Hansen TM. A double-blind comparative study of hydroxychloroquine and dapsone, alone and in combination, in rheumatoid arthritis. Scand J Rheumatol. 1993;22: 113–8.

65. Food and Drug Administration - FDA. FACT SHEET FOR HEALTH CARE PROVIDERS EMERGENCY USE AUTHORIZATION (EUA) OF CHLOROQUINE PHOSPHATE SUPPLIED FROM THE STRATEGIC NATIONAL STOCKPILE FOR TREATMENT OF COVID-19 IN CERTAIN HOSPITALIZED PATIENTS 2020 [Available from: https://www.fda.gov/media/136535/download.] Accessed 11 Apr 2020.

66. Jorge A, Ung C, Young LH, Melles RB, Choi HK. Hydroxychloroquine retinopathy - implications of research advances for rheumatology care. Nat Rev Rheumatol. 2018;14:693–703.

67. Yusuf IH, Sharma S, Luqmani R, Downes SM. Hydroxychloroquine retinopathy. Eye (Lond). 2017;31:828–45.

68. Petri M, Elkhalifa M, Li J, Magder LS, Goldman DW. Hydroxychloroquine blood levels predict Hydroxychloroquine retinopathy. Arthritis Rheumatol. 2020;72:448–53.

69. Sharma AN, Mesinkovska NA, Paravar T. Characterizing the adverse dermatologic effects of hydroxychloroquine: a systematic review. J Am Acad Dermatol. 2020. https://doi.org/10.1016/j.jaad.2020.04.024.

70. Ruzicka T, Sommerburg C, Goerz G, Kind P, Mensing H. Treatment of cutaneous lupus erythematosus with acitretin and hydroxychloroquine. Br J Dermatol. 1992;127:513–8.

71. Bahloul E, Jallouli M, Garbaa S, Marzouk S, Masmoudi A, Turki H, et al. Hydroxychloroquine-induced hyperpigmentation in systemic diseases: prevalence, clinical features and risk factors: a cross-sectional study of 41 cases. Lupus. 2017;26:1304–8.

72. Jallouli M, Frances C, Piette JC, du LT H, Moguelet P, Factor C, et al. Hydroxychloroquine-induced pigmentation in patients with systemic lupus erythematosus: a case-control study. JAMA Dermatol. 2013;149:935–40.

73. Tsankov N, Angelova I, Kazandjieva J. Drug-induced psoriasis. Recognition and management. Am J Clin Dermatol. 2000;1:159–65.

74. Sidoroff A, Dunant A, Viboud C, Halevy S, Bavinck JN, Naldi L, et al. Risk factors for acute generalized exanthematous pustulosis (AGEP)-results of a multinational case-control study (EuroSCAR). Br J Dermatol. 2007;157:989–96.

75. Chatre C, Roubille F, Vernhet H, Jorgensen C, Pers YM. Cardiac complications attributed to Chloroquine and Hydroxychloroquine: a systematic review of the literature. Drug Saf. 2018;41:919–31.

76. Thome R, Lopes SC, Costa FT, Verinaud L. Chloroquine: modes of action of an undervalued drug. Immunol Lett. 2013;153:50–7.

77. Baguet JP, Tremel F, Fabre M. Chloroquine cardiomyopathy with conduction disorders. Heart. 1999;81:221–3.

78. Nord JE, Shah PK, Rinaldi RZ, Weisman MH. Hydroxychloroquine cardiotoxicity in systemic lupus erythematosus: a report of 2 cases and review of the literature. Semin Arthritis Rheum. 2004;33:336–51.

79. Yogasundaram H, Hung W, Paterson ID, Sergi C, Oudit GY. Chloroquine-induced cardiomyopathy: a reversible cause of heart failure. ESC Heart Fail. 2018;5(3):372–5.

80. Tselios K, Deeb M, Gladman DD, Harvey P, Akhtari S, Mak S, et al. Antimalarial-induced cardiomyopathy in systemic lupus Erythematosus: as rare as considered? J Rheumatol. 2019;46:391–6.

81. Li EC, Esterly JS, Pohl S, Scott SD, McBride BF. Drug-induced QT-interval prolongation: considerations for clinicians. Pharmacotherapy. 2010;30:684–701.

16

Assessment of effectiveness of anakinra and canakinumab in patients with colchicine-resistant/ unresponsive familial Mediterranean fever

Ali Şahin[1] (iD), Mehmet Emin Derin[1*] (iD), Fatih Albayrak[1] (iD), Burak Karakaş[1] (iD) and Yalçın Karagöz[2] (iD)

Abstract

Introduction: Familial Mediterranean fever (FMF) is a hereditary auto-inflammatory disease characterized by recurrent fever and serosal inflammation. Anti-interleukin-1 (Anti-IL-1) treatments are recommended in colchicine resistant and/or intolerant FMF patients. This study aims to evaluate the efficacy of anakinra and canakinumab in FMF patients that are resistant/intolareted to colchicine or complicated with amyloidosis.

Methods: Between January 2014 and March 2019, 65 patients following-up at Sivas Cumhuriyet University (Medical Faculty Rheumatology-Internal Medicine Department) who were diagnosed with FMF according to the criteria of Tel-Hashomer were included in the study. The laboratory values and clinical features of patients and disease activities were recorded at least every 3 months, and these data were analyzed.

Results: Forty-one (63.1%) patients used anakinra (100 mg/day) and 24 (36.9%) patients used canakinumab (150 mg/8 week). The median duration of anti-IL-1 agents use was 7 months (range, 3–30). Fifteen (23.1%) cases were complicated with amyloidosis. Seven (10.8%) patients had renal transplantation. Overall, the FMF 50 score response was 96.9%. In the group that had a glomerular filtration rate (GFR) ≥ 60 ml/min/m^2, the median proteinuria decreased from 2390 mg/day (range, 1400–7200) to 890 mg/day (range, 120–2750) ($p = 0.008$). No serious infections were detected, except in one patient.

Conclusions: Anti-IL-1 agents are effective and safe in the treatment of FMF patients. These agents are particularly effective at reducing proteinuria in patients with GFR ≥ 60 ml/min/m^2, but less effective in cases with FMF associated with arthritis and sacroiliitis. Large and long follow-up studies are now needed to establish the long-term effects of these treatments.

Keywords: Anakinra, Canakinumab, Familial Mediterranean fever (FMF), Amyloidosis, Colchicine-resistant

Introduction

Familial Mediterranean fever (FMF) is a monogenic autoinflammatory disease characterized by self-limiting acute inflammatory attacks involving the peritoneum, synovium, pleura, and (rarely) pericardium, often accompanied by fever [1]. Turkey has the highest prevalence of FMF in any country in the world. The prevalence of FMF in Turkey shows regional characteristics. The prevalence rate is 0.25–0.88% in the Central Anatolia region, such as Sivas, Tokat, Erzincan, and Kastamonu [2, 3]. A Turkish FMF study group has reported that 90% of FMF patients in Turkey originate from the East and Black Sea and Central Anatolia regions [4]. The most severe complication of FMF is type AA amyloidosis. Nephrotic syndrome and end-stage renal failure tend to occur within 5–10 years in untreated FMF-associated amyloidosis patients [5]. The basic treatment goal for FMF is to prevent the attacks and to minimize the subclinical inflammation between attacks. Specifically, the main treatment for amyloidosis and FMF

* Correspondence: eminderin@gmail.com
[1]Department of Internal Medicine – Rheumatology, Faculty of Medicine, Cumhuriyet University, Unit Sivas Cumhuriyet, 58140 Sivas, Turkey
Full list of author information is available at the end of the article

attacks is colchicine. Colchicine resistance in FMF patients is about 5–15% [6]. Patients who use maximum dose colchicine treatment (3 mg/day) for at least 6 months are considered resistant/unresponsive to colchicine if they had one or more attacks per month. Biological agents, such as anti-interleukin-1 (IL) agents, are indicated in these patients [7]. In Turkey, anakinra (recombinant IL-1 antagonist, kineret®, 100 mg/day/subcutaneous) and canakinumab (IL-1β antibody, ilaris® 150 mg/8 weeks/subcutaneous) are used as anti-IL-1 treatments. Rinolocept, which is another anti-IL-1 agent, is not available in Turkey. Treatments in Turkey can be used by obtaining an off-label consent from the Turkey Medicines and Medical Devices Institution (TICTK). The purpose of this study is to share our clinical evaluation of anti-IL-1 treatment for FMF patients who have colchicine resistance or intolerance.

Materials and methods

Between January 2014 and March 2019, 65 patients who were admitted to Sivas Cumhuriyet University Hospital Internal Medicine Rheumatology Department were included in the study.

Our department includes a total of about 800–1000 FMF patients. The enrolled patients, who were diagnosed with FMF according to the Tel-Hashomer Criteria, had colchicine resistance/intolerance and were being treated with anti-IL-1 (anakinra or canakinumab) treatment. The European League Against Rheumatism (EULAR) criteria and recommendations were used to define colchicine resistance [7]. Patients who received the maximally tolerated dose colchicine treatment (3 mg/day) for at least 6 months were considered resistant/unresponsive to colchicine if they had one or more attacks per month. Intolerance to colchicine or proteinuria were other indications of anti-IL-1 therapy. The factors for deciding whether to start anakinra or canakinumab treatments varied from patient to patient.

Data had been collected when the patients were called for their routine check-ups once every 3 months. For each visit, we recorded whether they had an FMF attack. Moreover, patients' global and physicians' global assessments of disease severity [on a visual analog scale (VAS), range 0 to 10], acute phase reactants, erythrocyte sedimentation rate (ESR), C reactive protein (CRP), complete blood count (CBC), liver and kidney function values, and 24-h urinary protein levels were retrospectively investigated and included in our data. Patients who used anti-IL-1 treatment for at least 3 months were included in the study. Patients who were followed up for at least 3 months but discontinued treatment or follow-up for any reason were also included in the study. The FMF-50 score was used for the evaluation of responses. When at least five of the six variables were reduced by more than 50%, the patient was considered to be responding to treatment.

Approval from the ethics committee of Cumhuriyet University Medical Faculty was obtained (decision no 2019–04/29). The study was carried out in accordance with the World Medical Association's Declaration of Helsinki. Patients' informed consents were obtained.

Statistical analysis

The SPSS 23.0 statistical program was used for the analysis of our data. The normality of the data was checked using the Kolmogorov-Smirnov statistical test. The independent sample t-test was used for the independent groups, which satisfy the parametric conditions. More than two groups were analyzed by the F test (ANOVA). If satisfied the homogeneity assumption, the Tukey test was used to analyze which groups were different from the others, whereas Tamhane's T2 test was used for the groups that did not satisfy the homogeneity assumption. If one or all of the assumptions were not met, the Mann Whitney U test was used for two independent groups, the Wilcoxon test for two conjugate groups, and the Kruskal Wallis test for more than two independent groups. For the significance test, a p-value smaller than 0.05 was used.

Results
Demographic and clinical characteristics

In total, 65 patients were involved in this study. The median age of the patients was 32 years (range, 17–60 years). Thirty-three (50.8%) patients were male, and 30 (49.2%) were female. Forty-one (63.1%) patients used anakinra (100 mg/day/subcutaneous) and 24 (36.9%) patients used canakinumab (150 mg/8 week subcutaneous). The median duration of drug use was 6 months (range, 3–30 months) for anakinra and 8 months (range, 3–25 months) for canakinumab. The demographic and clinical features of the patients are shown in Table 1. Fifty-six of 65 (86.7%) patients continued to be followed up. Twelve of the patients directly started with canakinumab (50%), eight patients continued with canakinumab due to an allergic reaction to anakinra, and four patients used canakinumab because of inadequate response to anakinra (possibly due to non-compliance with treatment). Except for eight patients who had colchicine intolerance, 57 (87.7%) patients continued to used colchicine (mean, 2 mg/day; range, 0.5–2.5 mg/day). The Mediterranean fever gene (MEFV) mutation analysis is shown in Table 1. The homozygous M694 V mutation was the most frequent mutation, detected in 29 (44.6%) of the patients.

Treatment response

Before the treatment, the median FMF attack frequency over 3 months was three (range, 1–6), but was zero after

Table 1 Demographic and clinical features

Age		32 years (17–60)
Age of onset		18 years (3–46)
Sex		
Female	n: 32	49.2%
Male	n: 33	50.8%
Duration of use	n: 65 (100%)	7 month (3–30)
Anakinra	n: 41 (63.1%)	6 month (3–30)
Canakinumab	n: 24 (39.6%)	8 month (3–25)
Clinical Features		
Fever	n: 60	92.5%
Peritonitis	n: 61	93.8%
Erysipales LE	n: 18	27.7%
Amlyoidosis	n: 15	23.1%
Arthritis	n: 11	16.9%
Pleuritis	n: 20	30.8%
AxSpa	n: 9	13.8%
Renal trans	n: 7	10.8%
MEFV Mutation		
M694 V homozygous	n: 29	44.6%
M694 V heterozygous	n: 8	12.3%
M680I homozygous	n: 4	6.2%
E148Q homozygous	n: 1	1.5%
Compound	n: 16	24.6%
No	n: 3	4.6%
R761H heterozygous	n: 1	1.5%
Others	n: 3	4.6%
Indications of Anti-IL1 therapy		
Colchicine-Intolerant	n: 8	12.3%
Colchicine-Resistant	n: 46	70.8%
Proteinuria	n: 15	23.1%

All parameters are presented as median (min–max) or number (%). *LE* like erythema, *AxSpa* axialspondyloarthropathy

treatment (range, 0–1) ($p = 0.00$). There was a statistically significant improvement in the physician's VAS, ESR, CRP, and attack duration with anti-IL-1 treatment (Table 2). We found that 63 (96.9%) of the patients achieved FMF-50 scores (Table 3). There was no significant difference in efficacy when comparing anakinra and canakinumab ($p > 0.05$).

The median proteinuria was 3.2 g/day (range, 0.5–11.2 g/day) before the treatment, and decreased to 1.85 g/day (range, 0.1–12.2) after treatment ($p = 0.140$). Based on GFR values, there was a statistically significant change in proteinuria response. The group with GFR ≥ 60 ml/dk/m² before the treatment had 2390 mg/day (range, 1400–7200 mg/day) proteinuria, which decreased to 890 mg/day (range, 120–2750 mg/day) ($p = 0.008$). On the other hand, the median proteinuria decreased from 4472 to 3960 mg/day (range, 2050–12,200 mg/day) for the group with GFR < 60 ml/min/m². This difference was not statistically significant ($p = 0.345$). When the effect on proteinuria was investigated, the other factors (diets, the using of angiotensin-receptors inhibitors or blockers and blood pressure control etc.) of all patients were similar in both groups.

Side effects

Allergic reactions were observed in eight (19.5%) patients who used anakinra, and severe neutropenia was observed in one patient (2.4%). Another patient (2.4%) was diagnosed with Multiple Sclerosis after 2 years of anakinra use. In the group that used anakinra, one (2.4%) patient who also had polyarteritis nodosa (PAN) and sacroiliitis died due to sepsis. Mild infections of the upper respiratory tract and urinary tract were reported by 7–30% of the patients. There was no significant difference in the rate of side effects when comparing anakinra and canakinumab ($p > 0.05$). Although the glomerular filtration rate (GFR) increased during the treatment period, this difference was not statistically significant (Table 2).

Pregnancy and other conditions

We found that two patients continued to use anakinra during their pregnancy, and there were no problems during pregnancy, birth, or with the child.

We switched to another biological medicine for five (7.6%) patients (four canakinumab, one anakinra). Two out of five patients had stage-three sacroiliitis. Even though the FMF attack frequency decreased for these patients, we switched to tumor necrosis factor (TNF) inhibitor treatments due to their high Bath Ankylosing Spondylitis Disease Activity Index (BASDAI) scores. Although one (2.4%) patient used anakinra (100 mg/day) regularly for 3 months, knee arthritis continued at a rate of twice per month. For this patient, we switched to tocilizumab, and knee arthritis responded to this treatment. We considered the wash-out period of anakinra and canakinumab when we started patients on tocilizumab. Complete remission was achieved for about 14 months in a patient who used canakinumab due to both peritonitis and peripheral arthritis attacks. However, the treatment was changed to tocilizumab because the number of attacks was once or more per month. One of the patients (2.4%) had end-stage kidney failure and had renal transplant due to inadequate response to the treatment (Table 4).

The median duration of anti-IL-1 treatment ($n = 6$ (85%) for anakinra; $n = 1$ (15%) for canakinumab) was 3 months (range, 3–26 months) for the seven (10.8%)

Table 2 Comparison of laboratory values and disease severity before and after Anti-IL-1 therapy

	Before treatment	After treatment	p
Attack frequency (per 3 months)	3 (1–6)	0 (0–1)	.00*
Patients-VAS (0–10 cm)	10 (9–10)	2 (0–3)	.00*
Physicians-VAS (0–10 cm)	9 (8–10)	1 (0–2)	.00*
ESR (mm/h)	33 (9–85)	29 (2–106)	.00*
CRP (mg/dl)	16 (1–80)	2 (1–12)	.00*
GFR (ml/min/m^2)	54 (13–180)	42 (10–174)	.592
Durations of attacks (hours)	48 (36–96)	8 (0–24)	0.0*
Proteinuria (mg/day)	3200 (0.5–11.2)	1850 (0.1–12.2)	0.140
GFR ≥ 60 ml/min/m^2	2390 (1400–7200)	890 (120–2.75)	0.008*
GFR < 60 ml/min/m^2	4472 (1950–11.2)	3960 (2050–12.2)	0.345

Values presented as median (minimum-maximum).*VAS* Visual Analogue Scale (0–10 cm), *CRP* C reactive protein, *GFR* glomerul filtration rate, *ESR* Erythrocyte Sedimentation Rate *: $p < 0.05$

patients with renal transplantation. No side effects or drug-interactions were observed.

Discussion

In this study, we present the results of 65 FMF patients treated with anti-IL-1 agents. We show that IL-1 inhibitors are effective and safe in patients with FMF who are colchicine resistant/intolerant or with amyloidosis. Approximately 5–10% colchicine resistance and 5–10% colchicine intolerance have been reported during FMF treatment [8]. The use of anti-IL-1 treatments has increased among patients with colchicine-resistance. Some previous studies have demonstrated the efficiency of these treatments. Akar et al. reported the response rate as 76.5% in the anakinra group and 67.5% in the canakinumab group in a total of 172 colchicine-resistant patients [9]. In the study by Kucuksahin et al., anti-IL-1 treatments significantly decreased the number of attacks in 26 colchicine-resistant patients with FMF. Moreover, the serum acute phase reactants of these patients returned to normal levels [10]. Kohler et al. achieved a 90% FMF-50 score with IL-1blocking therapy in 31 FMF patients [11]. In our study, we achieved a 96% FMF-50 response rates for the anti-IL-1 treatments, which is similar to previous studies. Currently, the prevention

Table 3 FMF-50 response criteria

Parameters	At least 50% reduction
Attack frequency	63/65 (96.9%)
Durations of attacks	63/65 (96.9%)
Patients VAS	64/65 (98.5%)
Physicians VAS	64/65 (98.5%)
CRP (at least 2 weeks after the last attack)	62/65 (95.3%)
Arthritis	9/11 (81.8%)

Values presented by % frequency. *VAS* Visual Analogue Scale, *CRP* C reactive protein

and decreasing effects of anakinra and canakinumab were recognized in FMF attacks.

However, additional amyloidosis and spondyloarthritis (SpA) diagnoses can lead to some issues in FMF treatment. Some studies have reported a decreasing effect of anti-IL-1 treatment in proteinuria. By biopsy, Topaloglu et al. reported that anti-IL-1 treatments reduced proteinuria but also resulted in renal damage in three patients with AID-associated amyloidosis [12]. Özçakar et al. reported a significant decrease in the amount of proteinuria and an increase in quality of life in six children with FMF-associated amyloidosis [13]. Another Varan et al. showed that anti-IL1 treatments significantly reduced the amount of proteinuria (from 1606 mg/day to 519 mg/day) [14]. Moreover, national data that was collected with 172 subjects demonstrated a significant decrease in proteinuria (5458.7 mg/24 h before and 3557.3 mg/24 h after) [9]. Instead, in these studies, patients were not sub-grouped, and their data was not analyzed regarding their GFR. In our study, anti-IL-1 agents significantly decreased the proteinuria in patients with GFR > 60 ml/min/m^2, while no significant reduction was seen in patients with GFR < 60 ml/min/m^2. Therefore, we emphasized that GFR would be a useful indicator to decide the proper treatment for these patients. Another option is tocilizumab, which is an IL-6 blocking agent that has been recently started to be used in the treatment of FMF-associated amyloidosis. Ugurlu et al. [15] reported a reduction effect of tocilizumab on proteinuria among 20 subjects. Additionally, in this study, only two patients had GFR < 50 ml/min/m^2; these patients were offered tocilizumab treatment and responded positively. Despite these positive outcomes, the small sample size of these studies and the lack of a randomized controlled trial (RCT) creates confusion around this topic. Also factors such as blood pressure control, use of angiotensin receptor blocker drugs or colchicine and diet have positive

Table 4 Characteristics and recent treatments/conditions of patients with anti-IL-1 therapy discontinuation for various reasons

	Age	Sex	Mutation	Dominant clinical features and the Reasons for Discontinuation of Anti-IL1 Treatment	Duration of Using Anti-IL-1 agents	Recent treatments/conditions
Patient 1	21	F	M694V homozygous	Amyloidosis Stage 5 CRD 11 g/day proteinuria	Increase of proteinuria, Progression of CRD	Anakinra/12 months	Renal tx
Patient 2	28	M	M694V heterozygous M680I heterozygous	PAN+sacroiliitis	Activation of PAN/high dose corticosteroid	Anakinra/12 months	Sepsis-died
Patient 3	25	M	M694V heterozygous M680I heterozygous	Sacroiliitis	refractory low back pain high BASDAI score	Canakinumab/4 months	Anti-TNF
Patient 4	24	M	M694V homozygous	Sacroiliitis	refractory low back pain high BASDAI score	Canakinumab/6 months	Anti-TNF
Patient 5	50	M	R761H homozygous	Sacroiliitis+polyarthritis	Refractory arthritis	Canakinumab/18 months (secondary non-responder)	Tocilizumab
Patient 6	19	M	M680I homozygous	Peripheral Arthritis	Refractory arthritis	Anakinra/3 months	Tocilizumab
Patient 7	49	M	M694V homozygous	Amyloidosis Stage 4 CRD 2.5 g/day proteinuria	Increase of proteinuria	Canakinumab/4 months	Tocilizumab
Patient 8	45	F	M694V heterozygous		Side effect	Anakinra/2 years	Multiple sclerosis-drug stop

PAN polyarteritis nodosa, *CRD* Chronic Renal Disease, *Renal tx* renal transplant, (*BASDAI*) Bath Ankylosing Spondylitis Disease Activity Index, *TNF* Tumour necrosis factor, *IL* interleukin

effects in decreasing proteinuria. However, it is not easy to evaluate them clearly.

There are many studies on anti-TNF agents in patients with colchicine resistant FMF or FMF associated with sacroiliitis or peripheral arthritis. However, none of these studies were RCTs. In one review, Koga et al. reported that 29 FMF patients in various studies had successful results with anti-TNF agents [16]. The efficacy of anti-TNF drugs in the treatment of colchicine-resistant FMF is not yet clear. EULAR recommends using anti-TNF therapy, especially in cases with FMF-associated SpA and peripheral arthritis [7]. Interestingly, according to a recently published study, the $M694V$ gene variations were seen five-times as often among Ankylosing Spondylitis (AS) patients compared to a healthy population, and this variant might be associated with AS. In the same study, the serum level of IL-1 was higher in AS patients. Therefore, the researchers emphasized that anti-IL-1 treatments would be an appropriate therapy in these patients [17]. However, in our study, ten patients had axialspondyloarthritis (AxSpA), and only half of these subjects had proper anti-IL-1 treatment. The treatments in other patients had to be replaced with other biological treatments, such as anti-TNF. Only one patient was excluded from the study. The efficacy of anti-IL-1 treatments on AS patients should be investigated through RCTs.

In terms of safety issues the number of patients and the duration of drug use can be considered as a limitation. During the study, we did not detect any serious infection or tuberculosis or malignancy. While allergic reactions are commonly seen as an adverse effect of anakinra, in a review of 27 studies published by van der Hilst et al., it was shown that there were no serious infections when using IL-1 blocking agents. In addition, allergic reactions had been reported in just 6.5% of patients [18]. In our study, 19.5% of allergic reactions were detected in patients using anakinra. In this study, a participant who was using additional steroid and immunosuppressive agents had sepsis and died. Therefore, identification of anakinra as the main factor responsible for this death is impossible. While seven renal transplant patients were offered anakinra and the other immunosuppressive, no severe infections or drug interactions were seen. The previous studies that were carried out with renal transplant patients showed no severe adverse effect or drug interactions [19]. Multiple sclerosis is a possible adverse effect of any biological medication, and it was observed in one patient in this study. The medication was discontinued, and the patient has been followed closely. To our knowledge, there are no data available in the literature about this scenario.

Anakinra is classified as Food and Drug Administration (FDA) Pregnancy Category B. Recently, multicenter pregnancy data and case reports of pregnant women who have been using anti-IL-1 have been published. Among thirty-one pregnant women who were using canakinumab or anakinra (eight and 23 respectively), only one patient experienced renal agenesis [20, 21]. In our study, two pregnant patients safely used anakinra treatment throughout their pregnancy, and no fatal or maternal complications were noted.

Also, to identify new mutations and epigenetic mechanisms, whole gene analysis should be done in refractory FMF patients.

The main limitation of our study is that it is an observational study. The efficacy of anti-IL-1 treatment should be shown with randomized controlled trials. Another limitation is that these off-labeled medications were offered as fixed doses. Long term follow-ups are crucial to identify the long-term and potential adverse effects of this medication. The serum level of amyloid A has not been measured in all participants; therefore, there was no evaluation of it.

Conclusion

As a conclusion, anti-IL treatments among colchicine-resistant patients with FMF continue to be used as an effective treatment. However, this treatment is less effective against proteinuria in patients with stage 4 or 5 kidney disease. In our study, anti-TNF and tocilizumab have provided more successful outcomes in participants with FMF associated arthritis and sacroiliitis. RCTs should be conducted to demonstrate the efficiency of the treatment in these clinical situations. Further studies are needed to determine the safety and long-term side effects of anti-IL-1 therapies.

Acknowledgements
Not applicable.

Authors' contributions
All authors have contributed equally to the development of the manuscript. All authors read and approved the final manuscript.

Author details
[1]Department of Internal Medicine – Rheumatology, Faculty of Medicine, Cumhuriyet University, Unit Sivas Cumhuriyet, 58140 Sivas, Turkey. [2]Department of Biostatistic, Medical Faculty, Sivas Cumhuriyet University, Sivas, Turkey.

References
1. Ozdogan H, Ugurlu S. Familial Mediterranean fever. Presse Med. 2019;48(1): e61–76. https://doi.org/10.1016/j.lpm.2018.08.014.
2. Onen F, Sumer H, Turkay S, Akyurek O, Tunca M, Ozdogan H. Increased frequency of familial Mediterranean fever in Central Anatolia, Turkey. Clin Exp Rheumatol. 2004;22(4 Suppl 34):S31–3.
3. Sari I, Birlik M, Kasifoglu T. Familial Mediterranean fever: an updated review. Eur J Rheumatol. 2014;1(1):21–33. https://doi.org/10.5152/eurjrheum.2014.006.
4. Tunca M, Akar S, Onen F, Ozdogan H, Kasapcopur O, Yalcinkaya F, et al. Familial Mediterranean fever (FMF) in Turkey: results of a nationwide multicenter study. Medicine (Baltimore). 2005;84:1–11.

Assessment of effectiveness of anakinra and canakinumab in patients with colchicine-resistant/unresponsive...

135

5. Sethi S, Theis JD. Pathology and diagnosis of renal non-AL amyloidosis. J Nephrol. 2018;31(3):343–50. https://doi.org/10.1007/s40620-017-0426-6.

6. Gül A. Approach to the patients with inadequate response to colchicine in familial Mediterranean fever. Best Pract Res Clin Rheumatol. 2016;30(2):296–303. https://doi.org/10.1016/j.berh.2016.09.001.

7. Ozen S, Demirkaya E, Erer B, Livneh A, Ben-Chetrit E, Giancane G, et al. EULAR recommendations for the management of familial Mediterranean fever. Ann Rheum Dis. 2016;75(4):644–51. https://doi.org/10.1136/annrheumdis-2015-208690.

8. Hentgen V, Grateau G, Kone-Paut I, Livneh A, Padeh S, Rozenbaum M, et al. Evidence-based recommendations for the practical management of familial Mediterranean fever. Semin Arthritis Rheum. 2013;43:387–91.

9. Akar S, Cetin P, Kalyoncu U, Karadag O, Sari I, Cınar M, et al. Nationwide experience with off-label use of Interleukin-1 targeting treatment in familial Mediterranean fever patients. Arthritis Care Res. 2018;70(7):1090–4. https://doi.org/10.1002/acr.23446.

10. Kucuksahin O, Yildizgoren MT, Ilgen U, Ates A, Kinikli G, Turgay M, et al. Anti-interleukin-1 treatment in 26 patients with refractory familial mediterranean fever. Mod Rheumatol. 2017;27(2):350–5. https://doi.org/10.1080/14397595.2016.1194510.

11. Kohler BM, Lorenz H-M, Blank N. IL1-blocking therapy in colchicine-resistant familial Mediterranean fever. Eur J Rheumatol. 2018;5(4):230–4. https://doi.org/10.5152/eurjrheum.2018.18036.

12. Topaloglu R, Batu ED, Orhan D, Ozen S, Besbas N. Anti-interleukin 1 treatment in secondary amyloidosis associated with autoinflammatory diseases. Pediatr Nephrol. 2016;31(4):633–40.

13. Özçakar ZB, Özdel S, Yılmaz S, Kurt-Şükür ED, Ekim M, Yalçınkaya F. Anti-IL-1 treatment in familial Mediterranean fever and related amyloidosis. Clin Rheumatol. 2016;35(2):441–6.

14. Varan Ö., Kucuk H., Babaoglu H., Guven SC., Ozturk MA., Haznedaroglu, et al. (2019). Efficacy and safety of interleukin-1 inhibitors in familial Mediterranean fever patients complicated with amyloidosis. Mod Rheumatol, 29(2), 363–366. https://doi.org/10.1080/14397595.2018.1457469.

15. Ugurlu S, Hacioglu A, Adibnia Y, Hamuryudan V, Ozdogan H. Tocilizumab in the treatment of twelve cases with aa amyloidosis secondary to familial mediterranean fever. Orphanet J Rare Dis. 2017;12(1):105. https://doi.org/10.1186/s13023-017-0642-0.

16. Koga T, Migita K, Kawakami A. Biologic therapy in familial Mediterranean fever. Mod Rheumatol. 2016;26(5):637–41.

17. Li Z, Akar S, Yarkan H, Lee SK, Çetin P, Can G, et al. Genome-wide association study in Turkish and Iranian populations identify rare familial Mediterranean fever gene (MEFV) polymorphisms associated with ankylosing spondylitis. PLoS Genet. 2019;15(4):e1008038. https://doi.org/10.1371/journal.pgen.1008038.

18. van der Hilst JC, Moutschen M, Messiaen PE, Lauwerys BR, Vanderschueren S. Efficacy of anti-IL-1 treatment in familial Mediterranean fever: a systematic review of the literature. Biologics. 2016;10:75–80.

19. Trabulus S, Korkmaz M, Kaya E, Seyahi N. Canakinumab treatment in kidney transplant recipients with AA amyloidosis due to familial Mediterranean fever. Clin Transpl. 2018;32(8):e13345. https://doi.org/10.1111/ctr.13345.

20. Youngstein T, Hoffmann P, Gül A, Lane T, Williams R, Rowczenio DM, et al. International multi-Centre study of pregnancy outcomes with interleukin-1 inhibitors. Rheumatology (Oxford, England). 2017;56(12):2102–8. https://doi.org/10.1093/rheumatology/kex305.

21. İlgen U, Küçükşahin O. Anakinra use during pregnancy: report of a case with familial Mediterranean fever and infertility. Eur J Rheumatol. 2017;4(1):66–7.

17

Epidemiological, clinical and immune factors that influence the persistence of antiphospholipid antibodies in leprosy

Sandra Lúcia Euzébio Ribeiro[1*], Helena Lúcia Alves Pereira[1], Antonio Luiz Boechat[2*] (iD), Neusa Pereira Silva[3], Emilia Ionue Sato[3], Maria das Graças Souza Cunha[4], Luiz Fernando de Souza Passos[1] and Maria Cristina Dos-Santos[2]

Abstract

Introduction: Antiphospholipid antibodies (aPL) are described in individuals with leprosy without the clinical features of antiphospholipid antibody syndrome (APS), a condition involving thromboembolic phenomena. We have described the persistence of these antibodies for over 5 years in patients with leprosy after specific treatment.

Objectives: To determine whether epidemiological, clinical and immunological factors played a role in the long-term persistence of aPL antibodies in leprosy patients after multidrug therapy (MDT) had finished.

Methods: The study sample consisted of 38 patients with a diagnosis of leprosy being followed up at the Dermatology and Venereology Outpatient Department at the Alfredo da Matta Foundation (FUAM) in Manaus, AM. ELISA was used to detect anticardiolipin (aCL) and anti-β_2 glycoprotein I (anti-β_2GPI) antibodies. Patients were reassessed on average of 5 years after specific treatment for the disease (MDT) had been completed.

Results: Persistence of aPL antibodies among the 38 leprosy patients was 84% (32/38), and all had the IgM isotype. Mean age was 48.1 ± 15.9 years, and 23 (72.0%) were male. The lepromatous form (LL) of leprosy was the most common ($n = 16$, 50%). Reactional episodes were observed in three patients (9.4%). Eighteen (47.37%) were still taking medication (prednisone and/or thalidomide). Mean IgM levels were 64 U/mL for aCL and 62 U/mL for anti-β_2GPI. In the multivariate binary logistic regression the following variables showed a significant association: age ($p = 0.045$, OR = 0.91 and CI 95% 0.82–0.98), LL clinical presentation ($p = 0.034$; OR = 0.02 and CI 95% = 0.0–0.76) and bacterial index ($p = 0.044$; OR = 2.74 and CI 95% = 1.03–7.33). We did not find association between prednisone or thalidomide doses and positivity for aPL ($p = 0.504$ and $p = 0.670$, respectively). No differences in the variables vascular thrombosis, pregnancy morbidity, diabetes, smoking and alcoholism were found between aPL-positive and aPL-negative patients.

Conclusion: Persistence of positivity for aPL antibodies was influenced by age, clinical presentation and bacterial index. However, further studies are needed to elucidate the reason for this persistence, the role played by aPL antibodies in the disease and the B cell lineages responsible for generation of these antibodies.

---

* Correspondence: sandraler04@gmail.com; alboechat@ufam.edu.br
[1]Department of Clinical Medicine, Federal University of Amazonas, Faculty of Health Sciences, Rua Afonso Pena, 1053, Praça 14, Manaus, AM, Brazil
[2]Department of Parasitology, Federal University of Amazonas, Immunochemistry Laboratory, Av General Rodrigo Otavio, 6200 Coroado I, Manaus, AM, Brazil
Full list of author information is available at the end of the article

Introduction

Antiphospholipid (aPL) antibodies are autoreactive immunoglobulins that are very closely related to each other and react with anionic phospholipids. Thrombosis is the most important clinical event for aPL associated syndrome. Various studies have shown aPL antibody positivity in infectious diseases [1–7] or after exposure to some drugs [8]. Under these conditions, aPL are not usually associated with the clinical complications attributed to antiphospholipid antibody syndrome (APS) [9], are often short-lasting and can disappear when the infection is treated [1, 10]. Studies of leprosy patients with aPL failed to identify an association between the presence of these antibodies and thrombotic manifestations [1, 2, 5, 7, 11, 12].

Various studies have reported aCL antibodies in leprosy patients in frequencies varying from 20 to 98% using ELISA, primarily in lepromatous leprosy [5, 11, 13–20]. In tuberculoid forms the positivity is lower and varies between 7 and 39.5% [16, 20].

The literature on positivity for anti-β_2GPI antibodies in leprosy patients is conflicting. Some authors [15, 19], reported low positivity (2.9% until 18%), while others [1, 2, 5, 11, 12], report values from 39 to 89%. IgM was the isotype most frequently found by various authors [1, 2, 5]. However, in patients with the multibacillary LL form, other authors failed to find a predominant isotype [11].

While short-term positivity for the aPL has been observed in patients with infectious diseases such as infectious mononucleosis [6] and hepatitis B [4], persistent positivity has been reported in leprosy in two studies: in one, five out of six patients were positive for anti-β_2GPI antibodies for 2 years after their initial assessment [11], and in another, 32 patients who had completed MDT were positive for aPL antibodies for more than 5 years after their initial assessment [7]. The present study therefore sought to identify which epidemiological, clinical and immune factors contribute to persistence of these antibodies.

Materials & methods
Study population

The study sample consisted of 38 patients, previously described [7] with a diagnosis of leprosy and positive for one of the antiphospholipid antibodies and were followed up at the Dermatology and Venereology Outpatient Department at the Alfredo da Matta Foundation (FUAM) in Manaus, a referral center for treatment of leprosy in the state of Amazonas, and agreed to take part in the study. Serum samples and clinical data of these patients were collected in two occasions (June 2004 to October 2006 [7] and May 2010 to November 2011), when the patients were assessed.

Blood samples and laboratory tests

To carry out the tests to detect aPLs and identify their classes (IgG or IgM), 20 mL of peripheral venous blood was collected in dry tubes from all the participants. After centrifugation, the sera were aliquoted and frozen at − 20 °C in the FUAM laboratory. They were then sent to the rheumatology laboratory at the Federal University of São Paulo (UNIFESP) and the immunology laboratory at the Federal University of Amazonas (UFAM), where the tests were carried out. The sera collected and tested in 2004 were retested in 2012 together with the sera collected in 2010 and 2011 using the same kits for aCL and for anti-β_2GPI antibodies used previously to validate the results of the earlier tests.

Anticardiolipin antibodies (aCL)

ELISA was used to measure aCL with plates prepared in-house according to a standardized protocol used in the UNIFESP rheumatology laboratory. The ELISA plates (Polysorp NUNC, USA) were first sensitized with 50 µL/well of bovine heart cardiolipin (Sigma-Aldrich, St. Louis, MO, USA) dissolved in ethanol at a concentration of 50 µg/mL and kept overnight at 4 °C. They were then blocked for 1 h with 10% adult bovine serum albumin (BSA) in PBS (BSA/PBS). Next, test and control sera diluted 1:50 in BSA/PBS were added to duplicate wells (50 mL/well), and the plates were incubated overnight at 4 °C. After three washes in PBS, alkaline phosphatase-labeled anti-human IgG or IgM (Calbiochem, La Jolla, CA, USA) diluted 1:4000 and 1:5000, respectively, was added (50 mL/well). After incubation for 90 min at room temperature, the plates were washed, p-nitrophenyl phosphate (PNPP) was added (50 µL/well) and the plates were then kept at room temperature in the dark for 30 min. Absorbances were read at 450 nm using a plate reader/spectrophotometer (Labsystems Multiskan MS). A standard curve was constructed using international standards (LAPL-GM100 IgG/IgM Calibrators, Louisville APL Diagnostics Inc., Doraville, GA, USA) and the corresponding equation determined. The mean absorbances of the samples were inserted in this equation to get the results in IgG antiphospholipid (GPL) and IgM antiphospolipid (MPL) units. Values above 20 GPL and 10 MPL, respectively, were considered to indicate positivity for IgG and IgM anti-aCL antibodies. These reference values were obtained by calculating the 95th percentile of 200 blood donor samples analyzed at the UNIFESP rheumatology laboratory.

Anti-β_2-glycoprotein antibodies (anti-β2-GPI)

IgG and IgM anti-β_2-glycoprotein I (anti-β_2GPI) antibodies were detected by ELISA using commercial kits (BINDAZYME Human Anti-β_2GPI IgG and Anti-β_2GPI IgM, The Binding Site, Birmingham, UK) in accordance with the manufacturer's instructions. The reaction was quenched by adding 100 mL of stop solution to each well, and absorbances were then read at 450 nm using a plate reader (Labsystems Multiskan MS).

A standard curve was plotted using the standards supplied with the kit, and the corresponding equation was then used to convert the absorbances of the samples to U/mL. Values above 20 U/mL and 10 U/mL, respectively, were considered to indicate positivity for IgG and IgM anti-β_2GPI antibodies.

Statistical analysis

The statistical analysis was performed with R version 2.14.0 (New Zealand). For the descriptive analysis the mean, median, standard deviation (SD) and minimum and maximum values were used for continuous variables and the proportions for categorical variables. The binomial test was used to assess differences in the distribution of the data.

To assess the possible factors that caused sera to test negative for aPL antibodies during the observation period, Pearson's chi-squared test was used for categorical variables and the Mann-Whitney test for continuous variables. Multivariate binary logistic regression was used in the first model, in which the dependent variable was the categorical variable aPL (1 = negative for aPL; 0 = positive for aPL) and the independent variables were gender (1 = male; 2 = female), age (continuous), lepromatous clinical presentation (1 = LL; 0 = other forms), prednisone use (1 = used; 0 = not used) and thalidomide use (1 = used, 0 = not used). In the second model, an adjustment was made for the different thalidomide or prednisone doses as continuous variables to determine whether they were associated with a change in reactivity from positive to negative. To assess whether the initial bacterial index affected positivity for the antibodies, binary logistic regression was used, with each antibody (aCL or anti-β_2GPI) included in the model as dependent variables and the initial bacterial index as the continuous independent variable. The Hosmer-Lemeshow test was used to assess the goodness of fit of the models. Logistic regression was performed with MiniTab® 16.

As the patients in this study were assessed at different times since they had been diagnosed with the disease, the hypothesis tested was that persistence of positivity for aPL would depend on the clinical presetnation of the disease (LL and the other forms, BT, BB and BV). The graphs were generated with GraphPad Prisma 6.02.

Results

Patient clinical and demographic features

The study sample consisted of 38 patients with a diagnosis of leprosy and positive aPL. Mean age was 46.42 ± 16.62 years. Twenty-eight (73.6%) of the patients were

male, and ten (26.3%) female. A test of proportions indicated that the difference in gender distribution was significant ($p = 0.005$). There are two main types of reactional episodes in Hansen patients. The Type 1 reactional episodes includes new skin lesions or neuritis and the Type 2 is mainly characterized by erythema nodosum leprosum (ENL). During the last clinical evaluation, no patients were observed with reactional episodes, however reactions were observed in four patients (10.5%) during the study. Among them four presented with erythema nodosum leprosum (ENL) and were taking thalidomide and prednisone, and one presented with neuritis and was taking prednisone (20 mg). Eighteen (47.37%) were using some medication, six were taking prednisone, four were taking thalidomide and eight both medications.

A significant difference was observed in the distribution of the clinical presentations in the 38 patients. The LL form was the most common clinical presentation ($p = 0.026$) and was found in 16 (50%) of the patients. The BT and BV forms were found in eight patients (25%) and seven patients (21.87%), respectively.

All 38 patients had completed MDT. Mean and median time between completion of MDT and blood collection was 87.00 and 67.50 months, respectively, with a maximum and minimum of 9 and 174 months. One patient had a relapse in 2009 but had already completed the treatment 9 months previously when the serum was collected. Mean and median time between the first and second collections were 66.89 and 66.10 months, respectively, with a minimum and maximum of 53.43 and 86.83 months.

Laboratory assessment of patients

The 38 sera positive for aPL antibodies in the first analysis (sera collected in 2004/2006) were retested at the same time with the sera collected in 2010/2011. All sera were tested for anti-β_2GPI antibodies, and for aCL antibodies (patients that were positive in 2004/2006). Of the retested sera, 37 (97.4%) remained positive for one of the aPLs and one (2.6%), who had previously been positive for anti-β_2GPI, was negative. At the new samples collected (2010/2011) 32 (84.2%) remained positive and six (15.8%) became negative.

aCL antibody was only detected in patients with the BV and LL clinical presentation. Of the nine patients positive for aCL antibody at the retest serum from 2004/2006, all of whom had the LL clinical presentation, two patients became negative in 2010/2011 sera. The anti-β_2GPI antibody was quantified in patients with the BT, BB, BV and LL clinical presentations both at the retest (serum from 2004) and in serum from 2010/2011. Positivity for this antibody was lower in the serum collected in 2010/2011 for all clinical presentations.

IgM was found more frequently than IgG in the three analyses of the sera. Of the nine patients retested for aCL antibody, seven were positive for IgM, and two for IgG and IgM. At the sera collected in 2010/2011, two became negative and seven remained positive for IgM. Of the 37 patients retested for the anti-β_2GPI antibody, 35 were positive for IgM, one was positive for IgG and IgM and one patient who had been positive for IgG became negative. Of the three patients who were positive for IgG and IgM, two became negative for IgG but remained positive for IgM. Thirty-one of the sera collected in 2010/2011 remained positive for anti-β_2GPI antibody, but only IgM was detected. Among patients positive for aCL antibodies the mean concentration of aCL antibodies was 74.3 U/mL in the retested serum in 2012 and 64.6 U/mL in the serum collected in 2010/2011. The concentrations of anti-β_2GPI antibodies were 67.7 and 62.5 U/mL, respectively.

Among nine patients positive for aCL antibodies at the retest, seven (77.8%) had IgM antibody titers > 40 U/mL (mean concentration = 88 MPL). Among seven, six (85.7%) still had IgM titers > 40 U/mL in 2010/2011 sera, with a mean aCL antibody concentration of 70.8 MPL. Anti-β_2GPI titers > 40 U/mL were found in 12/37 sera (32.4%) that were positive at the retest. One was IgG (159 U/mL), and 11 IgM. In the sera collected in 2010/2011 six of the 12 still had high concentrations.

Among patients positive for aPL antibodies with titers > 40 U/mL, the LL form was the predominant form among patients positive for anti-β_2GPI and aCL antibodies at the retest and in sera collected in 2010/2011. Among seven patients positive for aCL antibodies, six (85.7%) were also positive for anti-β_2GPI antibodies.

Considering the sera collected in 2010/2011, 32/38 (84.2%) were positive for aPL antibodies (aCL and anti-β_2GPI) and six (15.8%) were negative. Among 32, one was positive for the aCL antibody, 25 (78.1%) for the anti-β_2GPI antibody and six (18.8%) for both antibodies. We did not find difference on demographic and clinical characteristics between positive and negative individuals (Table 1). Similarly, no difference was observed regarding other clinical variables for these 38 patients between positive and negative individuals (Table 2). There was no association between demographic and clinical characteristics and titers for one of the aPL antibodies > 40 U/mL (eight – 25.0%) or ≤ 40 U/mL (24–75.0%), in the 32 patients. There was no difference in the frequencies of the clinical variables in patients with aPL antibody titers above 40 U/mL and in those with titers below 40 U/mL.

Table 3 shows that for the first multivariate binary logistic regression model (model 1), the variables age (p = 0.045, OR = 0.91 and 95% CI 0.82–0.98) and LL clinical presentation (p = 0.034; OR = 0.02 and 95% CI = 0.0–0.76) reduced the likelihood of patients becoming

Table 1 Demographic and clinical characteristics of the 38 leprosy patients according to aPL positivity or negativity on sera collected in 2010/2011

Variables	Serum aPL (2010/2011 collected sera)						p
	Negative		Positive		Total		
	n	%	n	%	N	%	
Gender							0.670*
Male	5	83.3%	23	71.9%	28	73.7%	
Female	1	16.7%	9	28.1%	10	26.3%	
Age	37.0 ± 18.2		48.1 ± 16.0		46.3 ± 16.6		0.075**
Length of treatment	81.2 ± 18.3		77.4 ± 36.5		80.0 ± 34.1		0.389**
Clinical presentations							0.081*
BT	1	16.7%	8	25.0%	9	23.7%	
BB	2	33.3%	1	3.1%	3	7.9%	
BV	2	33.3%	7	21.9%	9	23.7%	
LL	1	16.7%	16	50.0%	17	44.7%	
Reactional episodes							1*
Present	0	0.0%	1	3.1%	3	7.9%	
Absent	6	100.0%	31	96.9%	35	92.1%	
Current reactional episodes							1*
Present	1	16.7%	3	9.4%	4	10.5%	
Absent	5	83.3%	29	90.6%	34	89.5%	
Medication							0.188*
No	5	83.3%	15	46.9%	20	52.6%	
Yes	1	16.7%	17	53.1%	18	47.4%	
Prednisone							0.278*
No	0	0.0%	4	23.5%	4	22.2%	
Yes	1	100.0%	13	76.5%	14	77.8%	
Thalidomide							0.387*
No	0	0.0%	6	35.3%	6	33.3%	
Yes	1	100.0%	11	64.7%	12	66.7%	

* Chi-square test ** Mann-Whitney Test

negative for aPL antibodies. The likelihood of older patients becoming negative for aPL antibodies is lower. Prednisone or thalidomide use and dose did not influence the change from positive to negative reactivity for aPL antibodies even when the model was adjusted for the doses of these two drugs (model 2) (p = 0.504; p = 0.670, respectively).

Table 4 shows that the initial bacterial index influenced positivity for aCL antibodies (p = 0.043; OR = 2.75) and anti-β_2GPI antibodies (p = 0.044; OR = 2.46). The initial (diagnostic) and current bacterial indices were grouped according to whether the patient was positive or negative for aPL antibodies using the Kruskal-Wallis test (p < 0.0001) and Dunn's test for multiple comparisons. Figure 1 shows that the diagnostic and initial bacterial index is greater in individuals positive for aPL antibodies (p = 0.029 and 0.012, respectively).

Table 2 Clinical variables for the 38 leprosy patients broken down according to aPL antibody positivity or negativity at the sera collected in 2010/2011

Variables	Serum aPL (2010/2011 collected sera)						p-value
	Negative		Positive		Total		
	N	%	n	%	N	%	
Vascular Thrombosis							1*
No	6	100.0%	31	96.9%	37	97.4%	
Yes	0	0.0%	1	3.1%	1	2.6%	
Pregnancy Morbidity							1*
No	6	100.0%	31	96.9%	37	97.4%	
Yes	0	0.0%	1	3.1%	1	2.6%	
Diabetes							1*
No	6	100.0%	30	93.8%	36	94.7%	
Yes	0	0.0%	2	6.3%	2	5.3%	
Smoking							0.670*
No	3	50.0%	20	62.5%	23	60.5%	
Yes	3	50.0%	12	37.5%	15	29.5%	
Alcoholism							0.315*
No	5	83.3%	31	96.9%	36	94.7%	
Yes	1	16.7%	1	3.1%	2	5.3%	

*Chi-square test

Discussion

The sample in this study consisted of outpatients with various forms of leprosy at a referral center for leprosy in the state of Amazonas. Most of the subjects had lepromatous leprosy, did not present with reactions and had completed specific MDT a long time previously (mean 78.0 months). The interval between the first and second blood collection was 66.9 months on average.

Table 3 Results of multivariate binary logistic regression to assess probable factors causing leprosy patients to become negative for aPL antibodies

Predictor	95% CI	Odds ratio (OR)	p-value
Model 1			
Age	0.82–0.98	0.91	0.045
Gender	0.0–2.84	0.11	0.185
Lepromatous form	0.0–0.76	0.02	0.034
Prednisone use	0.0–4.88	0.09	0.237
Thalidomide use	0.01–14.7	0.44	0.647
Model 2			
Age	0.84–0.97	0.92	0.044
Female	0.0–2.16	0.08	0.134
Lepromatous form	0.0–0.92	0.03	0.044
Prednisone dose	0.71–1.18	0.92	0.504
Thalidomide dose	0.95–1.03	0.99	0.670

Table 4 Results of binary logistic regression to assess the influence of initial bacterial index on presence of aPL antibodies in 38 leprosy patients

Model	95% CI	Odds ratio (OR)	p-value
aCL vs. Initial Bacterial Index 1	1.03–7.33	2.75	0.043
Anti-β2GPI vs. Initial Bacterial Index 2	1.02–5.58	2.46	0.044
aPL vs. Initial Bacterial Index 3	1.03–7.33	2.74	0.044

According to some authors, aPL antibodies in leprosy are often transient and can disappear after treatment [1, 10]. However, in the previous study of our group, in which 158 leprosy patients were followed up, positivity for aPL antibodies was not affected by time since completion of MDT, and titers remained high for months and years afterwards. No evidence was found to suggest that the presence of aPL antibodies is a transient phenomenon [5]. A longitudinal study with these patients was therefore undertaken to assess the persistence of these autoantibodies, which was confirmed by the findings of the study [7]. In the present study, several factors that could contribute to this finding, such as the epidemiological, clinical and immune characteristics of the disease, were investigated comparing patients that were positive or negative for aPL antibodies. The predominance of males among the patients in our study agrees with the literature, according to which detection rates in most countries apart from some countries in Africa are twice as high in men as in women [21].

Because there was a trend toward a statistically significant association between some variables, such as clinical presentation ($p = 0.081$), age ($p = 0.075$) and treatment ($p = 0.188$), when $p < 0.2$ was used to indicate a trend toward statistical significance [22], we performed multiple logistic regression adjusted for gender. This revealed that persistence of positivity for aPL antibodies was influenced independently by age, bacterial index and the LL clinical presentation. The data show that more advanced age tends to increase the likelihood of the patient being positive for aPL antibodies, possibly because of cumulative exposure to antigens of mycobacteria and other bacteria or because of immune system aging, which prevents complete elimination of *M. leprae*. Persistence was observed predominantly in leprosy patients with the LL form, whose sera collected in 2010/2011 had titers greater than 40 U/mL (77.8% for aCL and 32.4% for anti-β2GPI).

The persistence of the IgM isotype suggests the T-cell independent nature of the response to these non-peptide antigens, which are recognized by B1 B and MZ B (splenic marginal-zone B) cells. These antigens generally

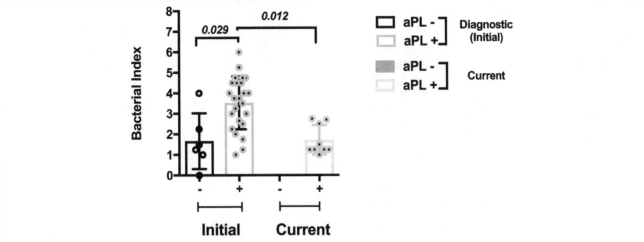

Fig. 1 Initial bacterial index (2004) and current bacterial index (2010/2011) according to positivity or negativity for aPL antibodies in 38 leprosy patients

include sugars and glycolipids that induce production of low-affinity IgM antibodies and rarely induce a class switch to IgG. Cardiolipin is a membrane phospholipid found in bacterial (including mycobacterial) membrane. Thus, it is probable that in the LL clinical presentations, which has a higher bacterial index, the *M. leprae* membrane phospholipids are recognized by B1 or MZ B cells as extracellular phase antigens at the bloodstream. Interestingly, the complement system can be activated by the presence of M. leprae in tissues, leading to the production of C3d, which is required for B-cell activation. It is also curious that bacteria in the intestine and urinary tract such as *Escherichia coli* contain cardiolipin in their membrane, suggesting that natural IgM aCL antibodies can be found in healthy individuals [23, 24].

Our results strongly indicate that the initial bacterial index influenced positivity for aPL antibodies. It is therefore reasonable to suppose that *M. leprae* persists in latent, or inactive, form in the human body even after treatment, particularly in individuals with the LL clinical presentations, who supposedly have a Th2 response. Latency is an acknowledged phenomenon in infections by mycobacteria, as suggested by the reactivation of tuberculosis when a "cured" infected person is severely immunosuppressed [25]. Spirochetes, bacteria of the genus Borrelia and viruses, particularly those in the family Herpesviridae, can also exhibit latency [26, 27]. The presence of reactional episodes and prolonged use of prednisone or thalidomide support persistence of the pathogen, albeit in inactive form, and suggest discrete interaction with the immune system. A noteworthy finding of the present study is that the treatment did not influence positivity and that the most important factor appears to be the bacterial load.

Some potential limitation of this study should be noted. Since this was an observational study in design,

the inference and causality are limited. Moreover, some marginal associations may not be significant due to the relatively small number of patients retested. New information was recorded for the patients that lost follow-up and were not evaluated for a second time. This could affect the sensitivity of the study to detect thrombosis and APS. However, the incidence rate for APS is expected to low for adults over 18-years old as 2.1% [28], and this probably did not affect the present results.

Conclusion
As in APS, IgM aPL antibodies are common in leprosy patients and persist for long periods in these individuals but without thromboembolic manifestations. Further studies are needed to elucidate the reason for this persistence, the role played by aPL antibodies in the disease and the B-lymphocyte lineages responsible for production of these antibodies. This knowledge would help to improve our understanding of the immunological mechanisms involved in the interaction between *M. leprae* and the human host.

Acknowledgements
Nothing to declare.

Authors' contributions
SLER design of the project, main responsible by ethics approval and data collection. HLAP: was co-responsible by data collection and design of the project. ALB: data analysis and interpretation. NPS: laboratory assays. EIS, NPS, LFSP and MCS: design of the project. SLER, ALB, MCS: writing of the manuscript. All authors read and approved the final manuscript.

Author details
[1]Department of Clinical Medicine, Federal University of Amazonas, Faculty of Health Sciences, Rua Afonso Pena, 1053, Praça 14, Manaus, AM, Brazil. [2]Department of Parasitology, Federal University of Amazonas, Immunochemistry Laboratory, Av General Rodrigo Otavio, 6200 Coroado I, Manaus, AM, Brazil. [3]Division of Rheumatology, Escola Paulista de Medicina, Federal University of São Paulo, São Paulo, Brazil. [4]Alfredo da Matta Foundation, Manaus, Amazonas, Brazil.

References

1. de Larrañaga GF, Forastiero RR, Martinuzzo ME, et al. High prevalence of antiphospholipid antibodies in leprosy: evaluation of antigen reactivity. Lupus. 2000;9(8):594–600.

2. Loizou S, Cazabon JK, Walport MJ, Tait D, So AK. Similarities of specificity and cofactor dependence in serum antiphospholipid antibodies from patients with human parvovirus B19 infection and from those with systemic lupus erythematosus. Arthritis Rheum. 1997;40(1):103–8.

3. Landenberg Von P, Lehmann HW, Knöll A, Dorsch S, Modrow S. Antiphospholipid antibodies in pediatric and adult patients with rheumatic disease are associated with parvovirus B19 infection. Arthritis Rheum. 2003; 48(7):1939–47.

4. Huh JY, Yi DY, Hwang SG, Choi JJ, Kang MS. Characterization of antiphospholipid antibodies in chronic hepatitis B infection. Korean J Hematol. 2011;46(1):36–40.

5. Ribeiro SL, Pereira HL, Silva NP, Souza AW, Sato EI. Anti-β2-glycoprotein I antibodies are highly prevalent in a large number of Brazilian leprosy patients. Acta Reumatol Port. 2011;36(1):30–7.

6. Ben-Chetrit E, Wiener-Well Y, Fadeela A, Wolf DG. Antiphospholipid antibodies during infectious mononucleosis and their long term clinical significance. J Clin Virol. 2013;56(4):312–5.

7. Ribeiro SLE, Pereira HLA, Silva NP, Sato EI, Passos LFS, dos MC S. Long-term persistence of anti-β2 glycoprotein I in treated leprosy patients. Lupus. 2014;23(12):1249–51.

8. Cervera R, Asherson RA. Clinical and epidemiological aspects in the antiphospholipid syndrome. Immunobiology. 2003;207(1):5–11.

9. Roubey RA. Immunology of the antiphospholipid antibody syndrome. Arthritis Rheum. 1996;39(9):1444–54.

10. Carreras LO, Forastiero RR, Martinuzzo ME. Which are the best biological markers of the antiphospholipid syndrome? J Autoimmun. 2000;15(2):163–72.

11. Arvieux J, Renaudineau Y, Mane I, Perraut R, Krilis SA, Youinou P. Distinguishing features of anti-beta2 glycoprotein I antibodies between patients with leprosy and the antiphospholipid syndrome. Thromb Haemost. 2002;87(4):599–605.

12. Forastiero RR, Martinuzzo ME, de Larrañaga GF. Circulating levels of tissue factor and proinflammatory cytokines in patients with primary antiphospholipid syndrome or leprosy related antiphospholipid antibodies. Lupus. 2005;14(2):129–36.

13. Furukawa F, Kashihara M, Imamura S, Ohshio G, Hamashima Y. Evaluation of anti-cardiolipin antibody and its cross-reactivity in sera of patients with lepromatous leprosy. Arch Dermatol Res. 1986;278(4):317–9.

14. Santiago MB, Cossermelli W, Tuma MF, Pinto MN, Oliveira RM. Anticardiolipin antibodies in patients with infectious diseases. Clin Rheumatol. 1989;8(1):23–8.

15. Hojnik M, Gilburd B, Ziporen L, et al. Anticardiolipin antibodies in infections are heterogenous in their dependency on beta 2-glycoprotein I: analysis of anticardiolipin antibodies in leprosy. Lupus. 1994;3(6):515–21.

16. Thawani G, Bhatia VN, Mukherjee A. Anticardiolipin antibodies in leprosy. Indian J Lepr. 1994;66(3):307–14.

17. Fiallo P, Nunzi E, Cardo PP. beta2-glycoprotein I-dependent anticardiolipin antibodies as risk factor for reactions in borderline leprosy patients. Int J Lepr Other Mycobact Dis. 1998;66(3):387–8.

18. Fiallo P, Travaglino C, Nunzi E, Cardo PP. Beta 2-glycoprotein I-dependence of anticardiolipin antibodies in multibacillary leprosy patients. Lepr Rev. 1998;69(4):376–81.

19. Elbeialy A, Strassburger-Lorna K, Atsumi T, et al. Antiphospholipid antibodies in leprotic patients: a correlation with disease manifestations. Clin Exp Rheumatol. 2000;18(4):492–4.

20. Repka JCD, Skare TL, Salles Jr G, Paul GM. Anticardiolipin antibodies in leprosy patients. Braz J Rheumatol. 2001;41(1):1–6.

21. Le Grand A. Women and leprosy: a review. Lepr Rev. 1997;68(3):203–11.

22. Riffenburgh RH. Statistics in medicine. 30th ed. London: Elsevier; 2012.

23. Milner ECB, Anolik J, Cappione A, Sanz I. Human innate B cells: a link between host defense and autoimmunity? Springer Semin Immunopathol. 2005;26(4):433–52.

24. Spencer JS, Brennan PJ. The role of mycobacterium leprae phenolic glycolipid I (PGL-I) in serodiagnosis and in the pathogenesis of leprosy. Lepr Rev. 2011;82(4):344–57.

25. Gupta A, Kaul A, Tsolaki AG, Kishore U, Bhakta S. Mycobacterium tuberculosis: immune evasion, latency and reactivation. Immunobiology. 2012;217(3):363–74.

26. Albert S, Schulze J, Riegel H, Brade V. Lyme arthritis in a 12-year-old patient after a latency period of 5 years. Infection. 1999;27(4–5):286–8.

27. White DW, Suzanne Beard R, Barton ES. Immune modulation during latent herpesvirus infection. Immunol Rev. 2012;245(1):189–208.

28. Duarte-Garcia A, Pham M, Crowson CS et al. The epidemiology of antiphospholipid syndrome: a population based study. Arthritis Rheum.

18

Incidence of Cytomegalovirus Antigenemia in patients with autoimmune rheumatic diseases: A 3-year retrospective study

Rebeka Paulo Santos[1] (iD), Edgard Torres dos Reis-Neto[1] (iD) and Marcelo Medeiros Pinheiro[1,2]* (iD)

Abstract

Objective: To determine the incidence of positive CMV antigenemia (CMV-Ag) in patients with autoimmune rheumatic diseases (AIRD) and to describe the outcomes of these patients.

Methods: From January 2011 to December 2014, a total of 443 patients with AIRD were enrolled in this retrospective analysis. Demographic, clinical and laboratory data, current clinical manifestations, organs affected by CMV infection, therapeutic management and outcomes were evaluated. The CMV-Ag was considered positive when one cell was detected at least.

Results: CMV-Ag was requested in 70 (15.8%) patients with suspicious CMV infection and was positive in 24 (34.3%). The incidence rate of positive CMV-Ag was 4.97% (95% CI 3.1–7.4%). Systemic lupus erythematosus (SLE) (59%), followed by ANCA-related vasculitis (18.2%) and rheumatoid arthritis (9%) were the diseases more associated with positive CMV-Ag. At the time of CMV infection, SLE patients had moderate to severe disease activity, with high frequency of positive anti-dsDNA antibody (69.2%) and complement consumption (61.5%), as well as high doses of corticosteroids and use of immunosuppressants. The main CMV sites involved were lung (45.5%), bone marrow (40.9%) and gut (27.3%). Mortality rate was 45.5%, especially in those with higher doses of daily oral corticosteroids (107 ± 55.4 mg vs. 71.7 ± 46.3 mg; $p = 0.07$) and lower number of lymphocytes ($309 \pm 368.2/mm^3$ vs. $821 \pm 692.9/mm^3$; $p = 0.06$).

Conclusions: Our data showed high incidence of CMV-Ag in AIRD patients, particularly those with SLE and greater disease severity. In addition, it was observed high mortality in these patients, highlighting the CMV infection should be included in differential diagnosis.

Keywords: Cytomegalovirus, Infection, Antigenemia, Autoimmunity, Incidence

Introduction

Cytomegalovirus (CMV) is related to opportunistic infections in immunocompromised patients with autoimmune rheumatic diseases (AIRD) [1, 2]. Several studies have highlighted its pathogenic role in triggering or hampering some AIRD [3]. In immunocompromised individuals, the reactivation of latent CMV infection may cause fever, chills, weight loss, asthenia, hematological disorders (anemia, leukopenia, and thrombocytopenia) or severe symptomatic organ involvement, including hepatitis, chorioretinitis, encephalitis, pneumonitis and digestive hemorrhage [4].

The CMV antigenemia (CMV-Ag) is the main method for the diagnosis of infection due its high sensitivity (91%) and specificity (95%), as well as early and fast detection and therapeutic monitoring by number of affected cells [3]. On the other hand, it has some limitations, such as neutropenia below $1000/mm^3$ (false-negative) and other tests should be necessary for a better diagnosis [5, 6].

There are some epidemiological data and management guidance addressed to immunosuppressed patients, including AIDS and after solid organ and bone marrow transplantation [7–11]. However, there is a lack of evidence in patients with AIRD and the recommendations

* Correspondence: mpinheiro@uol.com.br
[1]Division of Rheumatology, Universidade Federal de São Paulo, São Paulo, SP, Brazil
[2]Disciplina de Reumatologia, Escola Paulista de Medicina – Universidade Federal de São Paulo, Rua Leandro, Dupré, 204, conjunto 74, Vila Clementino, São Paulo, SP 04025-010, Brazil

for managing these patients are extrapolated from transplantation data [12].

Thus, the aim of this study was to evaluate the incidence of CMV-Ag and describe the main outcomes over time in AIRD patients.

Patients and methods
Patients
Patients admitted to the rheumatology service at a tertiary university hospital in São Paulo/ SP, Brazil, from 01/JAN/ 2011 to 31/DEC/2014, were analyzed and those with clinical CMV suspicion infection and positive CMV-Ag for one cell, at least, were included. A total of 443 patients with AIRD were enrolled in this retrospective analysis. Patients with other viral infections, including hepatitis B and C, HIV, and Epstein-Barr were excluded. The positive CMV-Ag was defined when one cell was detected at least.

Clinical evaluation
Demographic, clinical and laboratory data were recorded for all patients. Specific details of each AIRD and current clinical manifestations, including disease activity, organs affected by CMV infection, therapeutic management (initial and secondary prophylaxis) and outcomes were also explored. For assessment of disease activity were used the *Systemic Lupus Erythematosus Disease Activiy Index* (SLEDAI) for SLE [13] and *Birmingham Vasculitis Activity Score* (BVAS) for ANCA associated vasculitis [14].

Laboratory evaluation of the CMV viremia
CMV-pp65 antigen detection was undertaken by the monoclonal antibody indirect immunofluorescence (IF) method (CMV Brite Turbo Kit, IQ Products, Gronigen, The Netherlands). The number of leukocytes stained positive every 200,000 neutrophils in peripheral blood was then documented.

Quantitation of CMV-DNA was undertaken by real-time fluorescence quantitative polymerase chain reaction (RT-PCR-fluorecence) technology (CMV nuclei acid quantitative assay kit, TaqMan® Roche – FAM, Branchburg, USA) when available. The criteria for positive result was CMV-DNA ≥ 500copies/ml. Viral inclusion bodies found in the tissue biopsy, stained with hematoxylin-eosin, were also considered positive for CMV infection.

Definition of CMV disease and follow-up protocol
Patients with laboratory abnormalities (anemia, leukopenia, thrombocytopenia or liver enzymes) or clinical manifestations, such as fever, gut or eye symptoms or lung injury, excluding other infection causes, were considered as suspicious symptomatic for CMV infection. CMV disease was defined when the confirmation had been performed by biopsy and identification of positive viral inclusion corpuscles or immunohistochemistry of affected organ.

After treatment with antivirals, patients had CMV-Ag repeated weekly until becoming negative. This outcome was defined as improvement of CMV infection.

Statistical analysis
All analyses were proceeded using SPSS 20.0 (*IBM, New York, USA*). Shapiro-Wilk or Kolmogorov-Smirnov tests were applied to assess the normality of the variables. To compare continuous variables, Student-t test or Mann-Whitney test were used. Pearson and Spearman correlation tests were used to analyse the correlation between variables. Categorical data were analyzed by chi-square test or Fisher's exact test. Significant variables in the univariate analysis or correlation tests were used for tailoring the multivariate regression models in which the positive CMV-Ag was considered as dependent variable and all other as independent, in order to explore main prognostic factors. Besides, ROC analysis was performed to determine the absolute cut-off value of the positive CMV-Ag related to death. P value below 0.05 was set as significant.

This study was approved by the Ethics and Research Committee of Hospital São Paulo / Unifesp (506.406).

Results
From 443 patients with AIRD hospitalized in a tertiary university center, the CMV-Ag was requested to 70 (15.8%) patients with suspicious CMV infection and it was positive in 24 (34.3%).

Two positive CMV-Ag were excluded because one patient had cutaneous lupus (not systemic) and the other had Behcet's disease whose clinical manifestation of possible viral infection (acute diarrhea) was attributed later to adverse event by using of colchicine. Thus, 22 patients with AIRD and positive CMV-Ag were evaluated (Fig. 1). The incidence global rate of the positive CMV-Ag was 4.97% (95% CI 3.1 to 7.4%). Considering only lupus hospitalized patients, the CMV-Ag rate was 16.5% (95% CI 9.7 to 51.9%).

The main sites involved by CMV infection were lung, bone marrow and gut. Tables 1 and 2 show the main characteristics of AIRD patients with positive CMV-Ag. Lupus patients were younger than those with other AIRD (29.1 ± 13.4 years vs. 54.2 ± 21.1 years; $p = 0.03$). In addition, the majority of patients had high disease activity associated with severe infection, such as lupus patients (SLEDAI = 15.3 ± 9) and patients with ANCA-associated vasculitis (BVAS = 5.2 ± 3.8).

The length of hospital stay (11.5 ± 12 days) was long and there was a delay time between the beginning of symptoms and the CMV-Ag has been requested (7.8 ± 7.1 days). Besides, 16 (72.7%) patients had co-infections with other antimicrobial agents, such as *Candida albicans* and *Acinetobacter baumannii*, and there were five cases of polymicrobial infections.

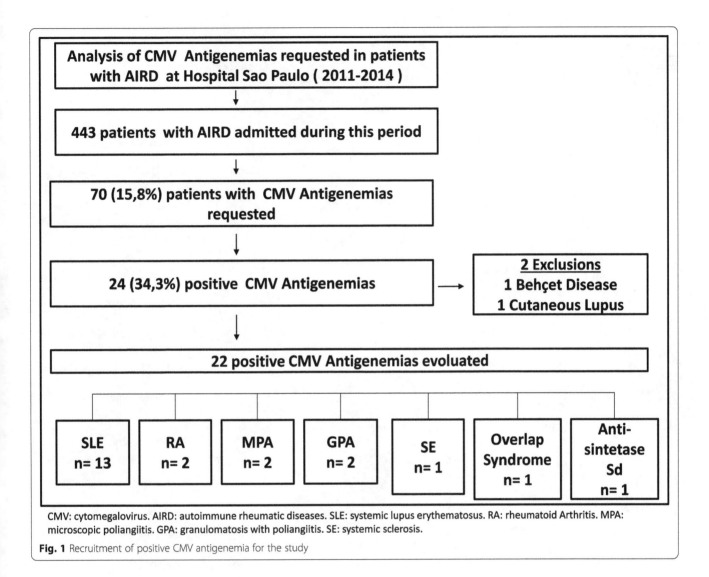

CMV: cytomegalovirus. AIRD: autoimmune rheumatic diseases. SLE: systemic lupus erythematosus. RA: rheumatoid Arthritis. MPA: microscopic poliangiitis. GPA: granulomatosis with poliangiitis. SE: systemic sclerosis.

Fig. 1 Recruitment of positive CMV antigenemia for the study

Regarding the treatment for AIRD, 19 (86.4%) patients used corticosteroid (up to 1 mg/ kg/ day of prednisone or equivalent) and 11 (50%) patients used other immunosuppressants drugs during hospitalization, including cyclophosphamide.

Concerning the treatment for CMV, 15 (68.2%) of them received ganciclovir. In general, these patients tended to have more positive cells than those untreated [16 (1–500) vs. 1 (1–4); $p = 0.05$]. Only three patients reported adverse events related to ganciclovir, including cutaneous and cytopenia reaction.

Lupus patients had greater number of positive CMV-Ag than other AIRD. These patients were using high doses of corticosteroids and had received methylprednisolone pulse therapy in the last 6 months prior to infection. Moreover, the median time of disease was only 12 months (0–276), suggesting higher likely of viremia and CMV involvement in early disease. They had higher predominance of joint, kidney and hematological involvement, as well as higher positivity for anti-dsDNA antibody (69.2%) and complement consumption (61.5%). Few lupus patients had cutaneous or neurological involvement.

The mortality rate was 45.4% (10 deaths in total: 4 in SLE patients; 3 in patients with ANCA-associated vasculitis, 1 patient had systemic sclerosis, 1 with RA and other with overlap syndrome). Three deaths were observed between the seven patients who did not receive specific treatment for CMV, although not significant.

After assessing the risk factors for death, there was no difference among patients who survived or died regarding to age, average number of positive cells on antigenemia, site of virus involvement, hospitalization, symptoms until the first CMV-Ag be requested and pulse therapy in the last 6 months. However, there was a tendency to higher doses of oral corticosteroids (107 ± 55.4 mg/day vs. 71.7 ± 46.3 mg/ day; $p = 0.07$) and lower number of lymphocytes when patients who died were compared to those who survived ($309 \pm 368.2/$ mm^3 vs. $821 \pm 692.9/$ mm^3; $p = 0.06$). Moreover, the surviving patients remained hospitalized for longer time than those who died (24.3 ± 23.9 days vs. 56.6 ± 35.1 days; $p = 0.017$) (Table 3).

Table 1 Clinical and laboratory data of 22 patients with autoimmune rheumatic disease (AIRD) and positive cytomegalovirus antigenemia

Patient	Age (years)/ Sex	AIRD	Immunosuppressive therapy in hospital	Lymphocyte Count (/μl)	Positive CMV antigenemia nuclei (/200.000PMN)	Sites involved by CMV infection	Symptoms	Outcome
1	67/F	SLE	CFA, PDN 130 mg/day	1311	32	Gut	Esophageal ulcers	Death
2	34/F	SLE	AZA, CFA, PDN 80 mg/day	1356	1	Lung	Cough, dyspnea, fever	Improvement
3	17/F	SLE	PDN 200 mg/day	444	2	Cytopenia	Neutropenia, Thrombocytopenia	Improvement
4	22/F	SLE	PDN 60 mg/day	695	5	Gut	Mouth ulcers	Improvement
5	21/F	SLE	PDN 60 mg/day	135	500	Cytopenia / Lung	Trombocyotpenia, Cough, dyspnea, fever	Death
6	25/F	SLE	PDN 180 mg/day	525	1	Lung	Cough, dyspnea, fever	Death
7	16/F	SLE	MP + CFA, PDN 50 mg/day	850	108	Cytopenia	Febrile neutropenia	Improvement
8	20/F	SLE	MP + CFA, PDN 60 mg/day	792	1	Gut	Esophageal ulcers	Improvement
9	38/F	SLE	PDN 60 mg/day	2751	2	Lung	Cough, dyspnea, fever	Improvement
10	30/F	SLE	CFA, PDN 60 mg/day	659	2	Cytopenia	Pancytopenia, fever	Death
11	25/F	SLE	MMF, MP, PDN 50 mg/day	853	164	Cytopenia	Anemia, Thrombocytopenia	Improvement
12	37/F	SLE	PDN 60 mg/day	80	46	Cytopenia /Gut	Anemia, diarrhea	Improvement
13	26/F	SLE	MP + CFA, PDN 90 mg/day	714	2	Lung	Cough, dyspnea	Improvement
14	77/F	SE	–	125	1	Cytopenia	Pancytopenia, fever	Death
15	29/M	Overlap Sd.	PDN160mg/day	246	16	Lung	Cough, dyspnea	Death
16	70/M	RA	MP, PDN 20 mg/day	77	1	Cytopenia	Pancytopenia, fever	Improvement
17	17/M	RA	PDN 160 mg/day	689	1	Lung	Cough, dyspnea	Death
18	42/F	MPA	PDN 100 mg/day	197	4	Lung	Cough, dyspnea, Fever	Death
19	77/F	MPA	PDN 100 mg/day	372	500	Cytopenia / Lung	Anemia, Leukopenia, Cough, Fever	Death
20	63/F	GPA	CFA, PDN 30 mg/day	857	9	Gut	Gastric ulcer	Improvement
21	58/M	GPA	AZA, MP, PDN 120 mg/day	213	73	Gut	Gastric ulcer	Death
22	55/F	Anti-sintetase Sd.	CFA, PDN 100 mg/day	975	7	Lung	Cough, dyspnea	Improvement

CMV cytomegalovirus, *SLE* Systemic Lupus Erythematosus, *SE* Systemic sclerosis, *Overlap syndrome* Systemic Lupus Erythematosus + Systemic sclerosis + polymyositis, *RA* rheumatoid arthritis, *MPA* microscopic polyangiitis, *GPA* granulomatosis with polyangiitis, *F* Female, *M*, Male, *AIRD* autoimmune rheumatic disease, *PDN* Prednisone, *AZA* Azathioprine, *MMF* mycophenolate mofetil, *CFA* Cyclophosphamide (pulse), *MP* Methylprednisolone (pulse), *MP + CFA* combined pulse: methylprednisolone and cyclophosphamide. a: Maximum dose during hospitalization. b: methylprednisolone pulse 1 g / day for 3 consecutive days

Table 2 Demographic and clinical data of 22 patients with autoimmune rheumatic disease (AIRD) and positive cytomegalovirus antigenemia

Female sex	19 (90%)
Age (years)[a]	39.4 ± 20.8
AIRD	
SLE	13 (59%)
ANCA-associated Vasculitis	4 (18.2%)
RA	2 (9%)
Systemic sclerosis	1 (4.5%)
Overlap syndrome	1 (4.5%)
Anti-sintetase syndrome	1 (4.5%)
Diagnosis AIRD[b] Time (months)	10.5 (0–276)
Hospitalization cause[a]	
Activity + Infection	11 (50%)
Infection only	8 (36.5%)
Activity only	3 (13.6%)
AIRD treatment	
Maximum dose of corticosteroids in hospital (mg/ day)[a]	87.7 ± 52.5
Corticosteroids dose above 1 mg /kg/ day[a]	19 (86.4%)
Methylprednisolone Pulse Therapy[a]	11 (50%)
Immunosuppressant medications[a]	11 (50%)
Site of CMV infection[a]	
Lung	10 (45.4%)
Cytopenia	9 (40.9%)
Gastrointestinal tract	6 (27.3%)
Hospitalization time[a](days)	41.9 ± 34.1
Hospitalization time until CMV-Ag be requested[a](days)	11.5 ± 12
Time of symptoms until CMV-Ag be requested[a](days)	7.8 ± 7.1
Time from the first positive CMV-Ag to specific treatment be started[a](days)	3.3 ± 3.1
Number of positive CMV-Ag nuclei after specific treatment	
With Ganciclovir[b]	15 (1–500)
No ganciclovir[b]	7 (1–4)
Co-Infections[a]	16 (72.7%)
Polymicrobial Infections	5 (22.7%)
CMV reactivation during hospitalization	0
Prophylaxis after standard Ganciclovir treatment	0

[a]Mean ± standard deviation; [b]Median (minimum and maximum); *AIRD* Autoimmune Rheumatic Diseases, *CMV-Ag* cytomegalovirus antigenemia, *SLE* Systemic Lupus Erythematosus, *RA* Rheumatoid Arthritis

Regarding absolute CMV-Ag, three (13.6%) patients had values above five cells and eight patients (36.4%) had values above 10 cells. However, none of these two cutoffs CMV-Ag had significant association with death or poor outcome.

Discussion

Our data showed high incidence of positive CMV-Ag in hospitalized patients with AIRD, as well as severe disease severity and poor prognosis, including death.

To our the best knowledge, this is the first study to highlight the incidence of positive CMV-Ag in hospitalized patients with severe AIRD, especially SLE and ANCA-associated vasculitis. Thus, it could not be compared with another retrospective studies no incidence data and heterogeneous prevalence (from 2 to 50%) [4, 8, 15, 16].

In addition to severity and high disease activity, it is worthy emphasizing that high doses of corticosteroids may have impaired the immune response in our patients [4, 17, 28]. Considering that over 95% of general

Table 3 Comparison of clinical and demographic characteristics of patients with positive cytomegalovirus antigenemia according to the outcome: survivor or death

	Death $n = 10$	Survivor $n = 11$	p
Age[b] (years)	44.3 ± 23.4	35.5 ± 18.3	0.32
Lymphocyte Count (/μL)[b]	447.2 ± 368.2	870.3 ± 692.9	0.06
CMV-Ag[b,c]	113 ± 205,2	29 ± 52.9	0.67
Oral glucocorticosteroids (mg/ day)[a,b]	107 ± 55.4	71.7 ± 46.3	0.07
Methylprednisolone Pulse Therapy, n			
Yes	3 (30%)	8 (72.2%)	0.19
No	7 (70%)	4 (36.6%)	
Hospitalization time[b]	24.3 ± 23.9	56.6 ± 35.1	0.017
Hospitalization time until CMV-Ag be requested (days)[b]	9.9 ± 14	12.9 ± 10.5	0.42
Time of symptoms until CMV-Ag be requested (days)[b]	7.9 ± 8.2	7.8 ± 6.4	0.77
Time from the first positive CMV-Ag to specific treatment be started (days) [b]	3.4 ± 2.6	3.3 ± 3.7	0.54
CMV suspicious cause, n			
Cytopenia	2 (20%)	4 (36.4%)	
Cytopenia e GIT	0 (0)	1 (9.1%)	
GIT	2 (20%)	3 (27.3%)	0.59
Pneumonia	4 (40%)	4 (36.3%)	
Cytopenia e Pneumonia	2 (20%)	0 (0)	

CMV-Ag: cytomegalovirus antigenemia, *b* mean ± standard deviation, *c* cels / 200.000polimorphonuclear. [a]Maximum corticosteroid dose during hospitalization. *GIT* gastrointestinal tract. Cutoff value of 10 positive cores for CMV antigenemia

population have immunological memory for CMV, likely these three aspects together could be involved for reactivation of latent viral infection [4, 12, 17, 18]. On the other hand, other authors found no association between CMV infection and immunosuppressive medications, especially corticosteroids [3, 8, 16].

The lung (45.5%) was the organ with the highest suspect involvement by CMV infection in our patients, confirming that the viral reactivation data in tracheal aspirates from immunosuppressed patients must be the main pathophysiologic mechanism, as well as pneumonitis reports and respiratory failure [21, 22]. However, it is important to state the possibility of pneumonia caused by multiple microbial agents. Cytopenia had the second place in frequency (40.9%), unlike recent retrospective report of 105 patients with SLE and active CMV infection related 81% of patients with some cytopenia [23]. The simultaneous involvement of various organs can also occur in immunosuppressed patients and was observed in 3 (13.6%) of our patients. Although the presence of cytopenia may constitute a simple and early warning for CMV infection in immunocompromised patients with AIRD, this finding was not specific, since it can also mean disease activity and toxicity to immunosuppressants.

Several mechanisms may explain the role of CMV and the onset of rheumatic disease or as a possible trigger, as well as its association with increased mortality in lupus patients [23]. Due to their broad cell tropism, CMV has

great variety of clinical manifestations in immunocompromised patients and can even be confused with the disease activity [3, 12, 19, 23, 25]. At diagnosis of CMV infection, SLE patients had higher incidence of hematologic, joint and kidney activity. Unlike cytopenias, articular and kidney involvement did not usually occur in reactivation of CMV infection and may be useful for the differential diagnosis between both clinical scenarios (infection vs. disease activity) [23].

Tasai et al. (2012) showed SLE patients infected by CMV had higher scores of SLEDAI, poor prognosis and increased mortality [12]. Our data confirm these interesting epidemiological features, since more than half of patients with positive CMV-Ag had SLE, particularly with early-onset disease and were youth. Thus, these findings address the role of CMV as trigger, as well as by collaborating on innate immunity and dysfunction of humoral and cellular immune response [4, 15, 24, 26, 27].

The diagnosis of CMV infection is not performed routinely by rheumatologists and there is no active search or specific treatment for patients with AIRD. Our study provides a new information about modern strategies headed for these patients. First of all, it is an alert to the presence of infection or co-infection with CMV, according to our high incidence of CMV-Ag in the first 10 days of hospitalization. Secondly, the red flag is the fast and sensible methodology for detecting suspicious cases of CMV infection in AIRD patients. Thirdly, the delay for requesting CMV-Ag and the risk of severe disease severity and higher mortality rate.

There are well-established recommendations for screening, treatment and prevention of CMV infection in immunocompromised patients with other conditions, such as cancer, AIDS and transplants [5, 7–11, 20]. However, there are a lack of information about management of AIRD patients, highlighting the relevance of current study and supporting the necessity for the development of specific protocols in this scenario.

In 2008, Takizawa et al. suggested the cut-off of 11.2 cells/ 200,000/ neutrophils as a significant value for distinguishing symptomatic and asymptomatic infections as well as higher positive predictive value for CMV infection and mortality in patients with AIRD [16]. As there is no consensus about the significant number of cells for AIRD patients, we considered at least one cell for the first investigation associated to clinical findings (fever plus cytopenias and/ or pulmonary infiltrates and/ or gut lesions and/ or hepatitis). However, in further re-analyses with several cut-off points, including 5 and 10 cells, we did not also find a significant CMV-Ag cut-off. Thus, our data confirm that, regardless age, duration of symptoms, number of positive cells, viral involvement site, the simple presence of CMV-Ag was associated with severe illness and higher risk of death, especially in those with shorter hospital stay and higher dose of corticosteroids.

Considering that AIRD hospitalized patients have multiple and complicated medical conditions, such as systemic inflammation, co-infections and renal failure, it is very difficult to assure the real direct cause of death and the multifactorial aspects altogether may occur among themselves.

Nonetheless, our study has some limitations. Firstly, it is related to CMV-Ag definition itself, because we cannot be sure that the presence of only one positive cell could be indicative of CMV infection. Secondly, is related to sample size, lack of control group and the heterogeneity of autoimmune diseases. Thirdly, we should not generalize our findings for outpatient patients or systematically request CMV-Ag for all hospitalized patients without a clinical suspicion. In addition, it is important to state that in any suspected case is need to confirm the CMV disease by histopathological analysis, for instance.

Although the survival patients with DRAI have kept imunossupression, none of them reactivated CMV over time (mean follow-up time 2 years), even without receiving prophylactic treatment with ganciclovir as suggested by protocols for transplanted patients. These new data emphasize that specific protocols are necessary for establishing appropriate diagnosis, treatment and monitoring CMV status in patients with AIRD, including prospective randomized controlled trials.

Conclusions
Our data showed high incidence of CMV-Ag in AIRD hospitalized patients, particularly early-onset lupus, severe disease activity, and higher mortality. Thus, the possibility of CMV infection should be included in differential diagnosis in AIRD patients.

Acknowledgements
None.

Author's contributions
All authors made substantial contributions to the acquisition of data, have been involved in drafting the manuscript revising it critically and approved the final manuscript.

References
1. Azuma N, Hashimoto N, Yasumitsu A, Fukuoka K, Yokoyama K, Sawada H, et al. CMV infection presenting as a Cavitary lung lesion in a patient with systemic lupus erythematosus receiving immunosuppressive therapy. Inter Med. 2009;48:2145–9.
2. Baldanti F, Lilleri D, Gerna G. Use of the human cytomegalovirus (HCMV) antigenemia assay for diagnosis and monitoring of HCMV infections and detection of antiviral drug resistance in the immunocompromised. J Clin Virol. 1998;11:51–60.
3. Yamashita M, Ishii T, Iwama N, Takahashi H. Incidence and clinical features of cytomegalovirus infection diagnosed by cytomegalovirus pp65 antigenemia assay during high dose corticosteroid therapy for collagen vascular diseases. Clin Exp Rheumatol. 2006;24:649–55.
4. Hanaoka R, Kurasawa K, Maezawa R, Kumano K, Arai S, Fukuda T. Reactivation of cytomegalovirus predicts poor prognosis in patients on intensive immunosuppressive treatment for collagen-vascular diseases. Mod Rheumatol. 2012;22:438–45.
5. Kotton CN. Management of cytomegalovirus infection in solid organ transplantation. Nat Rev Nephrol. 2010;6:711–21.
6. Drew LW. Nonpulmonary manifestations of Cytomegalovirus infection in immunocompromised patients. Clin Microbiol Rev. 1992;5:204–10.
7. Emery V, Zuckerman M, Jackson G, Aitken C, Osman H, Pagliuca A, et al. Management of cytomegalovirus infection in haemopoietic stem cell transplantation. Br J Haematol. 2013;162:25–39.
8. Kotton CN, Kumar D, Caliendo AM, Åsberg A, Chou S, Snydman DR, et al. Internacional consensus guidelines on the Management of Cytomegalovirus in solid organ transplantation. Transplantation. 2010;89:779–95.
9. Andrews PA, Emery VC, Newstead C. Summary of the British Transplantation Society guidelines for the prevention and management of CMV disease after solid organ transplantation. Transplantation. 2011;92:1181–7.
10. Whitley RJ, Jacobson MA, Friedberg DN, Holland GN, Jabs DA, Dieterich DT, et al. Guidelines for the treatment of Cytomegalovirus disease in patients with AIDS in the era of potent antiretroviral therapy. Arch Intern Med. 1998;158:957–69.
11. Lalonde RG, Bovivin G, Deschênes J, Hodge WG, Hopkins JJ, Klein AH. Et. al. Canadian consensus guidelines for the management of cytomegalovirus disease in HIV/AIDS. Can J Infect Dis Med Microbiol. 2004;15:327–35.
12. Tsai WP, Chen MH, Lee MH, Yu KH, Wu MW, Liou LB. Cytomegalovirus infection causes morbidity and mortality in patients with autoimmune diseases, particularly systemic lupus: in a Chinese population in Taiwan. Rheumatol Int. 2012;32:2901–8.
13. Gladman DD, Goldsmith CH, Urowitz MB, Bacon P, Bombardier C, Isenberg D, et al. Crosscultural validation and reliability of three disease activity indices in systemic lupus erythematosus. J Rheumatol. 1992;19:608–11.
14. Mukhtyar C, Lee R, Brown D, Carruthers D, Dasgupta B, Dubey S, et al. Modification and validation of the Birmingham Vasculitis activity score (version 3). Ann Rheum Dis. 2009;68:1827–32.
15. Lesprit P, Scieux C, Lemann M, Carbonelle E, Moday J, Molina JM. Use of the Cytomegalovirus (CMV) Antigenemia assay for the rapid diagnosis of primary CMV infection in hospitalized adults. Clin Infect Dis. 1998;26:646–50.
16. Takizawa Y, Inokuma S, Tanaka Y, Saito K, Atsumi T, Hirakata M, Kameda H, et al. Clinical characteristics of cytomegalovirus infection in rheumatic diseases: multicentre survey in a large patient population. Rheumatology. 2008;47:1373–8.

17. Kutza AST, Hackstein EMH, Kirchner H, Bein G. High incidence of active Cytomegalovirus infection among septic patients. Clin Infect Dis. 1998;26:1076–82.

18. Fujimoto D, Matsushima A, Nagao M, Takakura S, Ichiyama S. Risk factors associated with elevated blood cytomegalovirus pp65 antigen levels in patients with autoimmune diseases. Mod Rheumatol. 2013;23:345–50.

19. Eisenstein EM, Wolf DG. Cytomegalovirus infection in pediatric rheumatic diseases: a review. Pediatr Rheumatol. 2010;8:17.

20. Boeckh M, Boivin G. Quantitation of Cytomegalovirus: methodologic aspects and clinical applications. Clin Microbiol Rev. 1998;11:533–54.

21. Chilet M, Aguilar G, Benet I, Belda J, Tormo N, Carbonell JA, et al. Virological and immunological features of active cytomegalovirus infection in nonimmunosupressed pacientes in a surgical and trauma intensive care unit. J Med Virol. 2010;82:1884–391.

22. De Maar EF, Verschuuren EAM, Harmsen MC, The TH, Van Son WJ. Pulmonary involvement during cytomegalovirus infection in immunosuppressed patiens. Transpl Infec Dis. 2003;5:112–20.

23. Zhang J, Dou Y, Zhong Z, Su J, Xu D, Tang F, et al. Clinical characteristics and therapy exploration of active human cytomegalovirus infection in 105 lupus pacients. Lupus. 2014;0:1–9.

24. Nauclér CS. Autoimmunity induced by human cytomegalovirus in patients with systemic lupus erythematosus. Arthritis Res Ther. 2012;14:101–3.

25. Cunha BA, Gouzhva O, Nausheen S. Severe cytomegalovírus (CMV) community-acquired pneumonia (CAP) precipitaiting a systemic lúpus erytematosus (SLE) flare. Heart Lung. 2008;38:249–52.

26. Yoda Y, Hanaoka R, Ide H, Isozaki T, Matsunawa M, Yajima N, et al. Clinical evaluation of patients with inflammatory connective tissue diseases complicated by cytomegalovirus antigenemia. Mod Rheumatol. 2006;16:137–42.

27. Jih Su BY, Yu Su C, Fu Yu S, Jen Chen C. Incidental discovery of high systemic lupus erythematosus disease activity associated with cytomegalovirus viral activity. Med Microbiol Immunol. 2007;196:165–70.

28. Mori T, Kameda H, Ogawa H, Iizuka A, Sekiguchi N, Takei H, et al. Incidence of Cytomegalovirus reactivation in patients with inflammatory connective tissue diseases who are under immunosuppressive therapy. J Rheumatol. 2004;31:1349–51.

19

Could obesity be considered as risk factor for non-vertebral low-impact fractures?

Bruna Aurora Nunes Cavalcante Castro[1], Edgard Torres dos Reis Neto[1], Vera Lucia Szejnfeld[1], Jacob Szejnfeld[2], Valdecir Marvulle[3] and Marcelo de Medeiros Pinheiro[1]*

Abstract

Background: It has long been established that obesity plays a positive role against osteoporosis (OP) and low-impact fractures (Fx). However, more recent data has shown higher fracture risk in obese individuals. The aim of this study was to investigate the association between BMI, particularly obesity, OP and low-impact Fx in Brazilian women, as well as to evaluate the SAPORI (Sao Paulo Osteoporosis Risk Index) tool performance to identify low BMD according BMI category.

Methods: A total of 6182 women aged over 40 years were included in this cross-sectional analysis using data from two large Brazilian studies. All participants performed hip and spine bone mineral density (BMD) measurements and answered a detailed questionnaire about the presence of clinical risk factors (CRFs) related to low BMD and risk fractures. The World Health Organization (WHO) criteria were used to define obesity.

Results: Age-adjusted osteoporosis prevalence was 20.8, 33.6, 47 and 67.1% in obese, overweight, normal and underweight category, respectively. Obesity was present in 29,6% (1.830 women) in the study population and the likelihood of osteoporosis and low-impact Fx compared to a normal BMI in this subgroup was of 0.24 (95% CI 0.20–0.28; $p < 0.001$) and of 1.68 (95% CI 1.35–2.11; $p < 0.001$), respectively. However, the hip Fx likelihood was lower in obese compared with non-obese women (OR = 0.44; 95% CI 0.20–0.97). Using an originally validated cut-off, the SAPORI tool sensitivity was significantly hampered in overweight and obese women although the accuracy had remained suitable because of increasing in specificity.

Conclusions: The osteoporosis prevalence reduced as BMI increased and obesity was associated with low-impact Fx, regardless of the BMD measurements. Moreover, the SAPORI performance was impaired in obese women.

Keywords: Osteoporosis, Bone mineral density measurements, Low-impact fractures, Clinical risk factors, Obesity, BMI

Background

Obesity and osteoporosis (OP) are two major public health problems with increasing prevalence worldwide and high impact on morbidity and mortality [1–3]. Osteoporosis is a silent metabolic bone disease characterized by bone loss and microarchitectural deterioration and higher susceptibility to fragility fracture. It has a relevant global burden, including almost 9,000,000 new osteoporotic fractures worldwide, as well as disability, quality of life impaired and death [1, 4]. The World Health Organization (WHO) defines obesity when the body mass index (BMI) is higher than 30 kg/ m², with an abnormal or excessive fat accumulation and higher cardiovascular and metabolic risk [5].

According to the Brazilian Institute of Statistics and Geography over than 50% of population has been considered as overweight or obese, especially after 50 years [6]. Brazilian epidemiological studies also showed that the prevalence of osteoporosis and low-impact fractures is high [7–11].

BMI is an important aspect related to bone mineral density (BMD) measurements. Until recently, individuals with high BMI had some protection against fractures [12]. However, more recently epidemiological studies have shown that osteoporosis and obesity may coexist and could share complex pathophysiological

* Correspondence: mpinheiro@uol.com.br
[1]Rheumatology Division, Universidade Federal de São Paulo/Escola Paulista de Medicina (Unifesp/EPM), Rua Leandro Dupré, 204, conj. 74, Vila Clementino, São Paulo, São Paulo-SP CEP 04025-010, Brazil
Full list of author information is available at the end of the article

mechanisms, including genetic, environmental, and hormonal factors [12, 13].

The relationship between the BMI and the fracture risk is inverse and non-linear. Patients with BMI below 20 kg/ m^2 have higher risk and it is associated with low spine and hip BMD measurements. Nonetheless, only small decreases of fracture risk have been reported in individuals with BMI above 25 kg/ m^2 [14]. In addition, it has been hypothesized that obese individuals have inappropriately lower BMD than expected for their body weight, increasing the fracture risk [15–17].

Risk factors for fracture in obese individuals appear to be similar to those in non-obese populations, except some different patterns of falling [18, 19]. Several tools have been developed to estimate the individual risk of osteoporotic fracture [20, 21]. The SAPORI (Sao Paulo Osteoporosis Risk Index) is a Brazilian validated tool for identifying women at higher risk for low bone mineral density and osteoporotic fractures to recommend some BMD measurements. [22].

The aim of this study was to investigate the BMI relationship, particularly obesity, with OP and low-impact Fx in women aged over 40 years, as well as to evaluate the SAPORI performance in predicting low BMD, according to each BMI category.

Methods

Two largest Brazilian epidemiological databases were used for this particular analysis: São Paulo Osteoporosis Study (SAPOS) and Sao Paulo Osteoporosis Risk Index (SAPORI). The first one was a population-based epidemiologic study for the assessment of risk factors for low-impact fractures and low spine or hip BMD (T-score ≤ − 2 SD) in 7533 women aged over 40 years from São Paulo, Brazil. Briefly, a total of 4332 fulfilled the eligibility criteria and a detailed questionnaire addressing clinical risk factors (CRFs) for OP and Fx, including demographic and anthropometrical data; gynecological and hormonal information; personal medical history; previous fractures; family history of femur fracture (FHHF) after 50 years of age in first-degree relatives; and details about current lifestyle habits (smoking, regular physical activity in the previous 12 months and regular intake of dairy products) [7]. Regular physical activity was defined as any physical activity performed for more than 30 min and during three or more times per week, excluding routine activities of daily living. Low-impact fracture was defined as caused by a fall from one's own height or lower after 50 years of age. The information regarding these fractures was self-reported by the individuals [7, 22], including spine, hip and other non-vertebral fractures (humerus, distal forearm, ankle, pelvis, hands and feet). The categorization of dairy products daily intake was based on a frequency distribution

of 200 mL (no serving, up to three servings, and three servings or more). All of them performed spine and hip BMD measurements by DXA (DPX NT, GE-Lunar). The height (cm) and weight (kg) were measured with the subject wearing light clothes and no shoes [7].

The second one (SAPORI) was a study that aimed to validate a new tool to identify women under risk of low BMD using variables that were associated with higher risk for OP and Fx in the previous SAPOS study: age, weight, previous fracture, white color, current smoking, physical activity and family history of hip fracture. The SAPORI tool was subsequently validated in a second cohort of 1915 women from the metropolitan area of São Paulo. In both cohorts, the protocol for BMD measurements was the same and the sampling was considered representative of the Brazilian female population older than 40 years old, based on Brazilian Institute of Statistics and Geography (IBGE) [7, 22, 23]. Thus, the SAPORI tool had suitable performance to identify women with low bone mineral density (spine and hip) and low-impact fracture, with an area under the receiving operator curve (ROC) of 0.831, 0.724, and 0.689, respectively. The index or final score was obtained through simple mathematic equations. For instance, body weight contributes to 0.04 for each increase 1 SD hip BMD. Thus, the body weight is divided by 10 and then multiplied by 4. If the woman has already had any fracture, this simple risk factor contributes with 0.48 or 5 points for each 1 SD reduction. The other risk factors are counted in this way, according to the relevance of each one of them in the final regression model. Also, when the final value is greater or equal to zero it is considered as recommended screening for low bone mineral density [7, 22].

For this study, 65 patients (1%) were excluded because missing data totalizing 6.182 women. The BMI category was defined according to the WHO classification: underweight (BMI ≤ 18.5 kg/ m^2), normal weight (BMI 18.5–24.9 kg/ m^2), overweight (BMI 25–29.9 kg/ m^2), obesity (BMI ≥ 30 kg/ m^2) [24, 25]. Also, according to the WHO classification, osteoporosis was defined when T-score (lumbar spine and/or total hip) below − 2.5 standard-deviation (SD) and osteopenia if T-score between − 1.01 and − 2.49 SD [26]. T-scores were used for all population (women aged > 40 years), following the guidelines of the Brazilian Society of Clinical Densitometry (ABRASSO) [27].

The Research Ethics Committee of the Universidade Federal de São Paulo/ Escola Paulista de Medicina approved this study (CEP- 0406/2015).

Statistical analysis

Categorical data were shown as frequency and percentages and were compared using Chi-squared or Fisher's exact test as appropriate. Continuous data were reported as mean ± SD. Logistic regression models were used to

Could obesity be considered as risk factor for non-vertebral low-impact...

153

Table 1 Anthropometric data and clinical risk factors for osteoporosis and low-impact fractures of the population according to BMI

BMI categories	Total (N = 6182)	Underweight (N = 73; 1.2%)	Normal weight (N = 1902; 30.8%)	Overweight (N = 2377; 38.4%)	Obesity (N = 1830; 29.6%)	P
Weight (kg)	66.2 ± 13.0	41.1 ± 4.1	54.5 ± 6.0	65.3 ± 6.0	80.4 ± 10.9	< 0.001
Height (cm)	154.3 ± 6.3	154.0 ± 6.7	155.0 ± 6.5	154.1 ± 6.1	153.7 ± 6.3	< 0.001
BMI (kg/m^2)	27.8 ± 5.2	17.3 ± 1.0	22.6 ± 1.6	27.4 ± 1.4	34.0 ± 3.8	< 0.001
Age (years)	60.7 ± 9.8	60.7 ± 10.8	60.1 ± 10.5	61.2 ± 9.7	60.5 ± 9.2	< 0.001
White skin color (N, %)	4741 (76.8)	54 (74.0)	1508 (79.4)	1833 (77.2)	1346 (73.6)	< 0.001
Current use of HRT (N, %)	726 (11.7)	6 (8.2)	294 (15.5)	267 (11.2)	159 (8.7)	< 0.001
Current smoking (N, %)[c]	619 (10.0)	21 (28.8)	280 (14.7)	208 (8.8)	110 (6.0)	< 0.001
FHHF (N, %)	752 (12.2)	14 (19.2)	265 (13.9)	262 (11.0)	211 (11.5)	0.006
Premenopausal state (N, %)	489 (7.9)	5 (6.8)	180 (9.5)	166 (7.0)	138 (7.5)	0.02
Current physical activity (N, %)	1764 (28.5)	15 (20.5)	589 (31.0)	692 (29.1)	468 (25.6)	0.001
Calcium supplements intake (N, %)	925 (15.0)	22 (30.1)	407 (21.4)	335 (14.1)	161 (8.8)	< 0.001
Use of GCs (N, %)	59 (1.0)	1 (1.4)	25 (1.3)	20 (0.8)	13 (0.7)	0.239
DM (N, %)	478 (7.7)	1 (1.4)	61 (3.2)	187 (7.9)	229 (12.5)	< 0.001

Data are expressed as the estimated mean ± standard deviation or estimated percentage, as appropriate. P values are those of Student's t test for means or the chi-square test for proportions; Kruskal-Wallis test
BMI body mass index HRT hormone replacement therapy FHHF family history of hip fracture GCs glucocorticoids DM diabetes mellitus

evaluate independent predictors of low-impact Fx and osteoporosis, separately. Variables that showed some correlation (P value < 0.1, by the Chi-squared test) were entered into a forward/backward selection procedure (both with P value thresholds lesser than 0.05 to entry and retention). Variables included in the final multivariable model were: age, skin color, current smoking and physical activity, FHHF, menopausal status, hormone replacement therapy (HRT) in the last 12 months and diabetes mellitus. In this case, two final models were tested

Table 2 Characteristics of bone mineral density measurements and low-impact fractures, according to each BMI category

BMI category	Total N = 6182	Underweight N = 73	Normal weight N = 1902	Overweight N = 2377	Obesity N = 1830	P
Spine and femur BMD (n, %)						< 0.001
Normal	1316 (21.3)	3 (4.1)	244 (12.8)	473 (19.9)	596 (32.6)	
Osteopenia	2745 (44.4)	21 (28.8)	764 (40.2)	1106 (46.5)	854 (46.6)	
Osteoporosis	2121 (34.3)	49 (67.1)	894 (47.0)	798 (33.6)	380 (20.8)	
T-score						
Lumbar Spine	−1.49 (± 1.45)	−2.66 (± 1.40)	−1.89 (± 1.38)	−1.50 (± 1.37)	−1.07 (± 1.46)	< 0.001
Femoral neck	−1.54 (± 1.16)	−2.62 (± 1.25)	−1.93 (± 1.12)	−1.53 (± 1.07)	−1.11 (± 1.14)	< 0.001
Total femur	−0.80 (± 1.23)	−2.18 (± 1.12)	−1.37 (± 1.14)	−0.78 (± 1.08)	−0.17 (± 1.18)	< 0.001
BMD (g/cm^2)						
Lumbar Spine	1.000 (± 0.17)	0.859 (± 0.17)	0.952 (± 0.16)	0.999 (± 0.16)	1.059 (± 0.17)	< 0.001
Femoral neck	0.849 (± 0.15)	0.717 (± 0.14)	0.801 (± 0.14)	0.851 (± 0.14)	0.902 (± 0.14)	< 0.001
Total femur	0.910 (± 0.17)	0.746 (± 0.14)	0.843 (± 0.19)	0.911 (± 0.14)	0.985 (± 0.14)	< 0.001
Low-impact Fx (n, %)	756 (12.2)	10 (13.7)	234 (12.3)	280 (11.8)	232 (12.7)	0.81
Fracture sites (n, %)[b]						0.09
LL	276 (36.5)	2 (20.0)	76 (32.5)	108 (38.6)	90 (38.8)	
UL	318 (42.1)	7 (70.0)	97 (41.4)	118 (42.1)	96 (41.4)	
Spine	53 (7.0)	0 (0.0)	15 (6.4)	18 (6.4)	20 (8.6)	
Hip	46 (6.1)	0 (0.0)	17 (7.3)	21 (7.5)	8 (3.4)	
Others	63 (8.3)	1 (10.0)	29 (12.4)	15 (5.4)	18 (7.8)	

BMD bone mineral density BMI: body mass index Fx fracture LL lower limbs UL upper limbs BMD bone mineral density; P values are those of Student's t test for means or the chi-square test for proportions; Kruskal-Wallis test

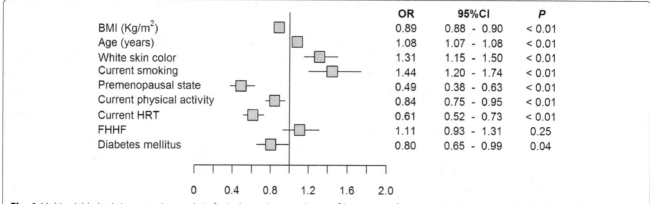

Fig. 1 Multivariable logistic regression analysis for independent predictors of low-impact fractures. OR: Odds Ratio; 95% CI: 95% confidence interval; BMI: body mass index; HRT: hormone replacement therapy; FHHF: familial history of hip fracture

using the BMI as continuous or by WHO categories. The SAPORI tool discriminative power (accuracy) was assessed by the area under receiver-operating characteristics (ROC) curve and performed in each BMI category, separately. P value < 0.05 was set as significant. Statistical analyses were performed using SPSS (version 20.0, Chicago, USA) and R software package (version 3.2, Vienna, Austria).

Results
Population
A total of 6182 women were included in this analysis. The mean age was 60.7 ± 9.8 years, with White (76.8%)

and postmenopausal (92.1%) predominance, although only 11.7% on HRT. The obesity prevalence was almost 30% (mean BMI $= 34 \pm 3.8$ kg/m^2) and only 1.2% was underweight (Table 1).

BMI and osteoporosis The OP prevalence was 20.8, 33.6, 47 and 67.1% in obese, overweight, normal and underweight BMI category, respectively (Table 2). After adjustments for the CRFs, the higher BMI had a protective role for OP (OR $= 0.89$; 95%CI 0.88–0.90; $p < 0.01$). In obese women, the likelihood for OP was lower (OR $= 0.26$; 95%CI 0.23–0.31; $p < 0.01$) than in underweight

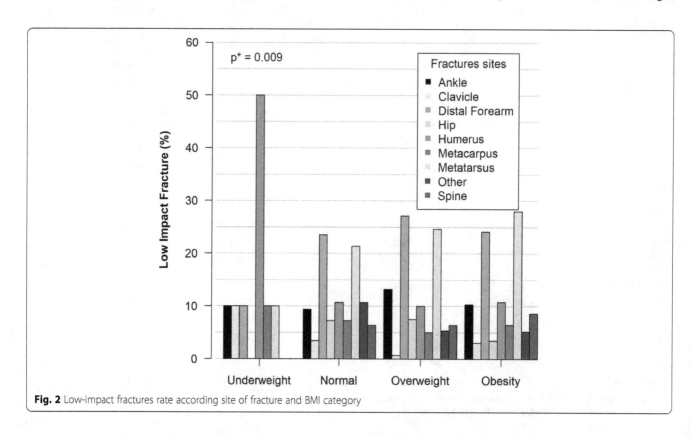

Fig. 2 Low-impact fractures rate according site of fracture and BMI category

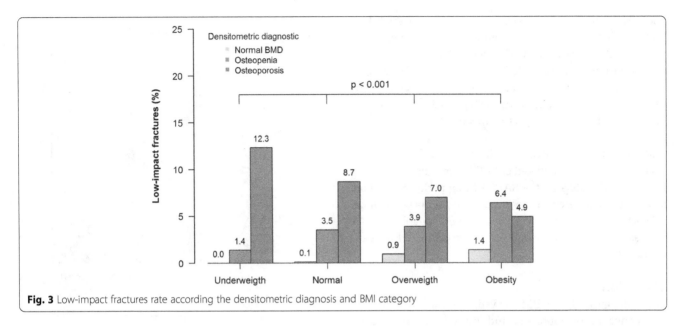

Fig. 3 Low-impact fractures rate according the densitometric diagnosis and BMI category

women (OR = 2.43; 95%CI 1.35–4.61; $p < 0.01$), if compared to normal weight group (Fig. 1).

BMI and low-impact fracture

Low-impact fractures were self-reported by 756 women (12.2%), but there was no significant difference was observed regarding each BMI category ($p = 0.81$). On the other hand, there was a significant difference when the skeletal site was analyzed ($p = 0.009$; Fig. 2). Non-vertebral fractures were the most prevalent (distal forearm: 24.9%, metatarsus: 24.5%), followed by spine (7%) and hip (6.1%). In underweight women, there was significantly higher

frequency of humerus and clavicle and the hip fracture was less common in obese women than non-obese group (7.4% vs. 3.4%; $p = 0.047$). Interestingly, obese and women with low-impact Fx had higher proportion of normal BMD than those with normal BMI (7.8% vs. 3.6%; $p < 0.001$; Fig. 3).

After several adjustments for CRFs and BMD measurements (T-score values), it was observed that increasing BMI, the fracture risk also rises (OR = 1.03; 95%CI 1.02–1.05; $p < 0.001$), regardless each BMI category. This finding highlights that obese individuals had higher fracture risk than other BMI category, regardless BMD measurements. In addition, age (OR = 1.03; 95%CI 1.02–1.04; $p < 0.001$)

Table 3 Logistic regression analysis to identify significant risk factors for low-impact fractures in women

	Model 1			Model 2		
	OR	95% CI	P	OR	95% CI	P
Age (years)	1.03	1.02–1.04	< 0.001	1.03	1.02–1.04	< 0.001
Premenopausal state	0.40	0.21–0.78	0.007	0.40	0.21–0.78	0.008
FHHF	4.18	3.46–5.06	< 0.001	4.21	3.48–5.09	< 0.001
Current use of HRT	1.16	0.89–1.52	0.25	1.16	0.89–1.52	0.25
White skin color	1.00	0.81–1.22	0.97	1.00	0.81–1.22	0.98
Current physical activity	1.00	0.84–1.21	0.92	1.00	0.83–1.20	0.92
Current smoking	1.15	0.86–1.54	0.32	1.16	0.87–1.55	0.30
Diabetes mellitus	1.30	0.98–1.73	0.06	1.32	0.98–1.72	0.06
T-score	0.58	0.53–0.63	< 0.001	0.58	0.53–0.63	< 0.001
BMI (continuous)	1.03	1.02–1.05	< 0.001			
BMI (categorical)						
Underweight				0.67	0.32–1.39	0.28
Normal weight				–	–	–
Overweight				1.22	0.99–1.49	0.05
Obesity				1.68	1.35–2.11	< 0.001

BMI body mass index *HRT* hormone replacement therapy *FHHF* family history of hip fracture *DM* diabetes mellitus

and FHHF (OR = 4.18; 95%CI 3.46–5.06; $p < 0.001$) had high predictive power for low-impact Fx. Nonetheless, higher BMD values (OR = 0.58; 95%CI 0.53–0.63; $p < 0.001$) and premenopausal status (OR = 0.40; 95%CI 0.21–0.78; $p < 0.007$) played a positive role against low-impact fracture (Table 3). In addition, diabetes mellitus had a tendency to be associated with low-impact Fx ($p = 0.06$).

SAPORI tool performance
Using an originally validated cut-off (greater or equal zero) for each BMI category, the SAPORI tool performance had sensitivity hampered in overweight and obese women (Fig. 4). However, the accuracy remained suitable, due to increase of specificity (AUC ROC above 0.7 in all BMI categories) (Fig. 5).

Discussion
Our data showed that BMI played a relevant role on the prevalence of osteoporosis and caused impairment of SAPORI tool performance. On the other hand, it did not affect the prevalence of fragility fractures, suggesting that obese women are at risk for having low-impact fractures, regardless BMD measurements.

Previous studies have shown a significant relationship between BMD measurements and BMI, where higher BMI increases BMD and losing weight reduces BMD measurements values [14, 17, 28]. Although there are some patients with osteoporosis, there are a significant number of low-impact fractures in our obese women group, as reported by recent meta-analysis [29]. These new findings are a paradigm break concerning the widespread belief that obesity is protective against fractures. However, it is worthy emphasizing that high BMI has a different influence on fracture risk according to skeletal site [30, 31]. Thus, the obesity becomes a risk factor for all low-impact non-vertebral fractures, except hip fractures [18, 32]. Another thing to be considered is higher ankle and humerus fracture risk in obese women observed by the Global Longitudinal Study of Osteoporosis [18] and a Spain based-population study [31], respectively. Regarding vertebral fractures, there are conflicting data [33–36].

Several mechanisms may be involved on fracture risk in obese individuals, including site-specific BMI effects, as well as falls, reduced physical mobility, muscular weakness and postural instability. Obesity may predispose to falling backwards or side-wards rather than forwards and combined to protective reactions impairment (e.g. an outstretched hand), causes higher rate of wrist fracture. The main reason for justifying the lowest prevalence of hip fracture in obese people is associated to fat and soft tissue padding distribution [37, 38].

Obese women with high values of spine or hip BMD measurements not necessarily is associated with lower risk of fragility fractures, because other aspects seem to

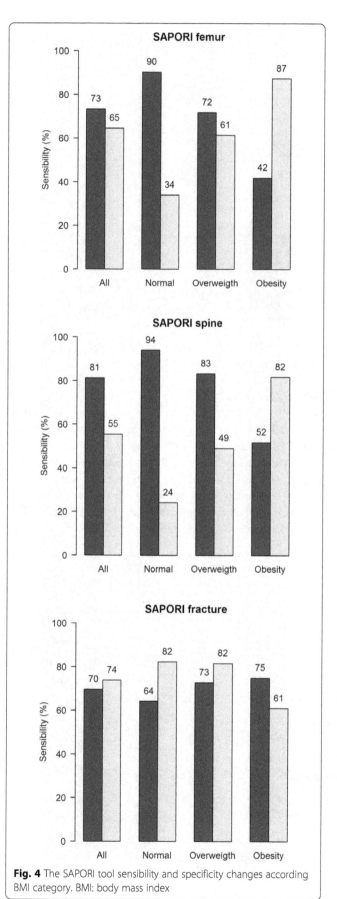

Fig. 4 The SAPORI tool sensibility and specificity changes according BMI category. BMI: body mass index

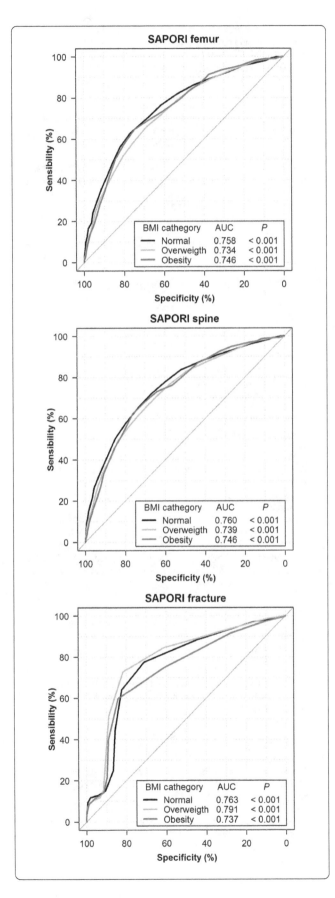

Fig. 5 SAPORI accuracy for low BMD and low-impact fractures according BMI. ROC curves of the SAPORI tool for low BMD (femur or spine) and low-impact fractures according BMI category. BMD: bone mineral density; BMI: body mass index; ROC: Receiver-operating characteristic

be involved [14, 29]. More recently, the fat-bone tissue axis has highlighted that low BMD measurements itself cannot explain higher fracture risk in obese individuals. Thus, aspects related to bone quality are pointed out as potential markers of bone strength in this scenario [38]. Considering these qualitative aspects, a similar parallel could be addressed to diabetes mellitus (DM), since is demonstrated higher spine and femur BMD measurements, but also higher non-vertebral fractures [39–41], where the resistance to insulin, hyperglycemia and higher advanced glycation end products levels on collagen bone fibers would cause lower bone strength and higher fracture risk. In addition, the diabetes-related complications, including poor balance and sight and peripheral neuropathy, may contribute to increased falling and fracture risk [41].

It is worthy emphasizing that although higher spine and hip BMD measurements have been observed in obese women with fractures, they may be inappropriately low for body weight, suggesting some lack of adaptive response [15, 16, 18]. Therefore, there is a growing awareness on how to identify bone fragility risk in obese individuals, considering that BMD measurements do not necessarily would cause higher fracture risk. Thus, other non-invasive methods to measure structural aspects of trabecular bone and cortical porosity, such as trabecular bone score (TBS) and high-resolution peripheral quantitative computed tomography (HR-pQCT), may have future applications for assessing the fragility fracture risk in obese individuals.

Numerous risk factors for osteoporosis and fractures have been used to develop several risk assessment tools, including the WHO Fracture Risk Assessment Tool (FRAX) algorithm, Q fracture algorithm and Garvan Fracture Risk Calculator, aiming to stratify individuals into 5- or 10-year fracture risk categories or to screen them for requesting BMD measurements. In general, the traditional CRFs for osteoporosis and fracture are similar between obese and non-obese women and it would not be necessary to individualize these indices regarding anthropometric data. Based on that, we decided to evaluate the SAPORI tool performance considering each BMI category. Interestingly, we demonstrated a significant impairment (50–60%) of its sensitivity when it was applied to obese group, suggesting that cut-off score adjustments are necessary in women with BMI above $30 \, kg/ m^2$. Although weight has been considered in several international screening tools, including OST, OSIRIS, ORAI, and

SCORE, none of them was separately tested according to BMI categories, and so, their sensitivity and specificity cannot be assured in obese patients [20, 22, 42–47].

Our study has some limitations, such as a cross-sectional design, lack of information about radiographic vertebral fractures and bone turnover markers, and inherent methodological problems concerning accuracy, precision and reliability of DXA measurements in obese [48]. On the other hand, it has several strengths, including a huge pioneer study to investigate specifically the relationship among anthropometric data, BMD measurements and fragility fractures, according to each BMI category, as well as to demonstrate the poorest tool performance to screen or to measure fracture or osteoporosis risk in obese.

Conclusions

In conclusion, our data highlighted obese women have the same prevalence of non-vertebral low-impact fractures than normal weight women, regardless spine or hip BMD measurements and traditional clinical risk factors, addressing that other bone and extra-skeletal aspects may be involved with bone fragility. For the first time, we demonstrated the performance of a screening tool is hampered in obese women, suggesting the necessity of calibrating the cut-off score, according to BMI category.

Acknowledgments
The authors thank to researchers of SAPOS (Sao Paulo Osteoporosis Study) and Sao Paulo Osteoporosis Index (SAPORI) for assistance and kindly have given their databases.

Authors' contributions
BANCC performed the data analysis and drafted the manuscript. VLS participated in the design of the study. ETR helped to data analysis. VM performed all statistical analysis. JS participated in the design of the study. MMP participated in the design of the study, helped with data analysis and in drafting of the manuscript. All authors have read and approved the final manuscript.

Author details
[1]Rheumatology Division, Universidade Federal de São Paulo/Escola Paulista de Medicina (Unifesp/EPM), Rua Leandro Dupré, 204, conj. 74, Vila Clementino, São Paulo, São Paulo-SP CEP 04025-010, Brazil. [2]Radiology Department, Universidade Federal de São Paulo/Escola Paulista de Medicina (Unifesp/EPM), São Paulo, Brazil. [3]Statistics Department, Universidade Federal de São Paulo/Escola Paulista de Medicina (Unifesp/EPM), São Paulo, Brazil.

References
1. Riggs BL, Melton LJ 3rd. The worldwide problem of osteoporosis: insights afforded by epidemiology. Bone. 1995;17(5 Suppl):505S–11S.
2. Stevens GA, et al. National, regional, and global trends in adult overweight and obesity prevalences. Popul Health Metr. 2012;10(1):22–2.
3. Swinburn BA, et al. The global obesity pandemic: shaped by global drivers and local environments. Lancet. 2011;378(9793):804–14.
4. Johnell O, Kanis JA. An estimate of the worldwide prevalence and disability associated with osteoporotic fractures. Osteoporos Int. 2006;17(12):1726–33.
5. WHO WHO. Obesity: Preventing and Managing the Global Epidemic; 2000.
6. Ence I. Antropometria e estado nutricional no Brasil :metodologia, índices e tendência secular; 2010.
7. Pinheiro MM, et al. Risk factors for osteoporotic fractures and low bone density in pre and postmenopausal women. Rev Saude Publica. 2010;44(3): 479–85.
8. Pinheiro Mde M, et al. Risk factors for recurrent falls among Brazilian women and men: the Brazilian Osteoporosis Study (BRAZOS). Cad Saude Publica. 2010;26(1):89–96.
9. Lopes JB, et al. Osteoporotic fractures in the Brazilian community-dwelling elderly: prevalence and risk factors. J Clin Densitom. 2011;14(3):359–66.
10. Copes RM, et al. Obesity and Fractures in Postmenopausal Women: A Primary-care Cross-Sectional Study at Santa Maria, Brazil. J Clin Densitom. 2015;18(2):165–71.
11. Pinheiro MM, et al. Clinical risk factors for osteoporotic fractures in Brazilian women and men: the Brazilian Osteoporosis Study (BRAZOS). Osteoporos Int. 2009;20(3):399–408.
12. Felson DT, et al. Effects of weight and body mass index on bone mineral density in men and women: the Framingham study. J Bone Miner Res. 1993;8(5):567–73.
13. Gimble JM, et al. Playing with bone and fat. J Cell Biochem. 2006;98(2):251–66.
14. De Laet C, et al. Body mass index as a predictor of fracture risk: a meta-analysis. Osteoporos Int. 2005;16(11):1330–8.
15. Premaor MO, et al. Risk factors for nonvertebral fracture in obese older women. J Clin Endocrinol Metab. 2011;96(8):2414–21.
16. Premaor MO, et al. Obesity and fractures in postmenopausal women. J Bone Miner Res. 2010;25(2):292–7.
17. Gnudi S, Sitta E, Lisi L. Relationship of body mass index with main limb fragility fractures in postmenopausal women. J Bone Miner Metab. 2009; 27(4):479–84.
18. Compston JE, et al. Obesity is not protective against fracture in postmenopausal women: GLOW. Am J Med. 2011;124(11):1043–50.
19. Himes CL, Reynolds SL. Effect of obesity on falls, injury, and disability. J Am Geriatr Soc. 2012;60(1):124–9.
20. Rubin KH, et al. Risk assessment tools to identify women with increased risk of osteoporotic fracture: complexity or simplicity? A systematic review. J Bone Miner Res. 2013;28(8):1701–17.
21. Rubin KH, et al. Comparison of different screening tools (FRAX(R), OST, ORAI, OSIRIS, SCORE and age alone) to identify women with increased risk of fracture. A population-based prospective study. Bone. 2013;56(1):16–22.
22. Pinheiro MM, et al. Development and validation of a tool for identifying women with low bone mineral density and low-impact fractures: the Sao Paulo Osteoporosis Risk Index (SAPORI). Osteoporos Int. 2012;23(4):1371–9.
23. Available from: http://www.ibge.gov.br/home/estatistica/populacao/censo2010/default.shtm. Acessed 13 April, 2016.
24. Organization, W.H. Obesity and overweight. 2013 [cited 2013 18/08/2013].
25. Global Database on Body Mass Index: an interactive surveillance tool for monitoring nutrition transition. Geneva, Switzerland: WHO, 2004.; Available from: http://apps.who.int/bmi/index.jsp?introPage5intro_3.html Acessed 3 February 2014.
26. Kanis JA, et al. The diagnosis of osteoporosis. J Bone Miner Res. 1994;9(8): 1137–41.
27. Brandao. C.M., et al., [2008 official positions of the Brazilian Society for Clinical Densitometry--SBDens]. Arq Bras Endocrinol Metabol. 2009;53(1): 107–12.
28. Saarelainen J, et al. Body mass index and bone loss among postmenopausal women: the 10-year follow-up of the OSTPRE cohort. J Bone Miner Metab. 2012;30(2):208–16.
29. Johansson H, et al. A meta-analysis of the association of fracture risk and body mass index in women. J Bone Miner Res. 2014;29(1):223–33.
30. Gonnelli S, Caffarelli C, Nuti R. Obesity and fracture risk. Clin Cases Miner Bone Metab. 2014;11(1):9–14.
31. Prieto-Alhambra D, et al. The association between fracture and obesity is site-dependent: a population-based study in postmenopausal women. J Bone Miner Res. 2012;27(2):294–300.
32. Beck TJ, et al. Does obesity really make the femur stronger? BMD, geometry, and fracture incidence in the women's health initiative-observational study. J Bone Miner Res. 2009;24(8):1369–79.
33. Nevitt MC, et al. Risk factors for a first-incident radiographic vertebral fracture in women > or = 65 years of age: the study of osteoporotic fractures. J Bone Miner Res. 2005;20(1):131–40.
34. Pirro M, et al. High weight or body mass index increase the risk of vertebral fractures in postmenopausal osteoporotic women. J Bone Miner Metab. 2010;28(1):88–93.

35. Laslett LL, et al. Excess body fat is associated with higher risk of vertebral deformities in older women but not in men: a cross-sectional study. Osteoporos Int. 2012;23(1):67–74.
36. Compston J. Obesity and bone. Curr Osteoporos Rep. 2013;11(1):30–5.
37. Ishii S, et al. Pleiotropic Effects of Obesity on Fracture Risk: The Study of Women's Health Across the Nation. J Bone Miner Res. 2014.
38. Zhao LJ, et al. Correlation of obesity and osteoporosis: effect of fat mass on the determination of osteoporosis. J Bone Miner Res. 2008;23(1):17–29.
39. de, L., II, et al., Bone mineral density and fracture risk in type-2 diabetes mellitus: the Rotterdam Study. Osteoporos Int, 2005. 16(12): p. 1713-1720.
40. Vashishth D, et al. Influence of nonenzymatic glycation on biomechanical properties of cortical bone. Bone. 2001;28(2):195–201.
41. Kurra S, Fink DA, Siris ES. Osteoporosis-associated fracture and diabetes. Endocrinol Metab Clin North Am. 2014;43(1):233–43.
42. Kanis JA, et al. The use of clinical risk factors enhances the performance of BMD in the prediction of hip and osteoporotic fractures in men and women. Osteoporos Int. 2007;18(8):1033–46.
43. Hippisley-Cox J, Coupland C. Predicting risk of osteoporotic fracture in men and women in England and Wales: prospective derivation and validation of QFractureScores. BMJ. 2009;339:b4229.
44. Cadarette SM, et al. Development and validation of the Osteoporosis Risk Assessment Instrument to facilitate selection of women for bone densitometry. CMAJ. 2000;162(9):1289–94.
45. Richy F, et al. Validation and comparative evaluation of the osteoporosis self-assessment tool (OST) in a Caucasian population from Belgium. QJM. 2004;97(1):39–46.
46. Sedrine WB, et al. Development and assessment of the Osteoporosis Index of Risk (OSIRIS) to facilitate selection of women for bone densitometry. Gynecol Endocrinol. 2002;16(3):245–50.
47. Lydick E, et al. Development and validation of a simple questionnaire to facilitate identification of women likely to have low bone density. Am J Manag Care. 1998;4(1):37–48.
48. Patel R, et al. Long-term precision of DXA scanning assessed over seven years in forty postmenopausal women. Osteoporos Int. 2000;11(1):68–75.

20

Virtual reality therapy for rehabilitation of balance in the elderly

Juleimar Soares Coelho de Amorim[1,4]*, Renata Cristine Leite[2], Renata Brizola[2] and Cristhiane Yumi Yonamine[3]

Abstract

Virtual reality therapy (VRT) has clinical indications in rehabilitation programs for the elderly; however, there is still no consensus on the recovery of body balance. The objective of this review was to summarize the effects of physical therapy interventions with VRT in the rehabilitation of balance in the elderly. The studies were identified via a systematic search in the databases PubMed, SciELO, LILACS and PEDro from 2010 onward. Clinical trials with interventions that involved VRT in the elderly were included in the study and were subjected to methodological quality analysis using the PEDro scale. A random effects meta-analysis of the studies that analyzed balance using the Berg Balance Scale and the Timed Up and Go (TUG) test was performed. Ten articles met the inclusion criteria, which presented variability in relation to the types of interventions used (70%) and the outcomes analyzed (60%). The mean duration of the interventions was 13.90 ($\pm$ 5.08) weeks, with at least two weekly sessions ($\pm$ 0.73). There were positive results in relation to improvements in both dynamic and static balance (70% of the studies), mobility (80%), flexibility (30%), gait (20%) and fall prevention (20%). A summary of the meta-analysis showed mean effects on the Berg scale (standardized mean difference [SMD]: -0.848; 95% CI: -1.161; -0.535) and the TUG test (SMD: 0.894; 95% CI: 0.341; 1.447). Individually, virtual reality is promising in rehabilitation programs for the elderly. The overall measures were sufficient to show beneficial effects of the therapy on balance in the elderly.

Keywords: Virtual reality exposure therapy, Postural balance, Rehabilitation, Physiotherapy modalities, Elderly

Background

The speed of population aging has led to challenges for the health system, especially with regard to interventions to maintain functional capacity and independence and to broaden the framework of rehabilitation professionals. Mobility, body balance (static and dynamic), gait, joint and lower limb muscle flexibility are indicated as musculoskeletal attributes that support functional capacity in the elderly [1]. The loss or decline of balance results in a major public health problem: falls. The imbalance results from interactions of the musculoskeletal, visual, and sensorimotor systems and related functional tasks that undergo changes with senescence, such as sarcopenia, proprioceptive alterations, joint stiffness, postural alignment, latency and temporal incoordination of muscle activation [1–4].

Orthopedic, rheumatologic and neurological diseases are responsible for compromising postural control and mobility, implying greater body oscillation. Similarly, healthy individuals may also suffer from balance disorders due to their own senescence, such as reduced neuromuscular response speed, motor planning, joint degeneration, bone density and sarcopenia. However, these changes should not result in bone fractures, soft tissue injuries or traumatic brain injury due to the occurrence of falls. Therefore, preventive and rehabilitative measures are necessary for the maintenance of the joint and musculoskeletal system [2–4].

Scientific evidence from the scope of physiotherapeutic rehabilitation points to kinesiotherapy for motor coordination, balance training, stretching, muscle strengthening and functional training as approaches capable of preventing functional capacity declines in the

* Correspondence: juleimar@yahoo.com.br
[1]Ciências da Reabilitação, Instituto Federal de Educação, Ciência e Tecnologia do Rio de Janeiro – IFRJ, Rio de Janeiro, RJ, Brasil
[4]Colina, Manhuaçu, Brazil
Full list of author information is available at the end of the article

elderly [5]. However, technological advances, including Virtual Reality Therapy (VRT), which employs games as a resource to help individuals with balance deficits through the use of electronic devices experienced by the "human-machine interface", have modernized the clinical practices of rehabilitation professionals [6–8].

VRT rehabilitation has received increasing attention from researchers and clinicians who recognize its benefits because of its therapeutic potential regarding falls prevention and balance rehabilitation [8, 9]. The easy applicability, the stimuli to the sensory and motor systems and the playful character of the therapy offer a high degree of motivation, pleasure and instantaneous feedback on the execution of the tasks. Thus, VRT stimulates functional activities, promotes social interaction when administered collectively and may encourage the adherence of the elderly to rehabilitation programs [8–10].

The patient's movements are captured by a sensor bar or camera and are similar to those performed in daily life activities, facilitating motor recovery. These movements generally simulate sports practices, and to effectively perform the game, the patient is challenged to perform movements that strengthen the muscles, stimulate brain activity, improve sensory response and increase concentration, balance, motor coordination, motor control and gait efficiency [10].

Contradictory results have been reported in the literature, and VRT dissemination is still incipient [6, 7]. Evidence of the positive and negative effects of virtual reality can prod physiotherapists to broaden their scope of action in the provision of care during rehabilitation of the elderly. Therefore, a literature review can provide information on which domains of functional rehabilitation have demonstrated effective interventions using VRT. This therapy has not yet received a structured critique for improving body balance. Therefore, the objective of this review was to evaluate and synthesize the effects of physiotherapeutic interventions with VRT in balance rehabilitation of the elderly.

Materials and methods

The systematic review identified and selected studies published in Portuguese, English and/or Spanish. Four search themes were combined using the Boolean operators "AND" and "OR". The first search was on virtual reality therapy, combined in the title/abstract from the key words *"Virtual Reality Exposure Therapy"* or *"Video Game"* and *"Rehabilitation"* or *"Physical Therapy"* or *"Physiotherapy Modalities"*. Next, we identified the studies with samples of elderly individuals using the term *"Elderly"*. The third search included the outcomes *"Postural Balance"* and/or *"Proprioception"*. Finally, *"Clinical Trial"* studies were selected as the type of publication. All the keywords were extracted from the Health

Descriptors (Descritores em Saúde - DeCS), and the search adopted its equivalents in English and Spanish. The search was performed in the electronic databases MEDLINE via PubMed, EMBASE, SciELO, LILACS and PEDro. The search ended in August 2016.

Clinical trial and controlled or randomized clinical trial articles published from 2010 onward with sample compositions that contained elderly subjects and that used VRT as a method of balance rehabilitation were included. Studies with interventions that were not specific to physical therapy or that presented preliminary data, pilot studies, interventions for vestibular rehabilitation (dizziness, labyrinthitis, vertigo), review articles, case studies, theses and dissertations were excluded.

The materials were selected by two independent reviewers who analyzed the title, the abstract and then the text in full, in this sequence; in cases of disagreement, a third reviewer was asked for consensus. To analyze the methodological quality of the studies, the PEDro scale was used. This scale is a *checklist* widely used in the area of rehabilitation, elaborated by the database *Physiotherapy Evidence Database Research*, which is specific for studies that investigate the effectiveness of interventions in physical therapy [11]. The scale has a total score of 10 points, with scores ≥5 considered to be of high quality.

The following data were extracted from the studies from a form that was specifically developed to analyze the data, adjusted by authors' interest as recommended by the *Cochrane Library* [12]: information about the author, year of publication, research objective, sample composition (size, diagnoses and age group), evaluation instruments, intervention measures (combined VRT or VRT alone), comparison, randomization process, intention-to-treat analysis, loss control and sample calculation, blinding process, number of sessions, weekly frequency, mean duration of therapy and the main results found. The final evaluation of the quality of the evidence was verified by the GRADE (*Grading of Recommendations Assessment, Development and Evaluation*) System, which establishes a consensus about the quantification of the quality of the evidence and of the recommendation strength in high, moderate, low or very low levels [13].

Articles that presented complete data regarding the evaluation and results (means and standard deviations) of the body balance construct and that presented homogeneity in the outcome measure were combined to perform the random effects meta-analysis using Stata13.1 software (StataCop 2013. College Station, TX: StatCopLP). The standardized mean difference (SMD), its 95% confidence intervals and the effect size (Overall Z) were used to estimate the effectiveness of the VRT intervention, with a value of $p < 0.05$ being considered statistically significant. The heterogeneity of the studies was evaluated by the value of the I^2 statistics, the p-value obtained by the Cochran Q test, the tau-square estimate and the difference between means, and those with p values > 0.05 were considered homogeneous.

Results

The search resulted in 486 articles in the MEDLINE, EMBASE, SciELO, LILACS and PEDro databases, of which only 24 met the inclusion and exclusion criteria for reading in full. The final sample of studies consists of 10 articles, as summarized in Fig. 1.

The characteristics of the selected articles regarding the intervention and the outcomes and results are presented in Table 1. There was variability in relation to the type of intervention used and the outcomes analyzed, in which seven different types of interventions were verified (proprioceptive training, aerobic training, static and dynamic balance, muscle flexibility, yoga and strengthening). The mean sample size was 31.40 ($\pm$ 13.75) participants, with a minimum age of 62.22 ($\pm$ 4.41) years old and a maximum of 87.40 ($\pm$ 6.02) years old; eight (80%) studies performed interventions with the elderly without reporting specific diseases (healthy), one study (10%) was on Parkinson's disease, and one study (10%) was on diabetes mellitus. The mean duration of the sessions was 13.90 ($\pm$ 5.08) weeks, with a mean weekly frequency of

2.10 ($\pm$ 0.73) times and an average duration of 37 ($\pm$ 10.85) minutes.

Two studies (20%) analyzed the results by intention to treat, and 30% of the articles had post-intervention follow-up for a mean time of 4.66 weeks ($\pm$ 1.15). In all studies, there was randomization with a control group; 20% ($N = 2$) had a blinded evaluator, 30% ($N = 3$) used combination therapy, 80% referred to sample calculation ($N = 8$), and the mean score in the PEDro scale equal was to 6.80 ($\pm$ 1.135) points. The main instruments for measuring the outcomes were the Berg balance scale (60%, $N = 6$), *Timed Up and Go* (TUG) (60%, N = 6), unipedal support (40%, $N = 4$) and functional range (30%, $N = 3$) (Table 2).

The effectiveness of the intervention was present in 70% of the individuals who performed VRT, the main effects being improvements in balance (dynamic and static) (80%, $N = 8$), mobility and flexibility (30%, $N = 3$) and gait (20%, N = 2) and a reduction in falls (20%, N = 2). Table 2 shows the variation in the choice of instruments for measuring these outcomes. To systematize the results in relation to the main domains of balance and based on the proportion of studies that adopted specific instruments to assess the efficacy of the therapy, the balance and mobility outcomes were measured, respectively, using the Berg Balance Scale and the TUG

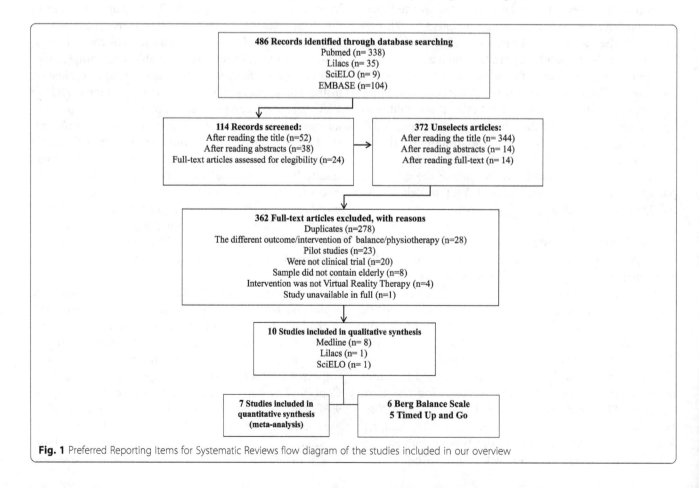

Fig. 1 Preferred Reporting Items for Systematic Reviews flow diagram of the studies included in our overview

Table 1 Characteristics of the articles included in the systematic review

Author/Year	Participants N (mean age)	Diagnosis	Outcomes	Intervention	Result	Conclusion
TREML, 2012 [15]	$N = 32$ CG = 16 (67.63 years old) EG = 16 (66.88 years old)	Healthy Elderly	Balance, mobility, flexibility and number of falls.	CG: proprioceptive training EG: proprioceptive training and Wii Fit Plus Games. Duration: 2 times a week, 10 sessions of 30 min.	POMA: $p = 0.018$ Unipedal support: $p = 0.018$ Anterior functional range: $p = 0.012$ Lateral functional range: $p = 0.012$ Berg Balance Scale: $p = 0.068$	VRT has been shown to be more efficient at conventional proprioceptive training in mobility, static balance and range.
RENDON, 2012 [8]	$N = 40$ CG = 20 (83.3 years old) EG = 20 (85.7 years old)	Elderly with risk of falls	Dynamic balance	CG: no intervention EG: stationary bicycle warm up and Wii Fit games. Duration: 3 times a week, 18 sessions of 35–45 min.	Balance confidence scale: $p = 0.04$	Authors reported improved dynamic balance, greater postural stability in the elderly and reduced risk of falls.
YEN, 2011 [18]	$N = 42$ CG = 14 (71.6 years old) GTC = 14 (70.1 years old) EG = 14 (70.4 years old)	Elderly with Parkinson's balance	Balance and functional capacity	CG: no intervention CTG: stretching and conventional balance training protocol EG: stretching, VRT balance board and games. Duration: 2 times per week, 12 sessions of 30 min.	Computerized posturography: $p > 0.05$	Both CTG and EG improved sensory integration for postural control. However, the demand for attention to postural control did not change after any VR or conventional treatment.
MUSSATO, 2012 [9]	$N = 10$ CG = 5 (65.6 years old) EG = 5 (66 years old)	Healthy Elderly	Balance and functional capacity	CG: no intervention EG: training with Nintendo Wii Fit accompanied by Balance Board and games. Duration: once a week, 10 sessions of 30 min.	Stabilometric platform variables after training with Wii Fit: $p > 0.05$ Unipedal support: $p = 0.01$ TUG: $p = 0.004$ (comparison between the pre- and post-intervention results of the EG) TUG: $p = 0.704$ (comparison between EG and CG)	The results did not show changes in stabilometric variables after treatment with Wii Fit. There was a significant difference between the pre- and post-intervention for the experimental group for both the Unipedal Support test and the TUG, but there was no statistical difference when compared with the control group.
LEE, 2013 [10]	$N = 55$ CG = 28 (74.29 years old) EG = 27 (73.78 years old)	Diabetes Mellitus	Balance and gait	CG: health education guidelines on diabetes EG: virtual reality and games. Duration: 2 times per week, 20 sessions of 50 min.	Unipedal support: $p = 0.001$ Gait cadence speed: $p = 0.001$ Falls efficacy scale: $p = 0.002$	After the training, the intervention group showed improvement in balance, decreased sitting and standing time, increased gait cadence and perceived falls.
SZTURM, 2011 [16]	$N = 27$ CG = 14 (81 years old) EG = 13 (80.5 years old)	Deficit of balance and mobility	Balance and gait	CG: conventional physiotherapy program for strengthening and balance sitting and standing. EG: rehabilitation with exercises of dynamic balance associated to games. Duration: 2 times per week, 16 sessions of 45 min	Berg Balance Scale: $p < 0.001$ Balance Confidence Scale: $p < 0.02$ Timed Up and Go: $p < 0.01$ Gait speed: $p = 0.20$	Improvement of the dynamic standing balance control (EG) compared with the conventional exercise program (CG). However, there was no statistically significant effect on gait.
BIERYLA, 2013 [17]	$N = 10$ CG = 5 (80.5 years old) EG = 5 (82.5 years old)	Healthy Elderly	balance	CG: no intervention EG: series of exercises and activities with games Duration: 3 times per week, 9 sessions of 30 min	Berg Balance Scale: $p = 0.037$ Fullerton Advanced Balance Scale: $p = 0.529$ Functional Reach Test: $p = 0.779$ Timed Up and Go: $p = 0.174$	Better balance results, with delayed effect for 1 month post-intervention on the Berg Balance Scale. No effects on the Advanced Balance Scale, range tests or TUG.
LAI, 2013 [20]	$N = 30$ CG = 15 (74.8 years old) EG = 15 (70.6 years old)	Healthy Elderly	Balance	CG: no intervention EG: VR therapy in the Xavix Measured Step System (XMSS) Duration: 3 times per week, 18 sessions of 30 min.	Berg Balance Scale: $p = 0.001$ Timed Up and Go: $p = 0.046$ Modified Falls Efficacy Scale: $p = 0.001$ Bipedal balance test on force platform: Eyes open: $p = 0.052$ Eyes closed: $p = 0.092$	Improved balance after 6 weeks of training; effects persisted partially after 6 weeks without intervention.

Table 1 Characteristics of the articles included in the systematic review *(Continued)*

Author/Year	Participants N (mean age)	Diagnosis	Outcomes	Intervention	Result	Conclusion
FRANCO, 2012 [14]	N = 32 CG = 10 (76.9 years old) GTP = 11 (77.9 years old) EG = 11 (79.8 years old)	Healthy Elderly	Balance	WFG: Guidance for balance and flexibility home exercises and intervention in Nintendo Wii Fit with games. MOB: group exercise sessions. CG: no intervention Duration: GTP: 2 times per week, 6 sessions of 10–15 min active play EG: 2 times per week, 6 sessions of 30–45 min	Berg's Balance Scale: $p = 0.837$ Tinetti's Balance Scale: $p = 0.913$ Quality of Life (SF-36): $p = 0.058$	No significant increase in balance in any outcome measures.
TOULOTTE, 2012 [19]	N = 36 G1 = 9 84.2 years old) G2 = 9 (72.2 years old) G3 = 9 (76.4 years old) G4 = 9 (71.8 years old)	Healthy Elderly	Balance	G1: Physical activities - strengthening exercises, proprioception, flexibility and static and dynamic balance. G2: Training with Wii Fit - Games. G3: Physical activities associated with Wii Fit training. G4: control group - watched television and board games Duration: once a week, 20 sessions of 60 min.	Tinetti scale: $p < 0.05$ for G1, G2 and G3 Unipedal support: $p < 0.05$ for G1 and G3. Modified position of center of gravity: $p < 0.05$ for G2 and G3.	Improvement in static balance. G1 and G3 improved dynamic balance.

*CG Control Group, EG Experimental Group, WFG Wii Fit Group, MOB Matter of Balance, TUG Timed Up and Go Group

Table 2 Studies included in the systematic review: analysis of the methodological quality, instruments and equipment to perform the therapy

Author/Year	PS	Outcome evaluation tools	Virtual Reality Therapy
TREML, 2012 [15]	7	Berg Balance Scale; Functional Range; Performance Oriented Gait and Balance Assessment; Unipedal Support	Nintendo Wii console associated with Balance Board and Wii Fit games
RENDON, 2012 [8]	6	TUG; Balance of Confidence Scale; Geriatric Depression Scale	Nintendo Wii console associated with Balance Board and Wii Fit games
YEN, 2011 [18]	7	Dynamic computerized posturography: Standing sensory organization test, sitting cognitive test and sensory organization test and standing cognitive test	Balance board, LCD monitor and a personal computer
MUSSATO, 2012 [9]	7	Stabilometric Platform (Baropodometry), Unipedal Support and TUG.	Nintendo Wii console associated with Balance Board and Wii Fit games
LEE, 2013 [10]	7	Unipedal Support, Berg Balance Scale, Functional Range, TUG, Sitting and standing up, Gait Rite System, Falls Efficacy Scale	PlayStation 2 with the EyeToy accessory: Play 1.2, 3" (Sony Computer Entertainment)
SZTURM, 2011 [16]	8	Gait Rite System, Berg Balance Scale, TUG, Balance Confidence Scale, modified version of the Clinical Test of Sensory Interaction and Balance	Pressure mat associated with computer games
BIERYLA, 2013 [17]	4	Berg Balance Scale; Fullerton Advanced Balance Scale; Functional Range and TUG	Nintendo Wii console associated with Balance Board and Wii Fit games
LAI, 2013 [20]	8	Berg Balance Scale; Falls Efficacy Scale, TUG and Force Platform for Static Balance	Xavix Measured Step System (XMSS)
FRANCO, 2012 [14]	7	Berg Balance Scale; Tinetti's Scale; Quality of Life Questionnaire - SF36	Nintendo Wii console associated with Balance Board and Wii Fit games
TOULOTTE, 2012 [19]	7	Unipedal Support; Tinetti's Scale and Wii Fit test	Nintendo Wii console associated with Balance Board and Wii Fit games

*PS PEDro Scale. TUG Timed Up and Go test

test. The study included 86 elderly subjects, with a difference of 3.76 (± 1.83) points in the scale; 64 individuals achieved an improvement of 2.16 (± 1.13) seconds in the test.

The meta-analysis for effectiveness of the intervention in improving the scores of the Berg Balance Scale was performed based on six articles [9, 10, 13–17] because the data were missing in 30%. The SMD of the studies was – 0.848, contained in a 95% CI of – 1.161 to – 0.535. The result refutes the null hypothesis and shows the efficacy in the rehabilitation of balance in the elderly through VRT.

Regarding the outcome of the Berg Balance Scale, the difference between means ($p = 0.000$) shows that there is a significant statistical difference in the final score of the scale between the pre- and post-intervention measures with VRT. There was no evidence of heterogeneity ($I^2 = 0.0\%$, $p = 0.666$, Chi^2: 3.03) between the studies. Table 3 presents the results with the synthetic measure of each study by comparing VRT with other therapies or placebo and shows the summary measure (SMD: -0.858; 95% CI:-1.161; – 0.535), which indicates improvement by 5.31 points in the final score (Z: 5.31, $p = 0.000$).

Likewise, five studies [9, 10, 15–17] analyzed the time of the TUG test using VRT in the experimental group. As measured by the meta-analysis summary measure (0.894) and its respective confidence interval (95% CI: 0.341, 1.447), the value of the I^2 statistics (46.4%, $p = 0.114$) and the tau-squared result (0.1715), the improvement obtained showed an absence of heterogeneity, low variability between studies and evidence of a statistically significant difference in test execution speed (Z: 3.17 s; $p = 0.002$) (Table 4). The evaluation of the quality of the evidence, performed through the GRADE System, showed low and very low recommendation of the VRT based on improvements in the parameters of the Berg Scale and the TUG test, respectively (Table 5).

Discussion

This systematic review shows a shortage of intervention studies in the elderly using VRT, likely related to the great challenges of working with technological tools that have a playful character, the novelty of these products in the therapeutic market, the low knowledge of physiotherapists about the benefits of VRT, the preferences of professionals and users, the development and standardization of games

Table 3 Standardized mean difference (95% CI) for the effect of virtual reality therapy on the Berg Balance Scale score, grouping data from six studies (N = 174)

Author, year	Therapy	Pre-Intervention			Post-Intervention			SMD (95% CI)	Study weight (%)	SMD, Random Effect Model, 95% CI
		Mean	SD	Total	Mean	SD	Total			
Treml, 2013	VRT vs proprioception	52.75	4.37	16	55.5	1.07	16	-0.864 (-1.591;-0.138)	18.57	
Lee, 2013	VRT vs health education	51.67	2.48	27	53.41	1.89	27	-0.791 (-1.341;-0.241)	32.45	
Szturm, 2011	VRT vs kinesiotherapy	47.0	13.8	13	53.2	12.4	13	-0.474 (-1.240;0.293)	16.70	
Bieryla, 2013	VRT vs placebo	50.0	2.82	4	53.0	1.4	5	-1.410 (-2.918;0.098)	4.31	
Lai, 2013	VRT vs placebo	50.53	4.75	15	53.87	3.56	15	-0.796 (-1.541;-0.050)	17.64	
Franco, 2011	VRT vs placebo	48.0	3.7	11	52.0	0.8	10	-1.460 (-2.434;-0.486)	10.33	
Total				86			86	**-0.848 (-1.161;-0.535)**	**100.0**	

Heterogeneity: $I^2 = 0.0\%$ (p = 0.696; $tau^2 = 0.000$)
Overall effect size (overall Z): Z = 5.31 (p = 0.000)

VRT: virtual reality exposure therapy; SD: standard deviation; SMD: standardized mean difference; CI: confidence interval. The mean of the measure used for evaluation refers to the score obtained (maximum 56 points).

to train functional tasks such as balance, gait and range and the design of clinical trials of high methodological quality [7].

Among the articles analyzed, the forms of intervention differed even in the presence of a similar outcome. Some studies were conducted with a more pragmatic therapeutic approach, with protocols varying according to the individual evaluation of the elderly [14, 18, 19]; others have established systematic, segmented and progressive protocols, including warm-up and isolated or combined exercises [8, 9, 15–17, 20]. Another study had a protocol associating practice at home with the clinical environment [10].

The beneficial effects of VRT presented by the studies included in this systematic review extended to the outcomes of the balance variables, including mobility, flexibility [15], gait cadence and fear of falls [10]. There seems to be agreement among the authors about the positive results in these components; however, the meta-analysis evidenced possible discrepancies in the sample composition and the interventions.

Table 4 Standardized mean difference (95% CI) for the effect of virtual reality therapy on the time (in seconds) of the *Timed Up and Go* (TUG) test, grouping data from five studies (N = 131)

Author, year	Therapy	Pre-Intervention			Post-Intervention			SMD (95% CI)	Study weight (%)	SMD, Random Effect Model, 95% CI
		Mean	SD	Total	Mean	SD	Total			
Mussato, 2012	VRT vs placebo	8.2	0.4	5	6.8	0.5	5	3.092 (1.135;5.050)	6.82	
Lee, 2013	VRT vs health education	11.48	2.31	27	9.78	1.58	27	0.862 (0.308;1.416)	31.72	
Szturm, 2011	VRT vs kinesiotherapy	8.0	1.0	13	5.1	3.7	13	1.052 (0.243;1.861)	23.30	
Bieryla, 2013	VRT vs placebo	12.8	1.9	4	11.2	2.61	4	0.686 (-0.677;2.049)	12.17	
Lai, 2013	VRT vs placebo	9.54	3.52	15	8.54	2.85	15	0.312 (-0.408;1.033)	26.00	
Total				64			64	**0.894 (0.341;1.447)**	**100.0**	

Heterogeneity: $I^2 = 46.4\%$ (p = 0.114; $tau^2 = 0.1715$)
Overall effect size (overall Z): Z = 3.17 (p = 0.002)

VRT: virtual reality exposure therapy; SD: standard deviation; SMD: standardized mean difference; CI: confidence interval. The mean of the measurement used to perform the test was in seconds.

Table 5 GRADE system quality of evidence analysis for the Berg Balance Scale and the Timed Up and Go (TUG) test

Quality assessment								Quality	Importance
Number of studies	Design	Serious limitations (risk of bias)?	Inconsistency of results (heterogeneity)?	Indirect evidence?	Inaccuracy?	Publishing bias?			
Berg Scale									
6	Quasi-experimental studies and RCTs	No	No	No	Very important	Sim		++ / ++++ Low	Critical
TUG Test									
5	Quasi-experimental studies and RCTs	No	Low	No	Very important	Sim		+++ / ++++ Very Low	Critical

TUG Timed Up and Go
GRADE Grading of Recommendations Assessment, Development and Evaluation

The study by Holden [7] systematically reviewed the literature on interventions using VRT for balance and motor skills specifically for neurological disorders in individuals over 45 years of age. The authors note that for body balance, the three studies reported significant improvements in performance. Another important meta-analysis reported no significant effect of VRT [21] compared with traditional physical therapy or no intervention. However, the authors' review did not include the electronic databases SciELO and LILACS as a search source on the use of games in balance recovery.

Specifically concerning the interventions with emphasis on the improvement of static balance, Mussato and collaborators [9] have noted that the effect is more sensitive to detection in the baropodometry test since it measures maximum peaks and not the mean oscillation amplitude of the body balance. The games selected for this study offered medial-lateral and anteroposterior imbalances, thus stimulating the recruitment of motor strategies and allowing greater variability in the displacements of the pressure center in the orthostatic posture [22].

For gait training, Lobo [23] points out games for the rehabilitation of weight transfer abilities between limbs, unipedal support, triple flexion and load acceptance during initial support. However, other important aspects, such as dissociation of waists, impulsion and continuous anterior displacement of the center of mass, are not possible through VRT since the step change occurs in a stationary manner, which would justify the fact that Szturm [16] did not obtain a positive effect on the gait speed. In conventional rehabilitation, the stimuli are offered by the equipment through active dynamic training, and the proprioceptive *inputs* are produced by the efferent route [15]. Visualization of the action on the display (visual *feedback*) and interaction with the game stimulate proprioceptive *inputs* in a static manner.

The benefits noted in the aspects of static balance, gait components and sensorimotor integration show that the games provide training conditions that favor an integration between cognitive and motor stimulation. More complex training involving dual tasks, such as cognition and motor activity, requires automatic control during movements since the focus of attention is on the game shown on the display, thus promoting motor function improvement when compared with conventional training [15, 24].

Regarding falls, the training approaches of the articles included in this review aimed to increase or restore the self-confidence of the elderly. Individually, studies showed the superiority of VRT in recovering body balance when compared with conventional interventions, with impacts on the self-efficacy of post-intervention falls and not necessarily on the reduction in the number of falls.

Based on the health problems, it was noted that the designs aimed at prevention of falls and other conditions were evaluated in patients with Parkinson's disease. The study by Yen [18] resulted in improved sensory integration for postural control; however, the demand for attention was not altered after any VRT. Santana [25] and Loureiro [26], in experimental studies without a comparison group, concluded that training using the Nintendo Wii Fit Plus platform proved to be useful for the rehabilitation of degenerative diseases regarding motor performance, flexibility, lower limb joint stiffness and functional independence, in addition to improving the motor learning ability due to the cognitive stimuli provided by the videogame. The activation of neural circuits and structures by virtual games can play a key role in transferring the immediate effects of games to long-term effects. Lai [20] did not attribute maintenance of improvement to VRT per se; after the end of the interventions, the elderly improved their balance and felt confident to engage in physical activity, which justifies maintaining good results regarding balance.

Some methodological aspects were observed in the included clinical trials that reduce the risk of bias and allow better measurements when systematically adopted by the studies. All of them reported randomization, with well-established selection criteria for the participants, to increase the significance of the data, restricting populations with similar characteristics and guaranteeing homogeneity of the samples. Only two of the studies analyzed blinded one of the evaluators, an important item to be considered since this principle is used to avoid systematic errors in the research. Another aspect is intention-to-treat analysis, which also avoids distortions caused by a loss of participants, which may interrupt the equivalence established by randomized selection, reflecting non-adherence to treatment and potential benefits in individuals receiving the treatment established by the study.

The studies sought to guarantee homogeneity of the samples from systematic methods of development of clinical trials, in which the absence of heterogeneity in the articles was confirmed in the meta-analysis. However, we emphasize that there was a discrepancy in the individual results, which can be attributed to the size of the sample, the intensity of the intervention and differences in the participants' baseline risks. It is observed that the sample size and the number of sessions in the studies that were not effective in the balance of the elderly showed lower averages than those of effective studies. In relation to statistical power, only three articles [8, 10, 18] performed the calculation, and it is not possible to state whether the absence of significant improvement due to the interventions in some studies occurred because of the lack of efficacy of the technique or because of the small sample size. The intervention protocol presented great variety regarding the number of sessions, weekly frequency, intervention time and isolated and/or combined exercises, and caution in decision making is required.

The literature evidenced dissent, and the dissemination of VRT was still incipient, which can also be demonstrated by the analysis of the quality of the evidence. According to evaluation criteria for recommending GRADE System evidence, the data selected to compose the meta-analysis may be influenced by publication bias, a tendency for published results to be systematically different from reality, as well as imprecision of the outcome measure and the sample size. Although there is a large body of literature on the role of physiotherapy in rehabilitating balance in the elderly and although studies published using VRT show positive results, the power of generalization is limited due to the samples sizes of the articles included in this review. Therefore, the results reflect a promising tool that requires more scientific investigations about the outcome to improve confidence in estimates of its effects. Future studies should specifically evaluate the types of protocol, as the need for advances in expanding the therapeutic armamentarium for rehabilitation practitioners is highlighted. To increase data reliability, new studies with sufficient sample size, better levels of evidence and methodological rigor are recommended in clinical trials demonstrating blinding techniques, intention-to-treat analysis, sample size and

number of sessions to establish specific protocols of treatment. As a limitation of this study, we highlight the difficulty in exploring other domains of balance rehabilitation of the elderly, given the limited number of clinical trials included limiting the subgroup analysis, in addition to restriction to literature in English, Spanish and Portuguese.

Systematic review of clinical research on physiotherapeutic interventions with VRT in the rehabilitation of balance in the elderly emphasized relevance through the scenario of population aging resulting in unfavorable structural and functional changes predisposing elderly people to falls. Therefore, the therapeutic approach based on virtual reality is another alternative, which may, in addition to promoting motor control stimuli, help in gait efficiency and body balance. Because VRT is a playful method, it can encourage the participation of these individuals in activities of balance rehabilitation. Evidence of the results of virtual reality can awaken physiotherapists to broaden the scope of action in the provision of care during the rehabilitation of the elderly.

Conclusion

This review synthesized the effects of virtual reality therapy. Individually, there was concordance in the analyzed clinical trials regarding the improvements of static balance, gait components, sensorimotor integration and self-efficacy of falls, with no significant relevance for dynamic balance, gait speed and reduction in the number of falls. The data set evaluated in the meta-analysis and the quality of evidence analysis indicate the effectiveness of VRT in the treatment of balance and mobility in the elderly, but further studies are needed. Implications for clinical practice require caution in decision making because of sample profiles, intervention protocols and outcome measures. Regarding implications for the research, due to the lack of homogeneity in the methodologies, interventions and study outcomes in the studies, systematic positive effects were demonstrated for the mobility outcomes. The findings on using virtual reality therapy for recovery and balance training seem promising. However, to make assertions regarding effectiveness, adjustments are still needed for future studies.

Authors' contributions

The individual contributions of authors should be specified following: JSCdA made substantial contributions to conception and design, analysis and interpretation of data; been involved in drafting the manuscript or revising it critically for important intellectual content; given final approval of the version to be published. RCL made substantial contributions to conception and design, acquisition of data and interpretation of data; been involved in drafting the manuscript or revising it critically for important intellectual content; given final approval of the version to be published. RB made substantial contributions to conception and design, acquisition of data and interpretation of data; been involved in drafting the manuscript or revising it critically for important intellectual content; given final approval of the version to be published.

CYY made substantial contributions to conception and design and interpretation of data; been involved in drafting the manuscript or revising it critically for important intellectual content; given final approval of the version to be published.

Author details
[1]Ciências da Reabilitação, Instituto Federal de Educação, Ciência e Tecnologia do Rio de Janeiro – IFRJ, Rio de Janeiro, RJ, Brasil. [2]Centro Universitário Filadélfia – UNIFIL, Londrina, PR, Brasil. [3]Saúde Coletiva, Centro Universitário Filadélfia – UNIFIL, Londrina, PR, Brasil. [4]Colina, Manhuaçu, Brazil.

References

1. Bruniera CAV, Rodacki ALF. Respostas estabilométricas de jovens e idosos para recuperar o equilíbrio após uma perturbação inesperada controlada. Rev Educ Fis UEM. 2014;25(3):345–51.

2. Meireles AE, Pereira LVS, Oliveira TG, Christofoletti G, Fonseca AL. Alterações neurológicas fisiológicas ao envelhecimento afetam o sistema mantenedor do equilíbrio. Rev Neurocienc. 2010;18(1):103–8.

3. Pícoli TS, Figueiredo LL, Patrizzi LJ. Sarcopenia e envelhecimento. Fisioter Mov. 2011;24(3):455–62.

4. Teixeira INAO, Guariento ME. Biologia do envelhecimento: teorias, mecanismos e perspectivas. Ciênc Saúde Coletiva 2010. 2016;15(6):2845–57.

5. Gontijo RW, Leão MRC. Eficácia de um programa de fisioterapia preventiva para idosos. Rev Méd Minas Gerais. 2013;23(2):173–80.

6. Keshner EA. Virtual reality and physical rehabilitation: a new toy or a new research and rehabilitation tool? J Neuroeng Rehabil 2004. 2016;3(1):8.

7. Holden MK. Virtual environments for motor rehabilitation: review. Cyberpsychol Behav. 2005;8(3):187–211.

8. Rendon AA, Lohman EB, Thorpe D, Johnson EG, Medina E, Bradley B. The effect of virtual reality gaming on dynamic balance in older adults. Age Ageing. 2012;41(4):549–52.

9. Mussato R, Brandalize D, Brandalize M. Nintendo Wii® e seu efeito no equilíbrio e capacidade funcional de idosos saudáveis. Rev Brasil Ciência Mov 2012. 2016;20(2):68–75.

10. Lee S, Shin S. Effectiveness of virtual reality using video gaming. Diabetes Technol Ther. 2013;15(6):489–96.

11. Shiwa SR, Costa LOP, Moser ADL, Aguiar IC, Oliveira LVF. PEDro: a base de dados de evidências em fisioterapia. Fisioter Mov. 2011;24(3):523–33.

12. Higgins JPT, Green S. Cochrane handbook for systematic reviews of interventions 4.2.6 [updated September 2006]. In: The Cochrane Library, Issue 4. Chichester: John Wiley & Sons, Ltda; 2006.

13. Brasil. Ministério da Saúde. Diretrizes metodológicas: elaboração de pareceres técnicos-científicos. 3rd ed. Brasília: Ministério da Saúde; 2011. 80p.: il.

14. Franco JR, Jacobs K, Inzerillo C, Kluzik J. The effect of the Nintendo Wii fit and exercise in improving balance and quality of life in community dwelling elderls. Technol Health Care. 2012;20(2):95–115.

15. Treml CJ, Kalil Filho FA, Ciccarino RFL, Wegner RS, Saita CYS, Corrêa AG. O uso da plataforma Balance Board como recurso fisioterápico em idosos. Revbrasgeriatrgerontol. 2012;16(4):759–68.

16. Szturm T, Betkler AL, Moussavi Z, Desai A, Goodeman V. Effects of an interactive computer game exercise regimen on balance impairment in frail community-dwelling older adults: a randomized controlled trial. Phys Ther. 2011;91(10):1449–62.

17. Bieryla KA, Dold NM. Feasibility of Wii fit training to improve clinical measures of balance in older adults. Clin Interv Aging. 2013;8:775–81.

18. Yen CY, Lin KH, Hu MH, Wu RM, Lu Tw LCH. Effects of virtual reality-augmented balance training on sensory organization and attentional demand for postural control in people with Parkinson disease: a randomized controlled trial. Phys Ther. 2011;91(6):862–74.

19. Toulotte C, Toursel C, Olivier N. Wii fit® training vs. adapted physical activities: which one is the most appropriate to improve the balance of independent senior subjects? A randomized controlled study. Clin Rehabil. 2012;26(9):827–35.

20. Lai CH, Peng CW, Chen YL, Huang CP, Hsiao YL, Chen SC. Effects of interactive video-game based system exercise on the balance of the elderly. Gait Posture. 2013;37(4):511–8.

21. Booth V, Masud T, Connell L, Bath-Hextall F. The effectiveness of virtual reality intervention in improving balance in adults with impaired balance compared with standard or no treatment: a systematic review and meta-analysis. Clin Rehabil. 2014;28(5):419–31.

22. Ricci NA, Gazzola JM, Coimbra IB. Sistemas sensoriais no equilíbrio corporal de idosos. Arq Bras Ciên Saúde. 2009;34(2):94–100.

23. Lobo AM. Efeito de um Treinamento em Ambiente Virtual Sobre o Desempenho da Marcha e Funções Cognitivas em Idosos Saudáveis. 2013. 112 f. São Paulo: Dissertação (Mestrado em Psicologia) - Universidade de São Paulo; 2013.

24. Silva, K. G. Efeito de um Treinamento com o Nintendo Wii® Sobre o Equilíbrio Postural e Funções Executivas de Idosos Saudáveis – Um Estudo Clinico Longitudinal, Controlado e Aleatorizado. 2013. 128 f. Dissertação (Mestrado em Psicologia) - Universidade de São Paulo, São Paulo, 2013.

25. Santana CMF, Lins OG, Sanguinetti DCM, Silva FP, Angelo TDA, Cariolano MGWS, Câmara SB, Silva JPA. Efeitos do tratamento com realidade virtual não imersiva na qualidade de vida de indivíduos com Parkinson. Revbrasgergerontol. 2015;18(1):49–58.

26. Loureiro APC, Ribas CG, Zotz TGG, Chen R, Ribas F. Viabilidade da terapia virtual na reabilitação de pacientes com doença de Parkinson: estudo-piloto. Fisioter. Mov. 2012;25(3):659–66.

21

Panniculitides of particular interest to the rheumatologist

Thâmara Cristiane Alves Batista Morita[1,5*] (ID), Gabriela Franco Sturzeneker Trés[1], Maria Salomé Cajas García[2], Ilana Halpern[1], Paulo Ricardo Criado[1,3] and Jozelio Freire de Carvalho[4]

Abstract

The panniculitides remain as one of the most challenging areas for clinicians, as they comprise a heterogeneous group of inflammatory diseases involving the subcutaneous fat with potentially-shared clinical and histopathological features. Clinically, most panniculitides present as red edematous nodules or plaques. Therefore, in addition to a detailed clinical history, a large scalpel biopsy of a recent-stage lesion with adequate representation of the subcutaneous tissue is essential to specific diagnosis and appropriate clinical management. Herein we review the panniculitides of particular interest to the rheumatologist.

Keywords: Cutaneous polyarteritis nodosa, Erythema nodosum, Infective panniculitis, Lupus panniculitis, Panniculitis, Subcutaneous tissue, Vasculitis

Background

The panniculitides comprise a heterogeneous group of inflammatory diseases involving the subcutaneous fat. The basic unit of the subcutaneous fat is a cohesive collection of adipocytes called primary microlobule. An aggregation of primary microlobules, termed a secondary lobule, is surrounded by an easily discernible rim of connective tissue known as septum, which house the nerves, the lymphatic vessels, and the arteries and veins of the subcutis. Every adipocyte in the subcutaneous fat is encircled by a capillary [1].

This knowledge is crucial, once classification of the panniculitides is far too complex and often contradictory. From an academic point of view, in this review we have chosen to follow the three-step approach for histopathologic diagnosis of panniculitides. The first step is to classify them as mostly septal (Fig. 1) or lobular (Fig. 2) depending on where the inflammatory cell infiltrate is located. Secondly, is necessary to define if vasculitis is present or not. Finally, the third step is further characterizing the type of the inflammatory cell infiltrate and the presence and pattern of necrosis [2, 3]. Nevertheless,

different stages in the evolution of diseases and categories that are not exclusive may lead clinicians to confusion. Therefore, after that initial classification, efforts should be made to look for the additional histopathological findings that may be considered as clues to reach specific diagnoses.

The purpose of this review is to present a comprehensive clinic pathologic overview of the panniculitides of particular interest to the rheumatologist.

Main text
Primarily-septal panniculitides
Primarily-septal panniculitides without vasculitis

Erythema nodosum Erythema nodosum (EN) is the most common clinical form of panniculitis. In children, up to the age of 12 years, the female-to-male ratio is approximately equal, whereas in adults it occurs three to six times more often in woman, usually in the second and third decades of life. EN typically manifest by the sudden onset of multiple painful inflammatory, cutaneous and subcutaneous red nodules, which may assume a deep bruised appearance as they fade, and coalescence-forming plaques. The most common location are the anterior and lateral surfaces of the lower limbs, although the extensor surfaces of the forearm, the thighs, and the trunk may also be affected (Fig. 3a). Systemic symptoms

* Correspondence: thamaramorita@usp.br
[1]Faculdade de Medicina FMUSP, Universidade de Sao Paulo, Sao Paulo, SP, Brazil
[5]Private practice, Aracaju, SE, Brazil
Full list of author information is available at the end of the article

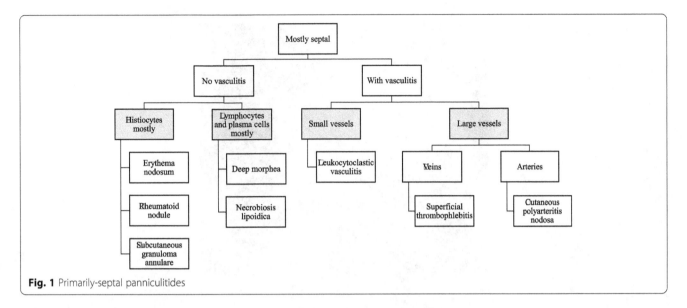

Fig. 1 Primarily-septal panniculitides

such as low-grade fever, fatigue, malaise, arthralgia, are present in more than 30% of the cases. The lesions never ulcerate and resolve spontaneously without leaving scars in approximately two to eight weeks [4, 5]. Currently, it is believed that EN migrans, subacute nodular migratory panniculitis, and chronic EN are clinical variants that may all be included within the spectrum of EN [6].

EN has been regarded a late type hypersensitivity reaction to several antigenic stimuli. The main etiologies are shown in Table 1 and may vary according to the geographic region. Streptococcal infection is a frequent cause of this panniculitis worldwide, especially in children; other potential infectious agents are represented by Epstein-Barr virus, Cytomegalovirus, *Yersinia spp.*, *Mycoplasma*, *Chlamydia*, *Histoplasma* and *Coccidioides*. Due to the elevated prevalence of tuberculosis in Brazil, *Mycobacterium tuberculosis* may be the most important factor in EN in our country. Drugs such as nonsteroidal anti-inflammatory drugs (NSAIDs), oral contraceptives, "biological" therapeutic agents (adalimumab, infliximab, imatinib, BRAF inhibitors, and immune checkpoint modulators) [7], and antibiotics, besides a wide group of conditions, which include sarcoidosis, pregnancy, autoimmune disorders, malignancies (mostly Hodgkin's disease), and enteropathies

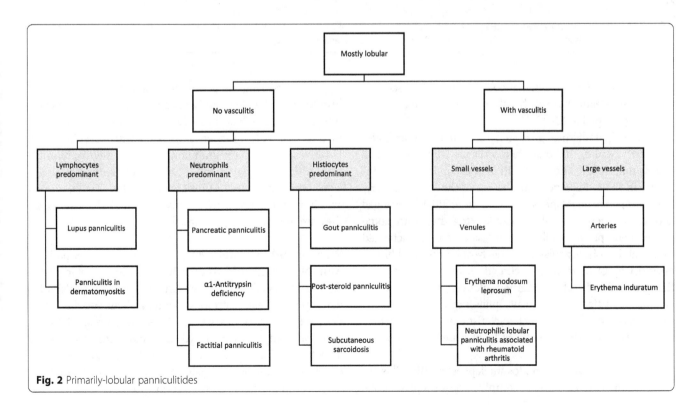

Fig. 2 Primarily-lobular panniculitides

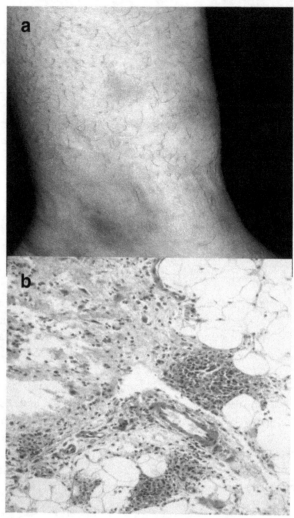

Fig. 3 Erythema nodosum. **a** Red nodules anterior on the anterior aspect of the lower limb. **b** Septal thickening with lymphohistiocytic infiltrate and formation of Miescher radial granulomas at the periphery of the subcutaneous fat lobule. H&E, 400x

(Crohn's disease and ulcerative colitis) can lead to secondary EN [8]. Meanwhile, nearly half of the cases are classified as having idiopathic EN [9, 10].

EN is the paradigm of predominantly septal panniculitides with no vasculitis, although hemorrhages within the small vessels may occur. The composition of the inflammatory infiltrate in the septa varies with the age of the lesion. In early lesions, sparse neutrophils are seen interstitially arranged and at the periphery of fat lobules, together with some foamy macrophages. Fully formed lesions are characterized by septal fibrosis, granulation tissue, lymphocytes and histiocytes, many of them multinucleated [2, 6]. Visualization of the so-called "Miescher radial granulomas", nodular aggregations of histiocytes and neutrophils radially surrounding small blood vessels, is quite characteristic in the histopathological evaluation (Fig. 3b) [4]. Fat lobules are reduced markedly in size.

In contrast, erythema nodosum leprosum (ENL) is an immune-mediated common complication of lepromatous

leprosy, occurring in about 50% of these patients. The histology of ENL lesions shows an intense perivascular infiltrate of neutrophils throughout the dermis and subcutis in a lobular pattern often associated with vasculitis [11]. However, macrophage granuloma without neutrophil infiltration occur in up to 35% of the patients. Foamy histiocytes containing large numbers of acid-fast bacilli, known as Virchow cells, are frequently seen in ENL lesions, as they are in lepromatous leprosy [12].

Rheumatoid nodule Almost one-third of the patients with rheumatoid arthritis exhibit skin lesions related to the disease, 98.3% of which are rheumatoid nodules (RNs). RNs develop in patients with long-standing rheumatoid arthritis (RA) and a higher disease activity score compared to patients without skin lesions. Rheumatoid factor positivity is detected in 75% of them. These nodules are commonly located on the metacarpophalangeal and proximal interphalangeal joints, on the olecranon process, and on the

Table 1 Etiologic factors in erythema nodosum

Infections	Pancreatic carcinoma
Streptococcal infections	**Medications**
Mycobacterium tuberculosis	Estrogens/oral contraceptive pills
Gastroenteritis due to *Yersinia, Salmonella, and Campylobacter*	Penicillin
Deep fungal infections: Blastomycosis, Histoplasmosis, Coccidioidomycosis, Sporotrichosis, Aspergillosis	Minocycline
Chlamydia pneumoniae	Sulfonamides
Chlamydia trachomatis	Halogens (bromides, iodides)
Mycoplasma pneumoniae infections	Salicylates
Cat-scratch disease	Chlorothiazides
Syphilis	Phenytoin
Infectious mononucleosis	Thalidomide
Herpes simplex	**Underlying disease processes**
Cytomegalovirus infections	Sarcoidosis (Lofgren's syndrome)
Hepatitis B (infection or vaccine)	Crohn's disease
Hepatitis C infection	Ulcerative colitis
Epstein–Barr virus	Behçet's disease
Protozoal infections: Toxoplasmosis, Ancylostomiasis, Amebiasis, Giardiasis, Ascariasis	Sweet's syndrome
Malignancy	Reiter's syndrome
Hodgkin's lymphoma	Takayasu's arteritis
Acute myelogenous leukemia	**Hormonal states**
Carcinoid tumor	Pregnancy

Main categories of etiologic factors are in boldface

proximal ulna; less frequently the palms, the back of the hands and, in bedridden patients, the occiput and ischium are affected. RNs are often asymptomatic, persistent, firm, and moveable in subcutaneous planes, characteristics that make them distinguishable from RNs mimickers, mostly tenosynovitis and bursitis nodules, that are softer, compressible and painful in the majority of the cases [13–16].

RNs have a distinctive histological appearance, resultant of an immune-mediated granulomatous process involving the deeper dermis and extending into the septa of the subcutaneous fat. They exhibit a well-defined palisading of elongated histiocytes around central collagen degeneration, with an intensely eosinophilic accumulation of fibrin in the center of the granuloma. Extensive fibrosis is prominent in old lesions. Accelerated rheumatoid nodulosis, a phenomenon that has been observed not only in patients on methotrexate therapy, but also during treatment with azathioprine, leflunomide, infliximab, and etanercept reveals the same histopathological findings of RNs [16–18]. Histopathologic differential diagnosis is made with subcutaneous granuloma annulare and necrobiosis lipoidica.

Deep morphea Morphea, or localized scleroderma, is a rare fibrosing disorder of the skin resulting from inflammation and deposition of collagen-rich extracellular matrix [19]. When sclerotic changes extend beyond the dermis to involve the subcutaneous tissue, the fascia or the superficial muscle, we refer to deep variant of circumscribed morphea (previously known as subcutaneous morphea or *morphea profunda*). In contrast, when there is exclusive deep fascia involvement, classification as eosinophilic fasciitis or Shulman's syndrome is more appropriate [20]. Clinically, deep morphea appears in the form of indurated plaques or nodules, frequently located on the upper part of the trunk close to the midline and on the lower limbs (Fig. 4a). The overlying skin may feel hardened and adherent to the underlying tissues; however, acute inflammatory signs, such as edema and erythema, are rarely observed [21–23]. The presence of deep sclerosis, in some cases perineural, may account for the presence of pain [19].

Morphea and systemic sclerosis cannot be differentiated by histopathologic examination. In the early stages, deep morphea shows perivascular infiltration in the reticular dermis that is predominantly lymphoplasmacytic, although eosinophils are found in one-third of the specimens, with swollen endothelial cells and thickened collagen bundles (Fig. 4b) [23]. Late morphea is characterized by dense collagen sclerosis, which produces thickened septa and fat lobule obliteration. Lipomembranous changes can also be observed [20, 24]. On the other hand,

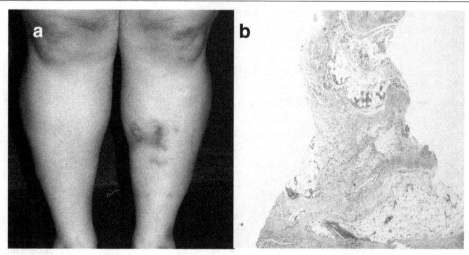

Fig. 4 Deep morphea. **a** Indurated plaque on the lower limb. **b** Thickening of the hypodermic septa by sclerotic collagen bundles, permeated by some lymphocytes and plasma cells, which extend to the periphery of the fat lobule. H&E, 100x

fibrous nodule formation in the setting of both systemic scleroderma and morphea consist histologically of mid dermal regions of fibrous tissue and inflammatory cells with increased mucin and decreased elastic fibers, indistinguishable from keloids [25].

Primarily-septal panniculitides with vasculitis

Cutaneous polyarteritis nodosa Polyarteritis nodosa (PAN) is a systemic necrotizing vasculitis that predominantly targets small and medium-sized muscular arteries. In adult patients, it is more common in male sex and the median age at presentation is 33 (19–71) years. Both genders are equally affected in children and the median age at disease onset is 11 (2–16) years [26, 27]. The pathway(s) leading to necrotizing inflammation of the blood vessels have not yet been completely unraveled. Immunological mechanisms seem to play a relevant role in the pathogenesis of PAN. Most of the cases are idiopathic; nevertheless, several triggers have been identified. Hepatitis B virus infection (HBV) is the most common and it is well known that patients with HBV-related PAN have more severe disease, even though its occurrence has largely decreased due to widespread vaccination [27]. PAN can also be associated with malignancies and others infectious agents, such as group A β-hemolytic *Streptococcus* [28, 29].

The most common manifestations are palpable purpura and reddish-purple subcutaneous nodules mainly located on the lower limbs; nevertheless, they may also include livedo racemosa, 'punched out' necrotic ulcers, *atrophie blanche*, and ultimately gangrene of digits, especially in children (Fig. 5a). Cutaneous PAN (C-PAN), also known as cutaneous arteritis since the 2012 Revised International Chapel Hill Consensus Conference, is a special form of

the disease restricted to the skin. Despite frequent relapses, cutaneous arteritis has a more benign course, milder constitutional symptoms and extra-cutaneous manifestations, which include arthritis, muscle pain and peripheral neuropathy, limited to the same area with overlying skin lesions [30, 31].

Skin biopsy is extremely useful for a definitive diagnosis. Cutaneous arteritis consists of a necrotizing vasculitis affecting small and medium-sized arteries within deep dermal or at the septa of the subcutaneous fat tissue. Fibrinoid degeneration involves all layers of the vascular wall, and internal elastic lamina disruption is detected (Fig. 5b). The histological changes can be divided into four stages (acute, subacute, reparative and healed), with a transition from a predominantly neutrophilic to lymphocytic infiltrate in the subacute and reparative stages. Then, vascular lumens become occluded by the fibrin thrombi with perivascular neovascularization in the healed stages [32, 33]. Direct immunofluorescence staining may show C3 and IgM deposits within vessels in the lesions [34]. Nodular vasculitis and thrombophlebitis are considered histopathologic differential diagnosis.

Primarily-lobular panniculitides
Primarily-lobular panniculitides without vasculitis

Gouty panniculitis Gouty panniculitis represents an extremely rare manifestation of gout, characterized by the deposition of monosodium urate crystals in the lobular hypodermis. The pathophysiology is currently poorly understood and serum uric acid level need not to be elevated to its development [35]. Gouty panniculitis may precede, appears concomitantly or years after the articular clinical expression of tophaceous gout. On physical examination, patients present with indurated, erythematous,

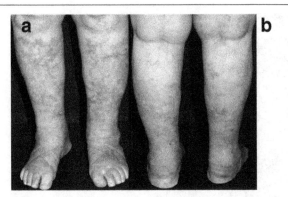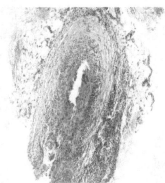

Fig. 5 Cutaneous polyarteritis nodosa. **a** Multiple infiltrated erythematous nodules mixed with livedo racemosa on the lower legs. **b** Vasculitis of medium-size-artery at the septa of the subcutaneous fat tissue. H&E, 200x

and irregular subcutaneous nodules or plaques, frequently painful, which can ulcerate and drain serous or opaque fluid. Lesions are located predominantly on the lower extremities, although they may be observed on upper extremities, torso, buttocks and scalp [36–38]. Skin biopsy reveals amorphous eosinophilic deposits in the deep dermis and subcutaneous tissue surrounded by a granulomatous reaction with macrophages and many multinucleated giant cells. Urate crystals causing lobular panniculitis show a needle-like shape and are doubly refractive under polarized light [39].

Post-steroid panniculitis This is a very rare panniculitis mostly described in childhood, but also in early adulthood, one to 10 days after cessation of systemic corticosteroid therapy. It has been suggested that a sudden decrease or withdrawal of high doses of corticosteroids either oral or intravenous may cause an increase in the ratio of saturated to unsaturated fatty acids, leading to crystal formation. The nodules tend to appear in those areas prone to accumulation of fat during steroid therapy such as the cheeks, jawline, arms and trunk, although it has also been reported on the legs. Usually there are no general symptoms [40, 41].

Characteristic histopathological findings consist of lobular panniculitis without vasculitis, with narrow strands needle-shaped clefts in radial arrangement within the cytoplasm of histiocytes, multinucleated giant cells, and the great majority of fat cells. The needle-shaped clefts represent negative images of crystals of triglycerides dissolved during tissue processing. These features are also seen in *sclerema neonatorum* and subcutaneous fat necrosis of the newborn. The lesions generally subside in weeks or months even without any treatment, leaving residual hyperpigmentation. If ulceration occurs in late stage, resuming steroid therapy may be indicated and then a slower and gradual decrease of the dose should be programmed [40, 41].

Lupus panniculitis Lupus panniculitis (LEP), also known as *lupus erythematosus profundus*, affects approximately 2% of the patients diagnosed with lupus erythematosus [42]. It can also appears concomitantly with discoid lupus erythematosus or subacute cutaneous lupus erythematosus (on the overlying skin or elsewhere), as well as an isolated phenomenon [43]. The development of LEP after an injury to the area, such as HPV vaccination, preceding trauma and injection site of adalimumab - a human monoclonal antibody to tumor necrosis factor (TNF)-α - has been previously described [44–47].

There is a predilection for the female sex. The mean age at diagnosis range from 28.5 to 32.9 years in different case series. In approximately two-thirds of the patients, the lesions are found on the head, mainly on the cheeks, and scalp. LEP involve predominantly the proximal part when affecting the limbs (Fig. 6a). The lateral aspect of the arms, the trunk, including the breasts, and the buttocks are commonly affected [43, 48, 49]. It presents clinically as deep subcutaneous nodules and erythematous to violaceous infiltrated plaques, which occasionally ulcerate and often resolve leaving depressed areas [42, 48]. A linear configuration of LEP has been sometimes reported, especially in children and adolescents [50]. Serologic abnormalities include antinuclear antibodies, usually at low titers, anti-double-stranded-DNA and anti-ENA-antibodies [51].

Histopathologic findings comprise a mostly lobular lymphoplasmacytic infiltrate, the presence of lymphoid follicles in the subcutaneous tissue, and hyaline fat necrosis (Fig. 6b). Epidermal and dermal changes typical of discoid lupus erythematosus, including epidermal atrophy, follicular plugging, vacuolar alteration, basement membrane thickening, and mucin deposition are observed in about one half to two-thirds of the patients in different case series. A positive lupus band test may be used to support a diagnosis of LEP. The predominant

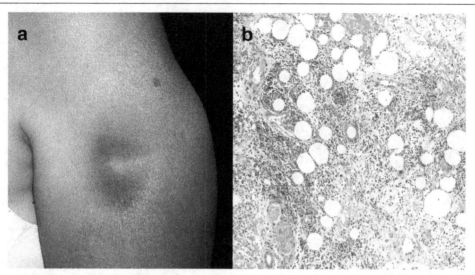

Fig. 6 Lupus panniculitis. **a** Depressed area involving the proximal part of the arm. **b** Extensive lobular infiltrate composed of lymphocytes. H&E, 200x

immune-deposit in direct immunofluorescence is IgM, and C3 and IgG are seen in half of the cases [43, 50].

The most troublesome differential diagnosis of LEP is subcutaneous panniculitis-like T-cell lymphoma, a subtype of non-Hodgkin lymphoma presenting with nodules, solitary or multiple, or deeply seated plaques mainly involving the legs, the arms and the trunk, that leave areas of lipoatrophy after regression. Systemic symptoms, such as fever, fatigue and weight loss are common. Although lymphoid nodules with germinal centers within fat cells are not pathognomonic of LEP, they are especially useful since their occurrence is not observed in cases of subcutaneous lymphoma, whilst rimming of fat lobules by lymphocytes and vascular invasion by atypical lymphocytes have been described in both entities. Immunohistochemistry is even more helpful in recognizing subcutaneous panniculitis-like T-cell lymphoma, revealing a cytotoxic T-cell phenotype consisting of CD3-positive, CD8-positive, CD4-negative lymphoid cells, coexpressing cytotoxic proteins granzyme B, TIA-1 and perforin [45, 49, 52]. Although rare, rheumatologists should be also aware of this malignancy, since there is one case report of subcutaneous panniculitis-like T-cell lymphoma in a patient receiving etanercept for rheumatoid arthritis [53].

Panniculitis in dermatomyositis Panniculitis is an usual finding in both juvenile and adult forms of dermatomyositis. It is characterized by a lobular infiltrate composed of lymphocytes and plasma cells. A certain degree of pseudomembranous changes, that refers to pseudocystic spaces lined with eosinophilic membranes in areas of fat necrosis, may be seen in a great number of panniculitides, besides those cases

related to dermatomyositis, including: sclerosing panniculitis, LEP, *erythema induratum* (EI), necrobiosis lipoidica, traumatic panniculitis, pancreatic panniculitis and subcutaneous sarcoidosis. There are reports of overlying dermal-epidermal vacuolar change and increased mucin deposition in the panniculitis associated with dermatomyositis resembling LEP [54, 55].

Neutrophilic lobular panniculitis The term neutrophilic (lobular) panniculitis refers to histopathological findings shared by a variety of cutaneous and systemic disorders, which includes pustular panniculitis associated with RA, pancreatic panniculitis, α1-antitrypsin deficiency panniculitis, subcutaneous Sweet syndrome, and factitious panniculitis [56, 57]. The most common form of panniculitis occurring in the setting of RA is EN [13]. However, rare cases of neutrophilic lobular panniculitis have also been reported in these patients. Cutaneous eruption manifests as tender erythematous nodules on the lower legs in which eventual ulceration and discharge of purulent material allow clinical distinction from EN (Fig. 7a). Histopathology in neutrophilic panniculitis associated with RA shows fat necrosis and neutrophilic dust in the subcutaneous tissue with surrounding fibrosis (Fig. 7b) [58].

Vemurafenib and dabrafenib were recently approved for the treatment of patients with unresectable or metastatic melanoma harboring the BRAF V600E mutation. Several cases of BRAF inhibitors-induced panniculitis have been reported within 7 days to 16 months after starting the medication. Joint pain and fever were associated with tender subcutaneous nodules on the upper or lower limbs, mostly the thighs, in 44 and 31% of the patients, respectively [7]. Histopathological investigation

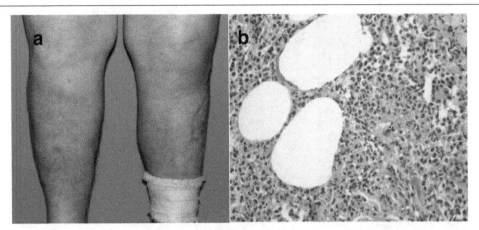

Fig. 7 Neutrophilic lobular panniculitis associated with rheumatoid arthritis. **a** Erythematous nodules on the anterior aspect of the legs. **b** Necrosis of adipocytes and intense infiltrate composed of neutrophils and histiocytes, in the lobules of the hypodermis. H&E, 400x

has shown mixed (both septal and lobular) panniculitis in some instances, but primarily lobular neutrophilic panniculitis usually predominates. Occasionally, small foci of fatty necrosis and some foamy macrophage are seen. Only in a few cases an inflammatory infiltrate surrounding blood vessel walls and focal erythrocyte extravasation were revealed, as did nonnecrotizing granulomas. Spontaneous resolution despite drug maintenance is possible; however, low-dose topical or systemic steroids and nonsteroidal anti-inflammatory drugs may be used for symptomatic treatment [7, 59]. Similarly, panniculitis has been reported as a rare side effect of specific inhibitors of tyrosine kinase activity ibrutinib, with marked activity in several B-cell malignant neoplasms, and dasatinib, used to treat chronic myeloid leukemia in chronic, blastic or accelerated phase that is resistant or intolerant to imatinib mesylate [60, 61].

Primarily-lobular panniculitides with vasculitis

Erythema induratum Erythema induratum (EI) has a female predominance and typically affects patients with some degree of obesity and venous insufficiency of the lower extremities. The disease presents with relapsing episodes of painless violaceous nodules on the calves and shins, but also on the buttocks and lower trunk, mostly during the winter. Lesions have a tendency to central ulceration and resolve spontaneously within a few months, leaving post inflammatory hyperpigmentation and occasionally atrophic pigmented scars (Fig. 8a). There are no accompanying systemic symptoms [62, 63].

EI occurs as hypersensitive immune reaction to *Mycobacterium tuberculosis*. As others tuberculids, which include lichen scrofulosorum and papulonecrotic tuberculid, although extremely rarely EI can be induced by tuberculin skin test, as well as by Bacillus Calmette–Guérin vaccine

even in children. Ziehl-Neelsen staining for acid-fast bacilli and mycobacterial culture usually result negative [64, 65]. However, there is one report in which *M. marinum* was isolated [66]. The most striking features of EI are strongly positive tuberculin purified protein derivative (PPD) with an induration greater than 20 mm and clearance of skin lesions with anti-tuberculosis therapy, which occurs within 1–6 months (mean, 2.1 months). Once diagnosis is suspected a skin biopsy should be obtained for histologic examination and polymerase chain reaction analysis for mycobacterial DNA [67].

Histopathological analysis reveals a predominant lobular panniculitis, with mild to moderate inflammation of the neighboring fibrous septa, which appear widened. At an early stage, the inflammatory infiltrate is mainly composed of neutrophils, with or without leukocytoclasis; whereas histiocytes and lipophages predominate in fully developed lesions. Some type of vascular damage is detected in 90% of the cases. The most common pattern identified is inflammation involving small venules of the center of the fat lobule; however, vasculitis involving large septal vessels can also be found, irrespectively of the stage of the lesion [68]. There are varying degrees of caseous and coagulative necrosis, and poorly developed granulomas (Fig. 8b) [69]. Although nowadays most authors use both terms indistinctly, nodular vasculitis usually refers to the nontuberculous variant of EI. There is one case report on a 28-year-old man who developed erythematous painful nodules on the lower legs, one year after starting etanercept for psoriasis. Physical examination and histologic manifestations were compatible to nodular vasculitis. Since the screening for infectious and auto-immune conditions was negative, the development of this panniculitis was attributed to TNF-α inhibitor treatment [70].

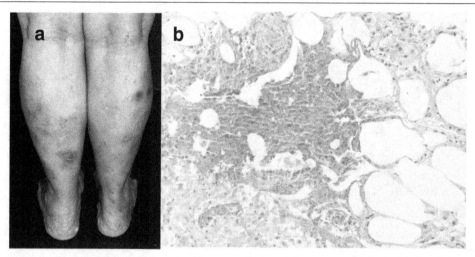

Fig. 8 Erythema induratum. **a** Erythematous nodules and atrophic scars in the legs. **b** Caseous necrosis in the lobules of the hypodermis. H&E, 400x

Panniculitis with crystals following etanercept injection According to Llamas-Velasco and Requena [71], panniculitis with lipid crystallization within adipocytes may be seen in several disorders, including crystal-storing histiocytosis, gouty panniculitis, post-steroid panniculitis, oxalosis and subcutaneous fungal infections by mucormycosis, zygomycosis or aspergillosis. These authors reported the first case of panniculitis with crystals induced by etanercept subcutaneous injection in a 62-year-old woman with severe psoriasis who developed an erythematous, slightly painful nodule on the skin of the anterior abdominal wall. The biopsy demonstrated a mostly lobular panniculitis with lymphocytic infiltrate, venulitis, as well as granulomas with foreign-body-type giant cells. Small radially arranged crystals surrounded by histiocytes were present at the interface between deep reticular dermis and subcutis. These crystals failed to stain with periodic acid-Schiff (PAS) and were slightly refractile under polarized light.

Mixed (septal and lobular) panniculitides

Infective panniculitis Infective panniculitis (IP) may occur as a primary infection by direct inoculation, as an extension from an underlying source of infection or secondarily via microbial hematogenous dissemination with subsequent infection of the subcutaneous tissue, induced by bacteria, mycobacteria, fungi, protozoa, or viruses. This type of panniculitis often manifests as multiple nodules predominantly found on the peripheral extremities, resembling EN (Fig. 9a). Other locations of involvement are possible such as the upper extremities, the gluteal region and the abdominal wall. However, the clinical picture can vary from infiltrated nodules with discharge or not to necrotizing ulcers depending on the organism involved, the

route of infection, the host immune response, and the duration of the lesion at the time of biopsy [72, 73].

There are many bacterial etiologic agents of IP. The more common of these include *Streptococcus pyogenes*, *Staphylococcus aureus*, *Pseudomonas* spp., *Mycobacterium* spp. (most of the cases of mycobacterial panniculitis being caused by nontuberculous mycobacteria), *Actinomyces*, *Nocardia* spp., *Borrelia burgdorferi*, and *Klebsiella* spp. When it comes to fungal infections that involve the subcutaneous fat, they can be divided into two major types: (1) panniculitis in the setting of a disseminated fungal infection and (2) classical subcutaneous mycosis (with the most important being mycetoma, chromoblastomycosis, and sporotrichosis), introduced into the subcutaneous tissue from the environment via inoculation. Cytomegalovirus has been rarely reported as a causative agent; immunocompromised patients were particularly affected, as in most of these IP [72, 73]. Similarly, there has been sporadic reports on parasitic organisms (Leishmania spp.; *Trypanosoma cruzi*; and Gnathostoma spp.) causing panniculitis [74].

Diagnosis is quite challenging, not only because of a nonspecific clinical presentation, but also due to its histologic findings, which can be indistinguishable from several types of panniculitides. Bacterial IP should be strongly considered when extensive suppurative panniculitis with perivascular, lobular, or mixed septal-lobular neutrophil-dominated infiltrate is present, which often extends into the dermis (Fig. 9b) [58, 72]. IP caused by atypical mycobacteria or deep fungal infection shows suppurative granulomas within the lobule, which consist of collections of neutrophils surrounded by epithelioid histiocytes [39, 73]. Borreliosis have been documented to show a histological picture mimicking LEP and subcutaneous panniculitis-like T-cell lymphoma, with a dense

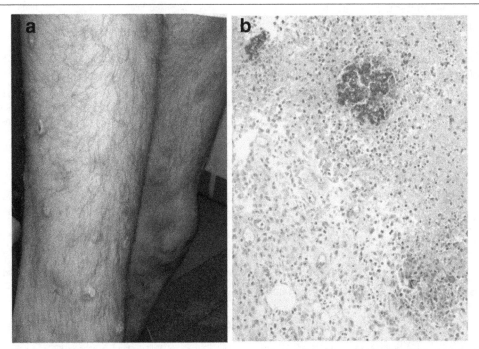

Fig. 9 Septic panniculitis in HIV positive male, caused by hematogenous dissemination. **a** Erythematous papules and ulcerated nodules on the lower limbs. **b** Basophilic areas corresponding to masses of microorganisms, with necrosis and infiltrate composed of neutrophils, eosinophils and histiocytes in the hypodermis. H&E, 200x

lymphocytic infiltrate of the subcutaneous tissue with scattered plasma cells [20]. Remarkably, besides typical cytomegalic inclusions localized predominantly within the endothelial cells of small vessels of the subcutaneous cellular tissue, skin biopsy of nodular lesions in panniculitis associated with cytomegalovirus infection may show septal involvement with abundant neutrophils, histiocytes, karyorrhexis and phagocytosis of cellular debris [75].

Regardless of the microorganism, vascular damage including necrotizing small vessel vasculitis involving arterioles and venules and/ or a thrombotic microangiopathy in the deep reticular dermis and subcutaneous fat (in secondary cutaneous infections) may be noteworthy [58, 76]. A high degree of clinical awareness is needed, since additional histological studies are necessary to identify the causative agent in many cases, including special stains (Gram, periodic acid-Schiff, Ziehl-Neelsen, methenamine-silver, anti–bacillus Calmette-Guerin antibody); cultures and molecular diagnostic techniques, like polymerase chain reaction PCR, especially in patients with preserved immune response [39, 72, 73].

Erythema nodosum-like lesions in Behçet's disease

EN-like lesions occur in 22.5 to 45.5% of the patients diagnosed with Behçet's disease (BD) [77, 78]. Nodular lesions are mostly present on the lower legs, but upper extremities may also be involved. They are histopathologically similar to those of conventional EN in approximately one-third of the cases, showing a mostly septal

panniculitis pattern, and an inflammatory infiltrate composed of neutrophils and various numbers of lymphocytes and histiocytes in the thickened septa of the subcutis. However, biopsy specimens with features of a panniculitis lobular or mixed septal and lobular in pattern, with variable degrees of lymphohistiocytic and neutrophilic infiltration, and clear evidence of vasculitis are even more common to be found [79, 80].

Vessels involvement is usually extensive and not limited to the areas of severe inflammation. It can be both of the venulitis or of the phlebitis type. The latter characteristically simulates C-PAN, as in superficial thrombophlebitis, and therefore must be clarified based on the investigation of the internal elastic lamina fiber by specific staining, such as Verhoeff van Gieson. Although the subcutaneous muscular veins in the lower legs usually have a compact concentric smooth muscle pattern with a round lumen and intimal elastic fiber proliferation due to the persistent hydrostatic pressure mimicking the characteristic features of arteries, the elastic fibers in the muscular layer are distributed between the bundled smooth muscle in veins, whereas the elastic fibers are scantly distributed in the medial muscular layer in arteries [81]. A variable degree of fat necrosis is frequently observed [79, 80].

Conclusion

Inflammation of the subcutaneous tissue is a dynamic process that shows different histopathologic findings at different stages of development. Even in the same stage of evolution, location and type of inflammation may vary among different cases of the same panniculitis; whereas similar histopathologic findings may be observed in panniculitides of different etiologies, for instance in superficial thrombophlebitis and C-PAN, or in EN and EI. In evaluating cases of panniculitidesis essential to know the associated changes outside the subcutis to establish a specific diagnosis.

Acknowledgements
The author's wish to acknowledge Alexandre Vargas, photographer from the Dermatology Department of Universidade de São Paulo.

Authors' contributions
TCABM wrote the manuscript in consultation with GFST. GFST contributed to the writing of the manuscript. MSCG designed the tables and figures. IH provided histopathological images and aided in describing histopathological findings of each panniculitis. PRC contributed to the design of the manuscript, provided clinical images and supervised the work. JFC conceived the idea of the manuscript and supervised the work. All authors read and approved the final manuscript.

Author details
[1]Faculdade de Medicina FMUSP, Universidade de Sao Paulo, Sao Paulo, SP, Brazil. [2]Instituto Dermatológico Professor Rubem David Azulay, Rio de Janeiro, RJ, Brazil. [3]Faculdade de Medicina do ABC FMABC, Santo Andre, SP, Brazil. [4]Instituto de Ciências da Saúde, Universidade Federal da Bahia (UFBA), Salvador, BA, Brazil. [5]Private practice, Aracaju, SE, Brazil.

References
1.   Segura S, Requena L. Anatomy and histology of Normal Subcutaneous fat, necrosis of adipocytes, and classification of the panniculitides. Dermatol Clin. 2008;26:419–24.
2.   Llamas Velasco M, et al. Clues in histopathological diagnosis of panniculitis. Am J Dermatopathol. 2018;40:155–67.
3.   Cascajo CD, Borghi S, Weyers W. Panniculitis. Am. J. Dermatopathol. 2000;22:530–49.
4.   Chowaniec M, Starba A, Wiland P. Erythema nodosum - review of the literature. Reumatologia. 2016;54:79–82.
5.   Requena L, Yus ES. Erythema Nodosum. Dermatol Clin. 2008;26:425–38.
6.   Requena L, Yus ES. Panniculitis. Part I. Mostly septal panniculitis. J. Am. Acad. Dermatol. 2001;45:163–83.
7.   Mössner R, et al. Erythema nodosum-like lesions during BRAF inhibitor therapy: report on 16 new cases and review of the literature. J Eur Acad Dermatology Venereol. 2015;29:1797–806.
8.   García-Porrúa C, et al. Erythema nodosum: etiologic and predictive factors in a defined population. Arthritis Rheum. 2000;43:584–92.
9.   Mert A, et al. Erythema nodosum: an experience of 10 years. Scand J Infect Dis. 2004;36:424–7.
10. Psychos DN, Voulgari PV, Skopouli FN, Drosos AA, Moutsopoulos HM. Erythema nodosum: the underlying conditions. Clin Rheumatol. 2000;19:212–6.
11. Negera E, et al. Clinico-pathological features of erythema nodosum leprosum: a case-control study at ALERT hospital, Ethiopia. PLoS Negl Trop Dis. 2017;11:1–13.
12. Sarita S, et al. A study on histological features of lepra reactions in patients attending the Dermatology Department of the Government Medical College, Calicut, Kerala, India. Lepr. Rev. 2013;84:51–64.
13. Ziemer M, Müller AK, Hein G, Oelzner P, Elsner P. Incidence and classification of cutaneous manifestations in rheumatoid arthritis. JDDG - J Ger Soc Dermatology. 2016;14:1237–46.
14. Ergun T, et al. Skin manifestations of rheumatoid arthritis: a study of 215 Turkish patients. Int J Dermatol. 2008;47:894–902.
15. Nakamura T, Inaba M, Yoshinaga T, Takaoka H, Iyama K. Nodules in patients with rheumatoid arthritis and methotrexate treatment. Mod Rheumatol. 2015;7595:1–2.
16. Tilstra JS, Lienesch DW. Rheumatoid Nodules. Dermatol Clin. 2015;33:361–71.
17. Wick MR. Granulomatous & histiocytic dermatitides. Semin Diagn Pathol. 2017;34:301–11.
18. Chua-Aguilera CJ, Moller B, Yawalkar N. Skin manifestations of rheumatoid arthritis, juvenile idiopathic arthritis, and Spondyloarthritides. Clin Rev Allergy Immunol. 2017. https://doi.org/10.1007/s12016-017-8632-5.
19. Walker D, Susa JS, Currimbhoy S, Jacobe H. Histopathological changes in morphea and their clinical correlates: results from the Morphea in adults and children cohort V. J Am Acad Dermatol. 2017;76:1124–30.
20. Shiau CJ, Abi Daoud MS, Wong SM, Crawford RI. Lymphocytic panniculitis: an algorithmic approach to lymphocytes in subcutaneous tissue. J Clin Pathol. 2015;68:954–62.
21. Bielsa Marsol I. Update on the classification and treatment of localized scleroderma. Actas Dermo-Sifiliográficas (English Ed). 2013;104:654–66.
22. Toledano C, et al. Localized scleroderma: a series of 52 patients. Eur J Intern Med. 2009;20:331–6.
23. Fett N, Werth VP. Update on morphea: Part I. Epidemiology, clinical presentation, and pathogenesis. J. Am. Acad. Dermatol. 2011;64:217–28.
24. Bielsa I, Ariza A. Deep Morphea. Semin Cutan Med Surg. 2007;26:90–5.
25. Evangelisto A, Werth V, Schumacher HR. What is that nodule?: a diagnostic approach to evaluating subcutaneous and cutaneous nodules. J Clin Rheumatol. 2006;12:230–40.
26. Erden A, et al. Comparing polyarteritis nodosa in children and adults: a single center study. Int J Rheum Dis. 2017;20:1016–22.
27. Sharma A, et al. Polyarteritis nodosa in North India: clinical manifestations and outcomes. Int J Rheum Dis. 2017;20:390–7.
28. Fain O, et al. Vasculitides associated with malignancies: analysis of sixty patients. Arthritis Care Res. 2007;57:1473–80.
29. Fathalla BM, Miller L, Brady S, Schaller JG. Cutaneous polyarteritis nodosa in children. J Am Acad Dermatol. 2005;53:724–8.
30. Pagnoux C, et al. Clinical features and outcomes in 348 patients with polyarteritis nodosa: a systematic retrospective study of patients diagnosed between 1963 and 2005 and entered into the French vasculitis study group database. Arthritis Rheum. 2010;62:616–26.
31. Nakamura T, et al. Cutaneous polyarteritis nodosa: revisiting its definition and diagnostic criteria. Arch Dermatol Res. 2009;301:117–21.
32. Furukawa F. Cutaneous Polyarteritis Nodosa: an update. Ann Vasc Dis. 2012;5:282–8.
33. Morimoto A, Chen K-RR. Reappraisal of histopathology of cutaneous polyarteritis nodosa. J Cutan Pathol. 2016;43:1131–8.
34. Kawakami T, Yamazaki M, Mizoguchi M, Soma Y. High titer of anti-phosphatidylserine-prothrombin complex antibodies in patients with cutaneous polyarteritis nodosa. Arthritis Care Res. 2007;57:1507–13.
35. Dahiya A, Leach J, Levy H. Gouty panniculitis in a healthy male. J Am Acad Dermatol. 2007;57:S52–4.
36. Weberschock T, Gholam P, Hartschuh W, Hartmann M. Gouty panniculitis in a 68-year-old man: case report and review of the literature. Int J Dermatol. 2010;49:410–3.
37. Ochoa CD, et al. Panniculitis: another clinical expression of gout. Rheumatol Int. 2011;31:831–5.
38. Forbess LJ, Fields TR. The broad Spectrum of urate crystal deposition: unusual presentations of gouty tophi. Semin Arthritis Rheum. 2012;42:146–54.
39. Requena L, Yus ES. Panniculitis. Part II. Mostly lobular panniculitis. J. Am. Acad. Dermatol. 2001;45:325–61.
40. Torrelo A, Hernández A. Panniculitis in Children. Dermatol. Clin. 2008;26:491–500.
41. Kim ST, et al. Post-steroid panniculitis in an adult. J Dermatol. 2008;35:786–8.
42. Tuffanelli DL. Lupus Erythematosus Panniculitis (Profundus). Arch. Dermatol. 1971;103:231.
43. Ng PP-L, Tan SH, Tan T. Lupus erythematosus panniculitis: a clinicopathologic study. Int J Dermatol. 2002;41:488–90.
44. Choi JY, Kim HS, Lee GY. Case of lupus erythematosus panniculitis triggered by human papillomavirus quadrivalent vaccine injection. J Dermatol. 2017;44:1420–1.
45. Castrillón MA, Murrell DF. Lupus profundus limited to a site of trauma: case report and review of the literature. Int J Womens Dermatol. 2017;3:117–20.
46. Durand A-L, et al. Anti-tumour necrosis factor α-induced lupus erythematosus panniculitis. J. Eur. Acad. Dermatol Venereol. 2017;31:e318–9.
47. Lee H, Kim DS, Chung KY. Adalimumab-induced lupus panniculitis. Lupus. 2014;23:1443–4.
48. Jacyk WK, Bhana KN. Lupus erythematosus profundus in black South Africans. 2006:717–21. https://doi.org/10.1111/j.1365-4632.2005.02770.x.

49. Park HS, Choi JW, Kim B, Cho KH. Lupus erythematosus panniculitis: Clinicopathological, Immunophenotypic, and molecular studies. Am J Dermatopathol. 2010;32:24–30.

50. Elbendary A, Griffin J, Li S, Tlougan B, Junkins-Hopkins JM. Linear Sclerodermoid lupus erythematosus Profundus in a child. Am J Dermatopathol. 2016;38:904–9.

51. Kündig TM, Trüeb RM, Krasovec M. Lupus profundus/panniculitis. Dermatology. 1997;195:99–101.

52. Willemze R. Cutaneous lymphomas with a panniculitic presentation. Semin Diagn Pathol. 2017;34:36–43.

53. Michot C, et al. Subcutaneous panniculitis-like T-cell lymphoma in a patient receiving etanercept for rheumatoid arthritis. Br J Dermatol. 2009;160:889–90.

54. Braunstein I, Werth VP. Update on management of connective tissue panniculitides. Dermatol Ther. 2012;25:173–82.

55. Polcari IC, Stein SL. Panniculitis in childhood. Dermatol Ther. 2010;23:356–67.

56. Cohen P, Subcutaneous R. Sweet's syndrome: a variant of acute febrile neutrophilic dermatosis that is included in the histopathologic differential diagnosis of neutrophilic panniculitis. J Am Acad Dermatol. 2005;52:927–8.

57. Nobeyama Y, Nakagawa H. Subcutaneous Sweet's syndrome and neutrophilic panniculitis. J Dermatol. 2014;41:861–2.

58. Chan MP. Neutrophilic panniculitis: algorithmic approach to a heterogeneous group of disorders. Arch Pathol Lab Med. 2014;138:1337–43.

59. Choy B, Chou S, Anforth R, Fernández-Peñas P. Panniculitis in patients treated with BRAF inhibitors: a case series. Am J Dermatopathol. 2014; 36:493–7.

60. Fabbro SK, Smith SM, Dubovsky JA, Gru AA, Jones JA. Panniculitis in patients undergoing treatment with the Bruton tyrosine kinase inhibitor ibrutinib for lymphoid leukemias. JAMA Oncol. 2015;1:684-6.

61. Assouline S, Laneuville P, Gambacorti-Passerini C. Panniculitis during dasatinib therapy for imatinib-resistant chronic myelogenous leukemia. N Engl J Med. 2006;354:2623–4.

62. Segura S, Pujol RM, Trindade F, Requena L. Vasculitis in erythema induratum of Bazin: A histopathologic study of 101 biopsy specimens from 86 patients. J Am Acad Dermatol. 2008;59(5):839–51.

63. Mascaró JM, Baselga E. Erythema induratum of Bazin. Dermatol Clin. 2008; 26(4):439–45.

64. Sekiguchi A, Motegi S, Ishikawa O. Erythema induratum of Bazin associated with bacillus Calmette-Guérin vaccination: implication of M1 macrophage infiltration and monocyte chemotactic protein-1 expression. J Dermatol. 2016;43(1):111–3.

65. Posada García C, et al. Erythema induratum of Bazin induced by tuberculin skin test. Int J Dermatol. 2015;54(11):1297–9.

66. Papathemeli D, Franke I, Bonnekoh B, Gollnick H, Ambach A. Explosive generalization of nodular vasculitis - Mycobacterium marinum challenges the paradigm. J Eur Acad Dermatol Venereol. 2016;30(12):e189–91.

67. Lighter J, Tse DB, Li Y, Borkowsky W. Erythema induratum of bazin in a child: evidence for a cell-mediated hyper-response to Mycobacterium tuberculosis. Pediatr Infect Dis J. 2009;28(4):326–8.

68. Segura S, Pujol RM, Trindade F, Requena L. Vasculitis in erythema induratum of Bazin: a histopathologic study of 101 biopsy specimens from 86 patients. J Am Acad Dermatol. 2008;59:839–51.

69. Gilchrist H, Patterson JW. Erythema nodosum and erythema induratum (nodular vasculitis): diagnosis and management. Dermatol Ther. 2010;23(4): 320–7.

70. Park S, et al. Nodular vasculitis developed during etanercept treatment in a patient with psoriasis. J Am Acad Dermatol. 2014;70:AB177.

71. Llamas-Velasco M, Requena L. Panniculitis with crystals induced by etanercept subcutaneous injection. J Cutan Pathol. 2015;42:413–5.

72. Morrison LK, Rapini R, Willison CB, Tyring S. Infection and panniculitis. Dermatol Ther. 2010;23:328–40.

73. Delgado-Jimenez Y, Fraga J, García-Díez A. Infective Panniculitis. Dermatol. Clin. 2008;26:471–80.

74. Norgan AP, Pritt BS. Parasitic infections of the skin and Subcutaneous tissues. Adv Anat Pathol. 2018;25:106–23.

75. Ballestero-Diez M, Alvarez-Ruiz SB, Aragues Montanes M, Fraga J. Septal panniculitis associated with cytomegalovirus infection. Histopathology. 2005;46:720–2.

76. Magro CM, Dyrsen ME, Crowson AN. Acute infectious id panniculitis/ panniculitic bacterid: a distinctive form of neutrophilic lobular panniculitis. J Cutan Pathol. 2008;35:941–6.

77. Davatchi F, et al. Behcet's disease in Iran: analysis of 6500 cases. Int J Rheum Dis. 2010;13:367–73.

78. Tursen U, Gurler A, Boyvat A. Evaluation of clinical findings according to sex in 2313 Turkish patients with Behçet's disease. Int J Dermatol. 2003;42:346–51.

79. Misago N, Tada Y, Koarada S, Narisawa Y. Erythema Nodosum-like lesions in Behçet's disease: a Clinicopathological study of 26 cases. Acta Derm Venereol. 2012;92:681–6.

80. Kim B, LeBoit PE. Histopathologic features of erythema nodosum-like lesions in Behcet disease: a comparison with erythema nodosum focusing on the role of vasculitis. Am J Dermatopathol. 2000;22:379–90.

81. Chen KR. The misdiagnosis of superficial thrombophlebitis as cutaneous polyarteritis nodosa: features of the internal elastic lamina and the compact concentric muscular layer as diagnostic pitfalls. Am J Dermatopathol. 2010; 32:688–93.

22

Poor obstetric outcomes in Indian women with Takayasu arteritis

Latika Gupta, Durga Prasanna Misra, Sakir Ahmed, Avinash Jain, Abhishek Zanwar, Able Lawrence, Vikas Agarwal, Amita Aggarwal and Ramnath Misra[*] ⓘ

Abstract

Introduction: Takayasu's arteritis (TA) affects young women in the childbearing age group. We studied obstetric outcomes in these patients before and after disease onset.

Methods: Women aged more than 18 years with Takayasu's arteritis (ACR 1990 criteria) were included. Demographic data, clinical features, disease activity using Indian Takayasu Arteritis clinical score (ITAS), Disease Extent Index for TA (DEI.TaK) and damage assessment using TA Damage score (TA), history of conception and maternal and fetal outcomes were recorded from hospital records and telephonic interview. Results are in median and IQR.

Results: Of the 64 women interviewed, aged 29 (24–38) years and disease duration 5 (4–10) years, 74 and 38 pregnancies had occurred before and after disease diagnosis in 29 and 20 women respectively. In eight, the diagnosis was made during pregnancy. Age at disease onset was 22 (18–30) years. Type 5 disease was the most common ($n = 32$, 59.3%), and an equal number of patients had Ishikawa's class I and II disease ($n = 26$, 40.6%). Median ITAS ($n = 44$) was 13 (7–16), DEI.Tak 12.5 (9–16.75) and TADS 8 (6.5–10). Twenty-five patients wanted to get pregnant, of which 8 (32%) did not do so because of their disease. Fifteen were unmarried of whom 6 did not marry due to disease. Obstetric outcomes were poorer in pregnancies that occurred after the onset of disease as compared with those before it (RR = 1.5, $p = 0.01$). Pregnancies after the onset of TA carried a very high risk of maternal [RR3.9 (1.8–8.5), $P < 0.001$] as well as fetal complications [RR = 2.0 (1.2–3.4), $p = 0.001$]. Hypertension was the most common maternal complication and occurred most often in the last trimester. The baby weight at birth was lower in pregnancies after disease (2.3 vs. 3.0, $p = 0.01$). Wong's score greater than or equal to 4 predicted lower birth weight ($p = 0.04$). ITAS, ITAS-A, DEI. Tak and TADS could not predict obstetric outcomes, and ITAS score exhibited moderate correlation with DEI. Tak ($r = 0.78$) and TADS ($r = 0.58$).

Conclusion: Women with TA suffer from extremely high risk of poor maternal and foetal outcomes. Wong's scoring can be useful to predict birth weight.

Keywords: Takayasu, Vasculitis, Pregnancy, Obstetric, Outcomes, Disease activity

Key messages

- Pregnancy in women with Takayasu's arteritis is associated with maternal and fetal morbidity
- Hypertension is the single most important complication
- Wong's score can predict outcomes in the neonate in TA

Introduction

Takayasu arteritis (TA) is a large vessel vasculitis predominantly found in Asian populations [1]. Recently various treatment options have come up, including multiple biologicals [2]. This, along with improved medical care, is bringing down mortality in this dreaded disease [3]. However, there is a lack of specific quality of life measures for Takayasu [4]. Thus, in the absence of specific measures, pregnancy outcomes could serve as an indirect measure of morbidity in this disease seen more often in females.

* Correspondence: rnmisra2000@gmail.com
Department of Clinical Immunology and Rheumatology, Sanjay Gandhi Postgraduate Institute of Medical Sciences, Lucknow 226014, India

Majorities of rheumatic diseases are more common in females, especially in the reproductive age group. Presence of rheumatic diseases often leads to lower fertility. This can be due to disease-related factors including drugs (impaired gonadal functioning, pregnancy loss, therapy-related avoidance of pregnancy) or due to psychosocial reasons (personal choice, depression leading to loss of libido, anxiety, altered self-image, etc) [5].

Takayasu is no different. It predominantly affects young women with a female to male ratio of 9:1. Most of the other vasculitis affect women beyond their reproductive years [6]. Still, overall fertility is reduced in vasculitis: pregnancy losses have been reported in around 10% of cases in granulomatosis with polyangiitis, up to 20% in eosinophilic granulomatosis with polyangiitis, 20–30% in Behçet's disease and up to 25–30% of TA in the developed world [7]. In a study in France, women with TA had a 13-fold higher risk of obstetric complications after diagnosis of pregnancy as compared to before [8]. Some studies have even shown no effect of TA on obstetric outcomes [9].

The scenario in India may be different [10]. In TA, it is well established that the pattern of vascular involvement differs by region with a plausible role of dynamic interactions of the genes with the environment. Vascular dynamics in pregnancy are likely to be differentially affected depending on vessel involvement. Type V with predominant abdominal aorta is most common in Indian patients [11].

The obstetric outcomes in Indian women are lesser known. The first series reported from India was from an institute in Northern India of 12 patients with 24 pregnancies (1979–1999, [12]. The authors followed this up with a second series (1999–2008) with 37 pregnancies in 15 women [13]. Another series is available from Eastern India which reported 16 patients with 29 pregnancies [14]. However, these were mostly Ishikawa Group IIa.

Also, the utility of outcome measures for disease activity such as ITAS [15] and DEI.TaK and for damage (TADS) [16] for prediction of pregnancy outcomes is unclear. A seminal paper by Wong et al. has suggested a score which can be used to predict fetal morbidity and gives room for pre-emptive escalated obstetric care [17].

Hence, we sought to explore the obstetric outcomes in patients with TA by comparing them in women who conceived before and after disease onset. In addition, the predictive value of ITAS, DEI. Tak, TADS and Wong's score were tested for association with obstetric outcomes.

Methods

This was a retrospective study in a cohort of patients from a single tertiary care centre in Northern India. Ethics permissions were taken from the institute ethics committee. All women with Takayasu's arteritis by 1990 ACR criteria, above 18 years of age, were recruited. Data on demographic parameters, clinical profile and comorbidities were collected from hospital records and supplemented by a personal or telephonic interview in July 2017. Patients with age of disease onset more than 40 years were excluded. Where available, angiography records, ITAS, ITAS-A (ITAS with acute phase reactants), DEI.TaK and TADS scores were retrieved from the records. Data from all sources were used to calculate the Wong's prognostic score for newborns (Table 1).

Outcomes included fertility and pregnancy outcomes. Fertility outcomes were early menopause (defined as presence of sustained amenorrhea for more than 1 year after attaining menarche, before 40 years of age), deferring pregnancy due to disease process, inability to conceive, and abstinence due to drugs or disease activity. Data on contraception use was also collected.

Pregnancy outcomes were divided into maternal and fetal outcomes. Maternal outcomes were flare of disease, hypertensive diseases of pregnancy, diabetes, abortions (spontaneous or induced), stillbirths and live-births. Fetal outcomes were prematurity, low birth weight, congenital anomalies, or neonatal deaths.

Data analysis was carried out using GraphPad Prism© 7 and SPSS© 20 software. Since data was mostly nonparametric, it was represented as median (Intra-quartile range: IQR). Fisher's Exact test for comparing proportions and Man-Whitney U test for comparing means were used. To estimate the effect of disease on various outcomes, the pregnancies before disease onset were taken as controls. The relative risk of different outcomes was calculated. Two mixed generalised models with age, duration of disease, diagnostic category, education status, place of residence, and age at conception as covariates was used to determine the factors influencing maternal and foetal outcomes respectively.

Table 1 Wong's prognostic scoring for neonate born to mother with Takayasu's arteritis

Score	Involvement of abdominal aorta	Trimester when treatment started	Highest Mean arterial pressure in 3rd Trimester	Super-imposed pre-eclampsia
0	No	1st	< 100	None
1	Yes	2nd	101–130	3rd Trimester
2	Yes + Renal involvement	3rd	> 130	1st-2nd Trimester

Results
Clinical profile of patients with TA
Sixty-four women with median age and disease duration 29 (IQR 24–38) years and 5 (4–10) years respectively were interviewed. Median age at menarche was 13 (12.5–15) years. Menstrual patterns were unchanged after the onset of disease. Five (7.8%) were post-menopausal. Median age at menopause was 44 (40–47.5) years. Table 2 highlights the demographic profile of the patients.

Social impact and conception
Fifteen of the 64 interviewed (23.4%) were unmarried, and six (40%) of them attributed it to the disease. Of those who were married, 25 wished to conceive, but 8 (32%) decided against due to the disease. One had infertility with no other cause found and the infertility was attributed to Takayasu by the treating physician.

Of the forty-nine married women, 32 had discussed contraceptive issues with their physicians. The others had declined due to personal preferences or lack of need. Barrier method was the most common ($n = 21$) mode of contraception.

Obstetric outcomes in TA
Seventy-four conception events occurred before the diagnosis of TA in 30 women while 38 were after the diagnosis in 26 women (Table 3).

Out of 38, there were 10 spontaneous abortions, 6 medical termination of pregnancy (MTP) and 19 live births (Fig. 1). Of the live births, 10 had foetal morbidity (Table 4). Six had low birth weight and one each had neonatal sepsis and meconium-stained liquor. Four of the six MTPs were advised due to inadvertent iatrogenic exposures (2 Methotrexate, 1 Azathioprine, and Computed tomogram (CT) scan done with foetus in utero) at another hospital and one due to uncontrolled hypertension while for the sixth one reason was unclear. Of maternal complications, hypertension was the most common, seen in 15 pregnancies of the 38, most often in the last trimester (Table 4). Of the 11 children whose birth weight was available, 6 had weighed normal at birth while 4 were of low birth weight and one was macrosomic.

Table 2 Demographic profile of interviewed patients

Characteristics	Women with TA ($n = 64$)
Age[a]	29 (24–38)
Disease duration[a]	5 (4–10)
Age of disease onset[a]	22 (18–30)
Clinical Profile	**N**
Type of TA (Angiographic)	
I	15 (23.4)
IIb	4 (6.2)
III	2 (3.1)
IV	1 (1.6)
V	32 (50)
Unknown	10 (15.6)
Ishikawa type	
1	11 (17.1)
2	26 (40.6)
3	12 (18.8)
Unknown	15 (23.4)
Outcome Measures ($n = 44$)	
ITAS	13 (7–16)
ITAS A	15 (7.25–18)
DEI.Tak	12.5 (9–16.75)
TADS	8 (6.5–10)

[a]in years [Median (IQR)]. For abbreviations (see text)

Table 3 Women with TA who conceived before or after the diagnosis

Characteristic	Patients with conception before the diagnosis of TA ($n = 30$)	Patients with conception concurrent or after the diagnosis of TA ($n = 26$)
Age[a]	40 (32–44.5)	30 (27–33.5)
Disease duration[a]	7 (4–14)	6.5 (3–11.8)
Age of disease onset[a]	30 (25–35)	23.5 (20.5–27.1)
Clinical Profile	N	
Type of TA (Angiographic)		
I	9 (30)	4 (15.4)
IIb	4 (13.3)	2 (7.7)
III	0	0
IV	0	0
V	15 (50)	16 (61.5)
Unknown	2 (6.7)	4 (16.7)
Ishikawa type		
1	5 (16.7)	4 (16.7)
2	14 (46.7)	10 (38.5)
3	6 (20)	4 (16.7)
Unknown	6 (20)	8 (30.8)
Outcome Measures ($n = 44$)		
ITAS	14 (7–17)	14.5 (9.3–17.8)
ITAS A	15.5 (7.3–20)	11 (2–20.5)
DEI.Tak	13 (9–17)	17 (12.5–19)
TADS	8 (6.5–11)	8 (7–10)

[a]in years [Median (IQR)]. For abbreviations (see text)

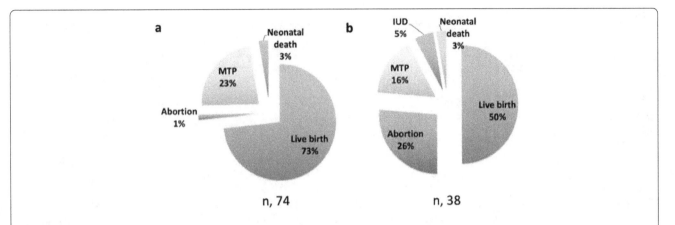

Fig. 1 Obstetric outcomes of conception before and after diagnosis of TA. **a** and **b** Obstetric outcome before and after the diagnosis of TA respectively. IUD, Intra-uterine death; MTP, Medical Termination of pregnancy; n, number of patients

Peripartum diagnosis of disease
Eight women had a diagnosis of TA during pregnancy, of which only 2 had prior (undiagnosed) symptoms.

Comparisons between obstetric outcomes before and after onset of TA
Obstetric complications were more common in pregnancies after the onset of TA as compared with those before (RR = 1.5, p = 0.01. Figure 1). Pregnancies after TA onset had higher maternal complications (RR = 3.9 (1.8–8.5),

Table 4 Maternal and fetal complications in conceptions before and after diagnosis of Takayasu arteritis

Obstetric outcomes	Before TA (n = 74, %)	After TA (n = 38, %)
Maternal complications		
Hypertension	1 (1.3)	15 (39.4)
Post-dated	0	2 (5.2)
Gestational Diabetes	0	2 (5.2)
Premature rupture of membranes	1 (1.3)	1 (2.6)
Prolonged labour	1 (1.3)	1 (2.6)
Jaundice	0	1 (2.6)
Polyhydramnios	0	1 (2.6)
Post-Partum Haemorrhage	2 (1.6)	0
Anti-Partum Haemorrhage	1 (1.3)	0
Fetal complications		
Low Birth Weight	2 (1.6)	6 (15.8)
Preterm	4 (5.4)	2 (5.2)
Congenital malformation	1 (1.3)	0
Meconium stained Liquor	1 (1.3)	1 (2.6)
Neonatal sepsis	0	1 (2.6)
Neonatal jaundice	1 (1.3)	0

P < 0.001) as well as fetal complications (RR = 2.0 (1.2–3.4), p = 0.001). Conception after the diagnosis of TA was more likely to result in abortions as compared to conception before TA diagnosis (RR 3.6, p < 0.0001).

Baby weight at birth was lower in pregnancies after disease diagnosis (2.3 kg vs 3.0 kg, p = 0.01). Wong's score ≥ 4 was associated with lower birth weight (p = 0.04). ITAS, ITAS A and TADS (n = 15) at baseline could not predict outcomes (Area under Curve - 0.5 & 0.7) and did not correlate with Wong's score.

In the multivariate analyses, age at disease onset, disease duration, type of TA, ITAS, or TADS were not associated with obstetric outcomes, including maternal or fetal complications individually or combined.

Discussion
Women with TA had poor obstetric outcomes, with increased risk of maternal as well as fetal complications. Hypertension was the most common maternal complication. Peripartum diagnosis was established in 12.5% of all cases. Angiographic type, disease activity measures like ITAS, DEI.Tak and damage score TADS could not predict pregnancy outcome. However, Wong's score envisaged neonatal outcomes.

Similar to our data, poor obstetric outcomes are seen in most series, though most lack a valid control group for comparison (Table 5) [8, 9, 12–14, 18–22]. Although hypertension is the most reported complication through most series, the percentages vary remarkably. While all prospective series describe hypertension in almost three fourths or more, all retrospective data sets (e.g. from Osaka and another multicentre from France), including the current one, describe HTN in 15–40% of women.

While most other studies describe live birth rates of around 80% (65–100%), our study had a lower percentage of live births (50%) [8, 9, 12, 13]. Implications from

Table 5 Comparison of obstetric outcomes in Takayasu arteritis across the world

Centre (year of publication)	No of Pregnancies	Hypertension	Fetal complications	Live birth- n (%)	Maternal mortality	Wong's scoring	Disease active	Controls	Conclusion
Wong et al., Hong Kong (1983) [17]	19	16 (84.2%)	9 (60%)	15 (78.9%)	1 (5.2%)- MI	Yes	0	Yes-TA before diagnosis	IUGR can be predicted by scoring system
PGI Chandigarh, India(2000) [12]	24	22 (91.7%)	9 (52.9%)	17 (70.8%)	0	No	NA	No	Abdominal vessel disease & delay in care predict poor outcomes
University de Estado, Brazil (2012) [18]	11	7 (63.6%)	7 (63.6%)	11 (100%)	0	No	0	No	Close monitoring with combined care is usedful; No disease activity seen during pregnancy
IPGMER, Kolkata, India (2012) [14]	29	29 (100%)	20 (86.9%)	23 (89.7%)	1 (5.8%)- CVA	Yes	NA	Yes-Healthy	Conception usually spontaneous, Disease not active
Osaka, Japan (2014) [19]	27	5 (18.5%)	4 (14.8%)	27 (100%)	0	No	3	No	Ishikawa stage II fares worse
Istanbul University, Turkey (2015) [20]	19	3 (16%)	1 (5.2%)	19 (100%)	0	No	2 (10.5%)	Yes-TA before diagnosis	TA pregnancies have favorable outcome
Multicentre Paris, France (2015) [21]	98	26 (27%)	13 (16.7%)	78 (79.6%)	0	No	6 (6.1%)	Yes-TA before diagnosis	Smoking and NIH score > 1 predict poor outcomes
CMC, Vellore, India [22]	16	7 (43.8%)	7 (43.8%)	16 (100%)	0	NA	4 (25%)	No	Good outcomes are seen in type V disease when in remission
Multicentric, Oslo, Norway (2017) [9]	37	17 (29.3)	12(32%)	25 (68)	0 (1 had stroke)	No	10(60%)	Yes-TA before diagnosis	Maternal and foetal outcomes were favourable.
Tel Aviv, Israel (2018) [23]	20	8/13 (61.5%)	9(45%)	13 (65%)	0	No	NA	No	Targeted treatment of high blood pressure emphasised
Ankara, Turkey (2019) [24]	22	8 (36.4)	18 (81.8%)	16 (72.7%)	0	No	5 relapsed during pregnancy	No	Almost half had disease relapse during pregnancy
Current study, Lucknow, India	38	15 (39.5%)	12 (63.2%)	19 (50%)	0	Yes	15 (7.25–18)[a]	Yes-TA before diagnosis	Wong's score useful, ITAS needs evaluation in larger cohort

MI myocardial infarction, *NA* Not available, *NIH* National Institute of Health indices index
[a]Median (IQR) CVA, cerebrovascular accident

the type of TA could be one factor although absence of uniform angiographic study in patients limits our ability to comment on that. In most other series angiographic type I and II predominate while our patients mostly had type V disease [8, 9]. This involvement of the abdominal aorta with or without renal artery involvement may be leading to pregnancy losses. Also noteworthy is that one-third (6 cases) had medical termination of pregnancy due to various reasons like unwanted pregnancy, conceived while on methotrexate, radiation exposure but only in one case reason was directly attributed to the disease (uncontrolled hypertension).

Poor obstetric care in a developing nation could be another reason. It has been previously shown from our hospital that women with inflammatory myositis, suffer from much poorer maternal outcomes than reported from other countries [10]. However, since the type of TA and consequently patterns of vascular involvement also differ geographically, it might be difficult to allocate attributability to poor outcomes from disease phenotype viz. a viz. socio-economic impact.

While Wong's score for prediction of outcomes in neonates of mothers with TA has been described way back in 1983, it not being used in routine practice [8, 9, 12, 13]. In our scenario, this may, in fact, be the best predictor for poor neonatal outcome. The study from eastern India also had found similar significance of the Wong score [14]. The other study from Chandigarh, India also found that abdominal aorta involvement (one of the components of Wong's score) portends poorer obstetric outcomes [13]. The fact that Wong's score > 4 predicted low birth weight suggest that this simple tool should find application in the clinic and rheumatologists and obstetrician should get together in this initiative to improve obstetric care in this morbid disease.

Another multicentre study from France found that (National Institute of Health) NIH score > 1 predicts poor prognosis [21]. Our data was limited, and we could not calculate the NIH score. However, the ITAS score or DEI.TaK or TADS score could not predict obstetric outcomes. This may be a type 2 error due to small numbers. But it is more likely that ITAS did not show a correlation because mostly the patients in remission had gotten pregnant. The fact that there was no correlation with the TADS score (as compared to the Wong score) seems to imply that abdominal aorta involvement and hypertension were better predictors than overall damage score. However, these need evaluation in a larger cohort. A recent study from India failed to establish utility of ITAS in 16 women although this could be as most women were in remission [22].

Peripartum onset of disease is seen in many autoimmune diseases [10, 24]. In TA which tends to be latent in a subset of individuals, the altered hemodynamics of pregnancy can lead to decompensation and consequent diagnosis. Our observations were comparable to those of others; although notably, only 25% of those diagnosed in the peripartum period had prior symptoms.

This study has the advantage of being one of the largest data set relating to obstetric outcomes from a single centre so far. The utility of TADS and DEI.TaK is being explored for the first time. However, the study has its limitations since data was collected retrospectively and used disease but not healthy controls for comparisons. The interviews can have a recall bias.

The results suggest that improved patient counselling and close watch for foetal well-being at a tertiary care centre should be provided to women of childbearing potential. Incorporation of Wong's score in the clinic can be useful to predict outcomes and institute higher priority care.

Conclusion

Women with Takayasu's arteritis suffer from 1.5-fold higher complications and poor maternal (RR 3.9) as well as fetal (RR 2.0) outcomes. Wong's scoring is useful to predict fetal outcomes.

Acknowledgements
None.

Authors' contributions
LG, DPM, SA, AJ and AZ co-wrote the manuscript and all authors have reviewed and approved it. LG, SA, and AZ compiled and analysed the data.

References
1. Misra R. Takayasu arteritis: a distinct syndrome of large vessel vasculitis: a view point by late Professor Paul bacon. Int J Rheum Dis. 2019;22(Suppl 1):49–52.
2. Misra DP, Wakhlu A, Agarwal V, Danda D. Recent advances in the management of Takayasu arteritis. Int J Rheum Dis. 2019;22(Suppl 1):60–8.
3. Seyahi E. Takayasu arteritis: an update. Curr Opin Rheumatol. 2017;29(1):51–6.
4. Sreih AG, Alibaz-Oner F, Easley E, Davis T, Mumcu G, Milman N, et al. Health-related outcomes of importance to patients with Takayasu's arteritis. Clin Exp Rheumatol. 2018;111(2):51–7.
5. Østensen M. Sexual and reproductive health in rheumatic disease. Nat Rev Rheumatol. 2017;13(8):485–93.
6. Machen L, Clowse MEB. Vasculitis and pregnancy. Rheum Dis Clin N Am. 2017;43(2):239–47.
7. Pagnoux C, Mahendira D, Laskin CA. Fertility and pregnancy in vasculitis. Best Pract Res Clin Rheumatol. 2013;27(1):79–94.
8. Comarmond C, Biard L, Lambert M, Mekinian A, Ferfar Y, Kahn J-E, et al. Long-term outcomes and prognostic factors of complications in Takayasu arteritis: a multicenter study of 318 patients. Circulation. 2017;136(12):1114–22.
9. Gudbrandsson B, Wallenius M, Garen T, Henriksen T, Molberg Ø, Palm Ø. Takayasu arteritis and pregnancy: a population-based study on outcomes and mother/child-related concerns. Arthritis Care Res. 2017;69(9):1384–90.
10. Gupta L, Zanwar A, Ahmed S, Aggarwal A. Outcomes of pregnancy in women with inflammatory myositis: a retrospective cohort from India. J Clin Rheumatol Pract Rep Rheum Musculoskelet Dis. 2019. [Epub ahead of print]. https://doi.org/10.1097/RHU.0000000000000996. PubMed PMID: 30720702..
11. Goel R, Danda D, Joseph G, Ravindran R, Kumar S, Jayaseelan V, et al. Long-term outcome of 251 patients with Takayasu arteritis on combination immunosuppressant therapy: single Centre experience from a large tertiary care teaching hospital in southern India. Semin Arthritis Rheum. 2018;47(5):718–26.
12. Sharma BK, Jain S, Vasishta K. Outcome of pregnancy in Takayasu arteritis. Int J Cardiol. 2000;75(Suppl 1):S159–62.
13. Suri V, Aggarwal N, Keepanasseril A, Chopra S, Vijayvergiya R, Jain S. Pregnancy and Takayasu arteritis: a single Centre experience from North India. J Obstet Gynaecol Res. 2010;36(3):519–24.
14. Mandal D, Mandal S, Dattaray C, Banerjee D, Ghosh P, Ghosh A, et al. Takayasu arteritis in pregnancy: an analysis from eastern India. Arch Gynecol Obstet. 2012;285(3):567–71.
15. Misra R, Danda D, Rajappa SM, Ghosh A, Gupta R, Mahendranath KM, et al. Development and initial validation of the Indian Takayasu clinical activity score (ITAS2010). Rheumatol Oxf Engl. 2013;52(10):1795–801.
16. Aydin SZ, Merkel PA, Direskeneli H. Outcome measures for Takayasu's arteritis. Curr Opin Rheumatol. 2015;27(1):32–7.
17. Wong VC, Wang RY, Tse TF. Pregnancy and Takayasu's arteritis. Am J Med. 1983;75(4):597–601.
18. de Jesús GR, Klumb EM, de Jesús NR, Levy RA. Pregnancy may Aggravate Arterial Hypertension in Women with Takayasu arteritis. Isr Med Assoc J. 2012;14(12):724–8.
19. Tanaka H, Tanaka K, Kamiya C, Iwanaga N, Yoshimatsu J. Analysis of pregnancies in women with Takayasu arteritis: complication of Takayasu arteritis involving obstetric or cardiovascular events. J Obstet Gynaecol Res. 2014;40(9):2031–6.
20. Alpay-Kanitez N, Omma A, Erer B, Artim-Esen B, Gül A, Inanç M, et al. Favourable pregnancy outcome in Takayasu arteritis: a single-centre experience. Clin Exp Rheumatol. 2015;33(2 Suppl 89):S-7-10.
21. Comarmond C, Mirault T, Biard L, Nizard J, Lambert M, Wechsler B, et al. Takayasu arteritis and pregnancy. Arthritis Rheumatol Hoboken NJ. 2015;67(12):3262–9.
22. David LS, Beck MM, Kumar M, Rajan SJ, Danda D, Vijayaselvi R. Obstetric and perinatal outcomes in pregnant women with Takayasu's arteritis: single Centre experience over five years. J Turk Ger Gynecol Assoc. 2019. https://doi.org/10.4274/jtgga.galenos.2019.2019.0115 [Epub ahead of print].
23. Kirshenbaum M, Simchen MJ. Pregnancy outcome in patients with Takayasu's arteritis: cohort study and review of the literature. J Matern-Fetal Neonatal Med Off J Eur Assoc Perinat Med Fed Asia Ocean Perinat Soc Int Soc Perinat Obstet. 2018;31(21):2877–83.
24. Tanacan A, Unal C, Yucesoy HM, Duru SA, Beksac MS. Management and evaluation of pregnant women with Takayasu arteritis. Arch Gynecol Obstet. 2019;299(1):79–88.

Anorectal diseases in patients with Antiphospholipid syndrome

E. Cunha[1], V. Guzela[2] , G. G. M. Balbi[3,4] , C. Sobrado[2] and D. Andrade[3*]

Abstract

Background: Hemorrhoid disease (HD) is one of the most common gastrointestinal complaints worldwide, affecting 4.4% of the general population in the United States. Since antiphospholipid syndrome (APS) may lead to intra-abdominal thrombosis, one may expect that this condition can impact the risk for HD development. Additionally, as APS patients are more prone to thrombosis and treatment with anticoagulants may increase risk of bleeding, one may also infer that rates of HD complications may be higher in this scenario. Nevertheless, no data in these regards have been published until now. The objective of the present study is to evaluate frequency of HD and describe its complications rates in antiphospholipid syndrome APS patients.

Methods: We consecutively invited patients who fulfilled APS criteria to undergo proctological examination. After examination, patients were divided in two groups, based on the presence of HD, and compared regarding different clinical manifestations and antiphospholipid profile. We performed the analysis of the data, using chi-square and Mann Whitney U when applicable and considering a significance level of 0.05. Multivariate regression analysis included age and variables with $p < 0.10$ in the bivariate analysis.

Results: Forty-one APS patients agreed to undergo proctological examination. All were female and overall median age was 43 (36–49). Seventeen (41.4%) patients were diagnosed with HD, with the following frequency distribution: 7 internal (41.2%), 4 external (23.5%) and 5 mixed hemorrhoids (29.4%). Of the internal hemorrhoids, 5 patients were classified as grade I (71.4%), 1 grade II (14.3%), and 1 grade IV (14.3%). Prior gestation ($p = 0.067$) and constipation ($p = 0.067$) correlated with a higher frequency of HD. In multivariate analysis, constipation remained as an important risk factor (OR 3.92,CI95% 1.03–14.2,$p = 0.037$). Five out of 17 patients (29.4%) reported anal bleeding, but it did not correlate with warfarin dose ($p = 0.949$). Surgical treatment was indicated for 10 patients (58.8%). Other anorectal findings were anal fissure, plicoma, condyloma and one chlamydial retitis.

Conclusion: We found an unexpected high frequency of hemorrhoids in APS patients, with a great proportion requiring surgical treatment.

Keywords: Antiphospholipid syndrome, Antiphospholipid antibodies, Rectal diseases, Anus diseases, Hemorrhoids, Hemorrhoidal disease

* Correspondence: danieli.andrade@hc.fm.usp.br
[3]Discipline of Rheumatology, Hospital das Clínicas/Faculdade de Medicina (HC-FMUSP), University of São Paulo, Av. Dr. Arnaldo 455, Third Floor, Room 3109, São Paulo 01246903, Brazil
Full list of author information is available at the end of the article

Background

Antiphospholipid syndrome (APS) is characterized by thrombosis and/or pregnancy morbidity, such as recurrent abortions, fetal loss and preterm birth, in the presence of antiphospholipid antibodies. Laboratory diagnosis is based on the persistent detection of lupus anticoagulant (LA), IgM or IgG anticardiolipin antibodies (aCL) in moderate to high titers and/or IgM or IgG anti-β2-glycoprotein I antibodies (aß2GPI) in titers over the 99th percentile [1].

Hemorrhoid disease (HD) is one of the most common gastrointestinal complaints worldwide, affecting 4.4% of the population in the United States. Its peak of incidence ranges from age 45 to 65 years, for both genders [2]. Anorectal symptoms may include bleeding, pain, prolapse, itching and/or soiling [3]. The most common complications of HD are thrombosis (especially in external hemorrhoids) and bleeding (especially in internal hemorrhoids) [2].

Hemorroids are characterized according to its origin relative to the dentate line, as: (1) internal (if proximal to this line), (2) external (if distal to this line), and (3) mixed (if both complexes are involved). Internal hemorrhoids can be further graded into four different stages (Goligher classification): grade I (1st degree or primary hemorrhoids) – prominent and engorged vasculature, no prolapse; grade II (2nd degree or secondary hemorrhoids) – prolapses with straining, spontaneous reduction; grade III (3rd degree or tertiary hemorrhoids) – prolapses beyond dentate line with straining and can only be reduced with manual maneuvers; and grade IV (4th degree or quaternary hemorrhoids) – evident prolapsed tissue, not reducible [3, 4].

There are several reported risk factors for the development of HD, including constipation, prolonged and/or frequent straining, obesity, increased intra-abdominal pressure, cirrhosis with ascites and pregnancy, all of them concurring to increase venous pressure and impair venous drainage [4]. Since APS may lead to intra-abdominal thrombosis, one may expect that this condition can impact the risk for HD development. Additionally, as APS patients are more prone to thrombosis and treatment with anticoagulants may increase risk of bleeding, one may also infer that rates of HD complications may be higher in this scenario. Nevertheless, no data in these regards have been published until now.

The primary objective of this study was to evaluate the frequency of HD and describe rates of HD complications in APS patients. We also recorded other anorectal diseases as an exploratory objective.

Methods

This is a cross-sectional study of HD and other anorectal diseases in APS patients. We consecutively invited patients who fulfilled Sydney criteria [1] and were frequently seen in our APS outpatient clinics to undergo proctological examination by an experienced colorectal surgeon. Anorectal symptoms were recorded only if they had a moderate to high frequency. Constipation was classified according to the Rome IV criteria. Clinical and serological data were obtained during visits and by chart review.

After examination, APS patients were divided in two groups, based on the presence of HD, and compared regarding different clinical manifestations and antiphospholipid profile.

We performed the analysis of the data, using chi-square and Mann Whitney U when applicable and considering a significance level of 0.05. Multivariate regression analysis included age and variables with $p < 0.10$ in the bivariate analysis.

This study was approved by the Ethics Committee of our institution (#2.368.484) and patients signed written informed consent, which have been archived in the Rheumatology department.

Results

Ninety-one APS patients were consecutively invited and 41 (45%) agreed to undergo proctological examination. Of those, all were female and overall median age was 43 (36–49). The most common causes for refusal to participate were: (1) patient considered proctological examination uncomfortable; and (2) absence of anal complaints.

Seventeen (41.4%) patients were diagnosed with HD, with the following frequency distribution: 7 had internal (41.2%), 4 external (23.5%) and 5 mixed hemorrhoids (29.4%). Of the internal hemorrhoids, 5 patients were further classified as grade I (71.4%), 1 as grade II (14.3%), 1 as grade IV (14.3%).

Patients diagnosed with HD were slightly older than those without HD (median 49 [39–53] vs. 41.5 [33.25–45]), even though this difference did not reach statistical significance.

Women with prior gestation ($p = 0.067$) and those with constipation ($p = 0.067$) showed a tendency for higher frequency of HD. In a multivariate analysis, constipation remained as an important risk factor (OR 3.92, CI95% 1.03–14.2, $p = 0.037$). Obesity, family history of HD, previous history of arterial or venous thrombosis, presence of lupus anticoagulant, anticardiolipin, anti-ß2-glycoprotein or triple positivity were not associated with a higher frequency of HD.

In the HD group, the most frequently reported signs were prolapse during defecation (88.2%), increased evacuation effort (64.7%) and anal discomfort (47.1%).

Regarding hemorrhagic complications of hemorrhoids, 5 out of 17 patients (29.4%) reported anal bleeding. Only two of all HD patients were not taking warfarin at the time of data collection; of those, one presented anal bleeding and the other did not. Anal bleeding did not correlate with warfarin dose in patients with HD ($p = 0.949$). No episode of thrombosed hemorrhoids was reported during proctological examination.

Surgical treatment was indicated for 10 patients (58.8%), due to internal hemorrhoid grade III or IV, mixed or external hemorrhoids.

Clinical and laboratory characteristics of each group are summarized and compared in Table 1.

Other anorectal findings were anal fissure ($N = 5$, 12.2%), plicoma ($N = 16$, 39%), condyloma ($N = 2$, 4.9%) and one chlamydial retitis ($N = 1$, 2.4%). Of the 2 condyloma patients, one was taking mycophenolate mofetil 500 mg BID and the other was on mycophenolate mofetil 1500 mg BID. The patient with chlamydial retitis was using azathioprine 100 mg QD and prednisone 30 mg QD.

Discussion

To the best of our knowledge, this is the first study about HD and other anorectal diseases in APS patients.

We found an unexpected high frequency of hemorrhoids (41.4%) in APS patients, if compared to the results of the largest published study in general population (prevalence of 4.4%) [2, 5].

Additionally, our patients were relatively young (median 43, interquartile range 36–49), when compared to peak incidence of HD (45–65 years) [2], what may suggest patients with APS are prone to develop HD earlier in life. Even though we cannot confirm this supposition without further prospective studies and matched healthy controls, the median age of our patients diagnosed with HD was 49 (interquartile range 39–53) and we did not find differences between ages of patients with or without HD in our sample.

Furthermore, 58.8% of our patients were referred to surgical treatment due to internal hemorrhoid grade III or IV, mixed or external hemorrhoids, suggesting that APS patients may have a more severe presentation of HD at the beginning and may require surgical interventions more often.

In our cohort, we identified that constipation correlated with a higher risk of HD, resembling the existing

Table 1 Clinical and laboratory characteristics of APS patients included, according to HD diagnosis

	Hemorrhoidal Disease ($N = 17$)	No Hemorrhoidal Disease ($N = 24$)	p-value
Demographic characteristics			
Female gender (N, %)	17 (100%)	24 (100%)	–
Age (Median, IQR)	49 (39–53)	41.5 (33.25–45)	0.09
Risk factors possibly related to HD			
Body Mass Index (Median, IQR)	29.9 (25.8–35.2)	28.57 (25.14–30.99)	0.223
Obesity (N, %)	8 (47.1%)	7 (29.2%)	0.241
Pregnancy (ever; N,%)	15 (88.2%)	15 (62.5%)	0.067
Constipation (N,%)	9 (52.9%)	6 (25%)	0.067
Family history of HD (N,%)	8 (47.1%)	7 (29.2%)	0.241
APS clinical and serological characteristics			
Arterial thrombosis (N,%)	7 (41.2%)	8 (33.3%)	0.607
Venous thrombosis (N,%)	11 (64.7%)	16 (66.7%)	0.896
Lupus anticoagulant (N,%)	13 (76.5%)	14 (58.3%)	0.130
Anticardiolipin (N,%)	4 (23.5%)	3 (12.5%)	0.355
Anti-ß2-glycoprotein I (N,%)	5 (71.4%)	7 (77.8%)	0.771
Triple positivity (N,%)	1 (5.9%)	1 (4.2%)	0.715
Anorectal symptoms/signs			
Rectal exteriorization during defecation	15 (88.2%)	13 (54.2%)	**0.021***
Increased evacuation effort	11 (64.7%)	11 (45.8%)	0.233
Anal discomfort	8 (47.1%)	4 (16.7%)	**0.035***
Pain during defecation	6 (35.3%)	9 (37.5%)	0.885
Anal burning	6 (35.3%)	4 (16.7%)	0.171
Plicoma	5 (29.4%)	11 (45.8%)	0.288
Bleeding	5 (29.4%)	3 (12.5%)	0.178
Anal itching	4 (23.5%)	5 (20.8%)	0.837
Anal Fissure	1 (5.9%)	4 (16.7%)	0.299

APS Antiphospholipid syndrome, *HD* Hemorrhoidal diseases, *IQR* Interquartile range. *$p < 0.05$

literature about risk factors for HD in other subgroups of patients [6, 7]. Nevertheless, we could not demonstrate an association between obesity and HD, what is in disagreement with other previously published studies [6, 8].

The cornerstone of APS treatment is anticoagulation therapy with vitamin K antagonists (VKA) and this is another point that needs consideration when treating HD in APS patients. One can anticipate that VKA may increase the risk of anal bleeding in those with HD and may limit surgical therapeutic options, due to increased risk of postoperative hemorrhage.

Five of our patients with HD diagnosis (29.4%) reported a past history of anal bleeding, but we were not able to check international normalized ratio (INR) of those using warfarin at the time of bleeding event. We tried to surpass this limitation using current dose of warfarin. However, we found no correlation between warfarin dose and history of anal bleeding.

Conservative measures are the mainstay treatment for HD in patients on anticoagulants [3]. A meta-analysis of 7 clinical trials comprising of 378 patients with hemorrhoids showed that fiber supplement had a consistent benefit of relieving symptom and minimizing risk of bleeding by approximately 50% [9]. However, even this strategy requires attention in APS patients. The amount of fibers consumed daily must be taken into account when prescribing VKA, as many of them also contain high levels of vitamin K. Therefore, increasing intake of fibers in diet can result in loss of efficacy of anticoagulant therapy indirectly. Patients should be instructed to consume constant doses of vitamin K and VKA dose should be adjusted to the level of vitamin K consumed daily [10].

Antithrombotic treatment has already been associated with increased risk of delayed hemorrhage after rubber band ligation (RBL) [2, 11]. RBL is one of the alternatives for treating HD. If RBL or other inpatient surgical procedures are necessary, physicians should consider withdrawing anticoagulant before these interventions [3, 12]. Since APS requires lifelong VKA use, heparin bridging is mandatory in this context [13]. Alternatively, some other technique may be preferred in this subset of patients, such as injection sclerotherapy or transanal hemorrhoidal dearterialization (THD), which have been described as safe in patients on anticoagulants [14, 15].

In addition to hemorrhoidal disease, the physician should be aware of other anorectal diseases, considering that anal fissure, condyloma and chlamydial retitis were found in our patient. As presented in the Results section, patients with condyloma and chlamydial retitis were using immunosuppression, which may have contributed to their occurrence.

Our study has several limitations. First, our sample is relatively small. Second, its cross-sectional design allows us only to suggest association, what needs to be confirmed in larger and prospective trials. Third, only 41 patients (45%) agreed to undergo proctological examination and one of the main reasons for refusal was that they had no anal symptoms. This may have introduced a selection bias and may have led to a higher than expected frequency and/or severity of HD. Finally, we enrolled both primary and secondary APS and, thus, we cannot exclude SLE as a contributing factor for our findings. Nonetheless, our study also has strengths: it provides insights about a condition poorly studied in APS; proctological examinations were performed by an experienced staff from specialized outpatient clinics with high patient volumes; and we provided description of our anorectal findings (including others besides HD), what may help future research.

Conclusions

We found an unexpected high frequency of hemorrhoids in APS patients, with a great proportion requiring surgical treatment. Physicians who work with APS should actively ask their patients regarding anorectal disease and refer to a colon and rectal surgeon whenever necessary.

Abbreviations
APS: Antiphospholipid syndrome; aCL: Anticardiolipin antibodies; aß2GPI: Anti-beta-2 glycoprotein I antibodies; BID: *Bis in die* (twice daily); HD: Hemorrhoidal disease; INR: International normalized ratio; QD: *Quaque die* (once daily); RBL: Rubber band ligation; THD: Transanal hemorrhoidal dearterialization; VKA: Vitamin K antagonists

Acknowledgements
Not applicable.

Authors' contributions
EC, GGMB and DA performed the clinical evaluation, and VG and CS performed the proctologic examinations of the patients. GGMB and DA analyzed the data and all authors contributed to the writing of the manuscript. The authors read and approved the final manuscript.

Author details
[1]Undergraduate student, Faculty of Medicine, University of São Paulo, São Paulo, SP, Brazil. [2]Discipline of Colorectal Surgery, Hospital das Clínicas/Faculdade de Medicina (HC-FMUSP), University of São Paulo, São Paulo, SP, Brazil. [3]Discipline of Rheumatology, Hospital das Clínicas/Faculdade de Medicina (HC-FMUSP), University of São Paulo, Av. Dr. Arnaldo 455, Third Floor, Room 3109, São Paulo 01246903, Brazil. [4]Discipline of Rheumatology, Hospital Universitário, Federal University of Juiz de Fora, Juiz de Fora, MG, Brazil.

References
1. Miyakis S, Lockshin MD, Atsumi T, Derksen RHWM, Groot PGDE, Koike T. International consensus statement on an update of the classification criteria for definite antiphospholipid syndrome. J Thromb Haemost. 2006;4(August 2005):295–306.
2. Sun Z, Migaly J. Review of hemorrhoid disease: presentation and management. Clin Colon Rectal Surg. 2016;29:22–9.
3. van Tol R, Kleijnen J, Watson A, Jongen J, Altomare D, Qvist N, et al. European society of ColoProctology: guideline for haemorrhoidal disease. Colorectal Dis. 2020;22:650 62.

4. Jacobs D. Hemorrhoids. N Engl J Med. 2014;371:944–51.

5. Johanson J, Sonnenberg A. The prevalence of hemorrhoids and chronic constipation: an epidemiologic study. Gastroenterology. 1990;98:380–6.

6. Lohsiriwat V. Treatment of hemorrhoids: a coloproctologist's view. World J Gastroenterol. 2015;21:9245–52.

7. Lee J, Kim H, Kang J, Shin J, Song Y. Factors associated with hemorrhoids in Korean adults: Korean national health and nutrition examination survey. Korean J Fam Med. 2014;35:227–36.

8. Loder P, Kamm M, Nicholls R, Phillips R. Haemorrhoids: pathology, pathophysiology and aetiology. Br J Surg. 1994;81:946–54.

9. Alonso-Coello P, Mills E, Heels-Ansdell D, López-Yarto M, Zhou Q, Johanson J, et al. Fiber for the treatment of hemorrhoids complications: a systematic review and meta-analysis. Am J Gastroenterol. 2006;101:181–8.

10. Klack K, de Carvalho JF. Dietetic issues in antiphospholipid syndrome. Rheumatol Int. 2013;33:823–4.

11. Nelson R, Thorson A. Risk of bleeding following hemorrhoidal banding in patients on antithrombotic therapy. Gastroenterol Clin Biol. 2009;33:463–5.

12. Lohsiriwat V. Hemorrhoids: from basic pathophysiology to clinical management. World J Gastroenterol. 2012;18:2009–17.

13. Saunders K, Erkan D, Lockshin M. Perioperative management of antiphospholipid antibody-positive patients. Curr Rheumatol Rep. 2014;16:426.

14. Yano T, Nogaki T, Asano M, Tanaka S, Kawakami K, Matsuda Y. Outcomes of case-matched injection sclerotherapy with a new agent for hemorrhoids in patients treated with or without blood thinners. Surg Today. 2013;43:854–8.

15. Atallah S, Maharaja G, Martin-Perez B, Burke J, Albert M, Larach S. Transanal hemorrhoidal dearterialization (THD): a safe procedure for the anticoagulated patient? Tech Coloproctol. 2016;20:461–6.

24

Position article and guidelines 2018 recommendations of the Brazilian Society of Rheumatology for the indication, interpretation and performance of nailfold capillaroscopy

Cristiane Kayser[1]* (iD), Markus Bredemeier[2], Maria Teresa Caleiro[3], Karina Capobianco[4], Tatiana Melo Fernandes[5], Sheila Márcia de Araújo Fontenele[6], Eutilia Freire[7], Lilian Lonzetti[8], Renata Miossi[3], Juliana Sekiyama[9] and Carolina de Souza Müller[10]

Abstract

Nailfold capillaroscopy (NFC) is a reproducible, simple, low-cost, and safe imaging technique used for morphological analysis of nail bed capillaries. It is considered to be extremely useful for the investigation of Raynaud's phenomenon and for the early diagnosis of systemic sclerosis (SSc). The capillaroscopic pattern typically associated with SSc, scleroderma ("SD") pattern, is characterized by dilated capillaries, microhemorrhages, avascular areas and/or capillary loss, and distortion of the capillary architecture. The aim of these recommendations is to provide orientation regarding the relevance of NFC, and to establish a consensus on the indications, nomenclature, the interpretation of NFC findings and the technical equipments that should be used. These recommendations were formulated based on a systematic literature review of studies included in the database MEDLINE (PubMed) without any time restriction.

Keywords: Capillaroscopy, Systemic sclerosis, Raynaud's phenomenon

Introduction

The microcirculation plays a crucial role in physiological processes. Comprising arterioles, capillaries, and venules, it is involved in thermoregulation, hemodynamic balance maintenance, the nutrient supply to cells, and removal of catabolites derived from cell metabolism. The capillary loops are vessels with a small diameter and are usually composed of one single layer of endothelial cells.

Nailfold capillaroscopy (NFC) is a reproducible, simple, low-cost, and noninvasive imaging technique that is used for morphological and functional analyses of the peripheral microcirculation. Because the microcirculation might be the primary site of abnormalities,

NFC is used for the diagnosis and evaluation of systemic sclerosis (SSc) spectrum disorders and for the differentiation between primary and secondary Raynaud's phenomenon (RP) [1]. Capillaroscopy evaluation of individuals with RP might contribute to the identification of an underlying disease, as well as to the assessment of disease progression [2–5]. Table 1 describes the main indications of NFC in rheumatology.

Although the role of NFC in the investigation of patients with RP and in the diagnosis of SSc is well established, different magnification equipment and a variety of definitions are used to describe the capillary morphology. In addition, there is no consensus on the parameters that should be analyzed or on the nomenclature to be used. These facts underscore the need to standardize the nomenclature, the indications and interpretation of NFC

* Correspondence: cristiane.kayser@unifesp.br
[1]Rheumatology Division, Escola Paulista de Medicina, Universidade Federal de São Paulo (UNIFESP), Rua Botucatu 740, 3° andar, São Paulo, SP 04023-062, Brazil
Full list of author information is available at the end of the article

Table 1 Main indications of capillaroscopy in rheumatology

Evaluation of individuals with Raynaud's phenomenon (RP)
Dermatomyositis (DM)
Mixed connective tissue disease (MCTD)
Systemic sclerosis (SSc)

findings and the technical equipment used to perform NFC [6].

The present recommendations were formulated to provide an orientation on the relevance, indications, technical equipment, nomenclature and the parameters that should be evaluated by NFC in rheumatology practice.

Methods

The present guidelines followed the criteria developed for systematic reviews. Evidence was collected according to an evidence-based medicine approach, which integrates clinical experience with the ability to critically analyze and rationally apply scientific information, thus improving the quality of medical care. The relevant clinical questions were formulated as per the PICO strategy (acrostic stands for "Patient," "Intervention," "Control," and "Outcome") by the authors, who are all professionally involved in performing nailfold capillaroscopy. The evidence to answer the clinical questions was collected according to the following steps: formulation of clinical questions, structuration of questions, search for evidence, critical evaluation and selection of evidence, presentation of results, and recommendations.

The formulation of structured questions allowed us to identify descriptors that served as a basis in the search for evidence in the MEDLINE–PubMed database. The abstracts of all the retrieved studies were analyzed. Following the application of eligibility (inclusion/exclusion) criteria, articles were selected to answer the questions, which led to the evidence forming the basis of the present guidelines. A manual search of the references cited in (narrative and systematic) reviews and selected studies was also performed. In addition, the references were manually updated until December 2017. The studies were categorized by grades of recommendation and strength of evidence according to the Oxford and GRADE classification systems, as shown in Table 2. The detail of the methods and results are described in the Additional file 1.

Results

What are the main indications of CAPILLAROSCOPY for rheumatic diseases?

Raynaud's phenomenon (RP)

RP is characterized by episodes of transient ischemia of the extremities, usually in response to cold or stress [7, 8]. It presents as a characteristic "triphasic" color pattern change, (pallor, cyanosis, and rubor) of the hands and feet. Population-based studies, which included several ethnic groups, estimated its prevalence as 3 to 20% as a function of the geographical location and local climate [7–11]. RP is classified as **primary,** or idiopathic, and **secondary**.

Primary RP manifests usually in young individuals (14 years of age, on average) and presents as symmetric and milder episodes, without necrosis, ulceration, or gangrene, in addition to the absence of any definite cause [1, 12]. In turn, secondary RP manifests in adults (generally ≥30 years old); episodes are more intense, painful, and associated with ischemic skin lesions that exhibit signs of microvascular abnormalities. Secondary RP is a common manifestation of autoimmune diseases, such as SSc, mixed connective tissue disease (MCTD), systemic lupus erythematosus (SLE), Sjögren's syndrome, dermatomyositis, and polymyositis [10, 11].

Investigations of RP by means of NFC are widely reported in the literature (**B**) [10] (**D**) [12]. NFC is an important method for the early detection of secondary RP and might further contribute to the characterization of clinical aspects and progression of the underlying disease (**B**) [13]. Several studies have found that the presence of abnormalities in the nailfold microcirculation on NFC is an independent risk factor for the development of autoimmune rheumatic disease (**B**) [14, 15].

A prospective study found that 20% of patients initially diagnosed with primary RP exhibited a transition to suspected or definite secondary RP during a 10-year follow-up (**B**) [16]. The frequency of such transitions might vary depending on the analyzed population (**C**) [17–19]. Another study conducted with 639 patients with primary RP found that 12.6% of the sample progressed into secondary RP after a mean time of 10.4 years. The main predictor of transition was an abnormal nailfold capillary pattern on NFC, with a positive predictive value of 47% (**A**) [17]. Based on the pattern assessed on nailfold videocapillaroscopy, 14.9% of patients ($n = 19$) in another prospective study were classified as secondary RP over a follow-up period of 29 ± 10

Table 2 Grade of recommendation and strength of evidence

A:	Experimental or observational studies with better consistency
B:	Experimental or observational studies with less consistency
C:	Case reports/uncontrolled studies
D:	Opinions without critical evaluation, based on consensus, physiological studies, or animal models

months. Interestingly, 4.6% of these patients exhibited a normal microcirculation pattern on NFC at the onset of the study (**B**) [18].

Finally, a study of adults with a history of isolated RP demonstrated, by means of a prognostic model, a correlation between abnormalities on NFC (microhemorrhages, giant loops, and number of capillaries) and progression into SSc spectrum disorders (**B**) [19].

Systemic sclerosis (SSc)

SSc is an autoimmune disease of unknown origin characterized by progressive vascular involvement, with subsequent chronic damage of several organs and systems, such as the gastrointestinal tract, lungs, heart, kidneys, and skin [20–22]. Due to its high morbidity and mortality, countless efforts have been devoted in recent years aiming at early diagnosis and early treatment of the disease, before organ damage becomes irreversible [23].

Typical microangiopathy in SSc includes dilated loops, giant loops, a reduced number of loops and avascular areas, microhemorrhages, neoangiogenesis and disorganization of the nailfold capillary architecture, which together are known as the "SD" (scleroderma) pattern (**B**) [24], (**C**) [25]. The "SD" pattern is found in 80 to 90% of SSc cases and also occurs in other autoimmune rheumatic diseases [26, 27].

These abnormalities might occur in the early stages of SSc, when the clinical manifestations are restricted to isolated RP. Progressive capillary loss is characteristic of the microvascular dysfunction in SSc and is associated with a higher disease severity (**B**) [28–30]. A study conducted with SSc patients found that the severity of organ involvement, such as the lungs, skin, and heart, was directly correlated to the pattern of microcirculation damage (**B**) [28]. Thus, NFC seems to be useful for clinical staging and to obtain prognostic information.

Dermatomyositis

Capillaroscopic findings in dermatomyositis characteristically include a reduction of capillary loops, dilated capillary loops, remarkably branched loops, and disorganization of the capillary architecture (**C**) [31, 32]. The typical "SD" pattern found in SSc exhibits variable rates (**B**) [33], (**C**) [32]. Capillaroscopic abnormalities are associated with the activity and severity of disease and interstitial lung involvement (**B**) [33]. Loop reduction is associated with the global activity of disease and hemorrhage with skin activity (**B**) [33].

Systemic lupus erythematosus (SLE)

The main abnormalities found on NFC among SLE patients are increased capillary tortuosity, elongated loops, focal areas of capillary loss, and increased visibility of the subpapillary venous plexus. Capillary rarefaction and

dilated loops are correlated with lung involvement (**C**) [34]. NFC abnormalities are more frequent among patients with SLE and RP (**B**) [35].

Mixed connective tissue disease (MCTD)

Several microcirculation abnormalities have been described among patients with MCTD, such as microhemorrhages and capillary disorganization. The pattern on NFC is similar to that of SSc; however, capillary rarefaction and giant capillaries are less frequent in MCTD (**C**) [36, 37].

Recommendation 1

Nailfold capillaroscopy is a method for the assessment of the microcirculation and represents a reliable tool for differential diagnosis between primary and secondary Raynaud's phenomenon.

The inclusion of NFC in examinations of patients with Raynaud's phenomenon is recommended to support or rule out its association with systemic sclerosis spectrum disorders, dermatomyositis, and mixed connective tissue disease.

What equipment might be used to perform CAPILLAROSCOPY?

By means of an optical magnification device and incident light, NFC enables direct evaluation of peripheral microcirculation structures. NFC might be performed with different devices, such as a **stereomicroscope, videocapillaroscope, dermatoscope,** and **ophthalmoscope**, which exhibit different sensitivities and specificities. Stereomicroscopy magnifies images up to 50 times and provides detailed information regarding the microcirculation; assessment of the entire nailbed enables widefield NFC. Videocapillaroscopy allows the storage of images and uses magnification up to 600 times, thus enabling exact measurements of individual capillaries using specific softwares [38].

A study analyzed videocapillaroscopy with 200x magnification and stereomicroscopy (10 to 25x magnification) among patients with RP. Both techniques were similar in diagnostic performance and reproducibility regarding the evaluation of several capillaroscopic parameters (number of capillaries/mm, capillary dimension, and microhemorrhages) (**B**) [39]. In this study, the diagnostic accuracy to discriminate patients with SSc from healthy individuals was similar for both techniques (**B**) [39]. Similarly to the data described above, the two methods exhibited a good correlation for capillary density among patients with SSc (**B**) [40].

Dermatoscopy is widely used in dermatology to investigate skin lesions, but the images have less magnification and poorer resolution. A prospective study designed to analyze the diagnostic performance of dermatoscopy with 30x magnification among patients with RP found good concordance compared with conventional capillaroscopy, with a sensitivity and specificity of 76.9 and 90.9% for the "SD" pattern, respectively (**B**) [41]. Similar findings were reported by other authors, who described good diagnostic accuracy of dermatoscopy for connective tissue diseases (**B**) [42].

Some authors have suggested the use of portable devices, such as the ophthalmoscope (**C**) [43]. In an observational study that analyzed nailfold abnormalities among SSc patients with an ophthalmoscope or dermatoscope (with polarized light and without immersion), Baron et al. found good reproducibility in the identification of dilated capillaries and giant capillaries. However, there was no concordance in the identification of avascular areas (**B**) [43].

Recommendation 2
Nailfold capillaroscopy is a complementary diagnostic method for evaluation of the microvascular structure. It might be performed with a stereomicroscope, videocapillaroscope, dermatoscope, or ophthalmoscope. The stereomicroscope and videocapillaroscope exhibit excellent reliability for the evaluation of capillaroscopic abnormalities, which suggests that any of them might be indistinctly used for assessment of peripheral microangiopathy among individuals with systemic sclerosis and Raynaud's phenomenon. The latter two (dermatoscope and ophthalmoscope) provide less magnified images of poorer quality. However, they might be used in services in which stereomicroscopy and videocapillaroscopy are not available. All these techniques are examiner-dependent, and they do not point, alone, to the diagnosis of disease.

What morphological parameters should be evaluated in NAILFOLD CAPILLAROSCOPY?
Only the morphological aspects of the distal row capillaries are evaluated using NFC. The capillaroscopic pattern is not established based on the evaluation of one single parameter but on a combination of numerical and morphological characteristics [44]. Table 3 describes the main morphological characteristics, which should be evaluated on NFC [44–46].

Table 3 Morphological parameters assessed on capillaroscopy

- Capillary architecture and organization
- Capillary morphology
- Capillary density (number of capillary loops per millimeter)
- Capillary size (including enlarged and giant capillaries)
- Microhemorrhages
- Avascular areas
- Neoangiogenesis

Capillary architecture and organization
Normally, the distal row of capillaries are orderly distributed in horizontal lines or palisade array on the periungueal region. This distribution is homogeneous and regular, and perpendicular to the nail edge (**B**) [44]. It is important to bear in mind that there are variations in NFC findings even among healthy individuals (**B**) [44, 45, 47].

Capillary morphology
Individual loops look like hairpins (**C**) [48]. Normal capillaries have an inverted "U" shape with a thinner arterial (afferent) side. Discrete abnormalities might be found in healthy individuals, such as tortuous or "meandering" loops (capillaries with limbs crossed upon themselves), branching, and few dilatation (**D**) [49, 50].

Capillary density
Is defined as the number of capillary loops per millimeter in each finger. It is one of the most significant parameters for the early identification of individuals at high risk for the development of autoimmune rheumatic diseases, especially the ones with RP (**B**) [44]. The average number of capillaries per millimeter is variable among studies, ranging from 7 to 12 capillaries/mm (**B**) [44, 45], (**C**) [51].

Capillary size
Several values and measurements are described in the literature relative to the capillary size. The most significant measurements that can be measured using videocapillaroscopy are the capillary width, diameter of the afferent (arterial) side, diameter of the efferent (venous) side, and diameter of the apical loop (**B**) [44, 53], (**C**) [52].

Enlarged and giant capillaries
According to Maricq et al., capillaries are considered to be dilated when all three loop sides—afferent, apical, and efferent—are 4 to 9 times larger than the normal diameters. Giant capillaries are extremely enlarged loops, with diameters 10 or more times larger than the normal adjacent loops (**B**) [54]. According to more recent classifications or software measurement of capillary size, giant capillaries are those with arterial, venous, or apical diameters over 50 μm (**B**) [55], (**C**) [27], (**D**) [56]. Capillaries with a diameter greater than 20 μm are defined as enlarged (**B**) [55].

Microhemorrhages
These are easily visible dark areas on the nailfold capillary bed, and they occur due to rupture of the capillary wall. Microhemorrhages might be focal or diffuse. Isolated microhemorrhages might occur in healthy individuals due to microtrauma [45]. In SSc and scleroderma

spectrum disorders, microhemorrhages usually exhibit a diffuse distribution and are close to dilated capillaries, which tend to become broken more easily.

Avascular areas

Avascular areas may be variably defined and can be focal or diffuse. As a rule, they are defined based on the number of capillaries per millimeter; diffuse devascularization is present when the number of capillaries per millimeter is ≤7. Alternatively, diffuse devascularization is defined as a distance larger than 500 μm between two adjacent loops (D) [56]. Avascular areas are also defined as the absence of two or more successive capillaries. They are attended by tissue hypoxia and occur in SSc spectrum disorders, in which case they are highly relevant because they are associated with the severity of the disease (B) [57], (C) [58]. Some authors quantify the extension of devascularization by means of a semiquantitative scale ranging from 0 to 3: 0–absence of avascular areas; 1–discrete devascularization (one or two avascular areas); 2–moderate devascularization (more than two avascular areas); 3–extensive and confluent devascularization areas (D) [56], (B) [39, 45].

Neoangiogenesis

Branched capillaries with a highly heterogeneous shape, usually due to capillary neoformation (angiogenesis), may occur among individuals with secondary RP (D) [54].

Recommendation 3

Nailfold capillaroscopy is a noninvasive, relatively easy to perform, complementary method for assessment of the microcirculation, and it demands training from examiners. As a rule, the main parameters to be assessed are as follows: capillary architecture and morphology, capillary density (number of capillaries per millimeter) and size,

presence of microhemorrhages, devascularization, and neoangiogenesis.

What are the normal parameters on NAILFOLD CAPILLAROSCOPY?

Among healthy individuals, loops are homogeneous in shape, exhibiting a homogeneous and regular array perpendicular to the nailbed (Fig. 1a). Discrete variations, such as tortuous and "meandering" loops and a visible subpapillary venous plexus, might occur, particularly among light-skinned individuals (B) [45]. Normal findings are described in Table 4.

Recommendation 4

Findings on normal nailfold capillaroscopy include a palisade array of capillaries, with a regular and homogeneous distribution, and the absence of devascularization areas. It is important to bear in mind the wide variability in morphology and size of the loops among healthy individuals, and even between the fingers of one and the same individual.

Which morphological abnormalities are present in the "SD" pattern?

The term "SD" (scleroderma) **pattern**, first described in 1980, alludes to a set of typical abnormalities on NFC found among patients with SSc (B) [26]. It is characterized by the presence of dilated and giant capillaries, a reduced capillary density, architectural distortion, morphological abnormalities in loops, microhemorrhages, and neoangiogenesis (Fig. 1b) [59, 60]. Structures might be blurred by edema, and anomalous connective tissue proliferation might occur [61]. In the early 2000's, capillaroscopic abnormalities were sequentially classified into three patterns based on the microcirculation involvement: "early" pattern, characterized by few dilated capillaries, small

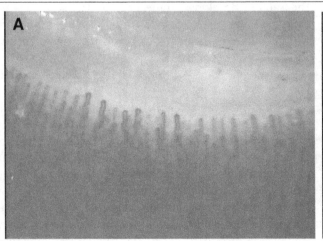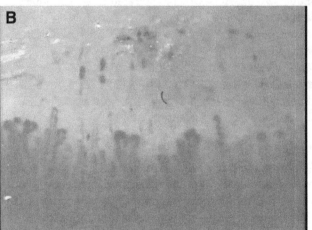

Fig. 1 Nailfold capillaroscopy showing a normal pattern (**a**) and a scleroderma pattern, characterized by the presence of enlarged and giant capillaries, reduced capillary density, and microhemorrhages (**b**)

Table 4 Normal morphological parameters on capillaroscopy

Capillaroscopic parameters	Normal pattern
Skin transparency and visibility	Capillaries are clearly visible
Pericapillary edema	Absent
Subpapillary venous plexus	Visible in > 30% of healthy individuals
Capillary architecture	Capillaries perpendicular to the nail edge
Capillary morphology	Inverted "U" shape
Capillary loop diameter	< 20 μm
Tortuosity	Normally absent
Dilated and giant loops	Absent
Neoangiogenesis	Absent
Microhemorrhages	Normally absent
Capillary density	7 to 12 capillaries/mm
Avascular areas	Absent
Capillary blood flow	Dynamic, without stasis

Adapted from Chojnowski et al., 2016[59] (**D**)

number of microhemorrhages, no evident capillary loss and relatively preserved distribution; "active" pattern, in which giant capillaries and microhemorrhages are frequent, and there is a discrete distortion of the capillary architecture; "late" pattern, with few or no giant capillaries, and the presence of neoangiogenesis and large avascular areas [24].

In addition to the aforementioned morphological abnormalities on NFC, the "SD" pattern includes histopathological and functional changes, such as endothelial edema, inflammatory infiltrates, and slower blood flow [49, 62].

Recommendation 5
The **"SD" pattern** on nailfold capillaroscopy exhibits dilated capillaries, a reduced density of the capillary loops, distortion of the capillary architecture, and microhemorrhages.

Should CAPILLAROSCOPY be indicated to all individuals with RAYNAUD'S phenomenon?
Under normal conditions, and also among individuals with primary RP, NFC exhibits regular capillary loops, some dilated capillaries eventually, and an absence of giant capillaries or avascular areas (**C**) [63]. Microcirculation abnormalities, such as increased capillary diameter, architectural disorganization, angiogenesis, and avascular areas, point to a possible connective tissue disease or secondary RP (**B**) [5, 64].

In a study that analyzed microvascular abnormalities among individuals with undifferentiated connective tissue disease (UCTD), RP was found in 52.5% of the sample (**B**) [65]. The most frequent microvascular abnormalities were giant capillaries, and dilated and irregular capillaries. The patients with UCTD but without RP exhibited unspecific microcirculation changes (**B**) [65].

A retrospective study was conducted with 67 patients to analyze the sensitivity, specificity, positive (PPV), and negative (NPV) predictive value of capillaroscopy for the diagnosis of connective tissue diseases (**B**) [2]. The sensitivity and specificity for the diagnosis of SSc was 89.4 and 80%, respectively, when the "SD" pattern was found on NFC. PPV and NPV for SSc was 68 and 94%, respectively (**B**) [2]. The sensitivity and specificity of SLE-related capillaroscopic patterns was 33 and 95.4%, respectively, with PPV of 71.4% and NPV of 80.7%. The sensitivity and specificity for diagnosis of dermatomyositis/polymyositis was 60 and 96.3%, respectively, with PPV 60% and NPV 96.3%. The sensitivity and specificity for diagnosis of MCTD was 20 and 100%, respectively, with PPV of 100% and NPV 93.1% (**B**) [2].

A prospective study performed to analyze the prognostic value of the "SD" pattern on NFC among individuals with primary RP ($n = 3029$) found that 37% of the sample developed some connective tissue disease (SSc, SLE, rheumatoid arthritis, Sjögren's syndrome, MCTD, dermatomyositis, polymyositis). The sensitivity, specificity, PPV, and NPV of the "SD" pattern in regard to SSc was 94, 92, 52, and 99%, respectively (**B**) [66].

Corroborating these findings, another prospective study investigated the contribution of NFC to the assessment of the progression of individuals with RP. The sample included 288 patients with primary RP, 11.8% of whom exhibited a transition from isolated RP to SSc, and 42 patients to other connective tissue diseases (**B**) [67].

Additionally, other authors reported that microcirculation abnormalities, such as avascular areas, giant capillaries, and distortion of the capillary architecture, were capillaroscopic predictors of connective tissue diseases among individuals with RP (**B**) [13].

It should be observed that normal NFC findings are diagnostic criteria for primary RP, as formulated by LeRoy et al. in 1992 (**B**) [68], and they are also included in the new diagnostic criteria suggested by Maverakis et al. in 2014 (**B**) [69].

Recommendation 6

Nailfold capillaroscopy is highly relevant for the differential diagnosis of connective tissue diseases among individuals with Raynaud's phenomenon. Among them, NFC exhibits considerable predictive value regarding the development of autoimmune rheumatic disease and, thus, it should be performed in all individuals with Raynaud's phenomenon.

What is the relevance of CAPILLAROSCOPY for the early diagnosis of systemic sclerosis?

Several studies have confirmed the relevance of NFC for the early diagnosis of SSc. This method was recently included in the classification criteria for SSc proposed by the American College of Rheumatology (ACR) and European League Against Rheumatism (EULAR), despite the lack of consensus on the technique to be used and the variables that should be analyzed (**D**) [70, 71]. Preliminary criteria for very early diagnosis of systemic sclerosis (VE DOSS) were also published. According to the latter, the main clinical characteristics of very early SSc are RP, positive autoantibodies (anticentromere and antitopoisomerase), and "SD" pattern on NFC (**D**) [72]. These parameters allow the identification of SSc patients in a very early stage of disease, allowing early treatment and represent a true "window of opportunity."

A study that analyzed morphological and functional microcirculation abnormalities among patients diagnosed with SSc found that in the early stages of disease, both widefield NFC and videocapillaroscopy allowed the detection of milder abnormalities, such as a higher capillary density, smaller number of giant capillaries, and smaller avascular areas, by comparison to patients with established disease (**B**) [73].

Prospective studies that assessed NFC performance in SSc demonstrated the pathophysiological sequence of microvascular damage (**B**) [28, 74].

Recommendation 7

Although there is no medication able to hinder the natural progression of disease, recent advances were made in the treatment of systemic sclerosis based on new drugs with effects on vascular remodeling, such as endothelin receptor antagonists, phosphodiesterase inhibitors, and prostanoids. Therefore, optimization of diagnosis in early stages of disease, including identification of milder structural abnormalities, might provide an opportunity to prevent the progression of systemic sclerosis. Within this context,

nailfold capillaroscopy is useful for the early diagnosis of disease.

Is the "SD" pattern specific for systemic sclerosis? Do other diseases exhibit this pattern?

Present in approximately 80 to 90% of SSc cases, the "SD" pattern can, however, also be found among patients with other autoimmune rheumatic diseases, such as dermatomyositis and MCTD (**C**) [26], (**D**) [75]. A study analyzed the predictive value of the "SD" pattern for the diagnosis of SSc in a cohort of unselected patients. The results showed a sensitivity, specificity, PPV, and NPV of 71, 95, 84, and 90%, respectively (**B**) [76].

A prospective observational study with more than 3000 patients and 5.3-year follow-up found that the "SD" pattern on NFC was significantly associated with SSc. The "SD" pattern was detected in 94% of the patients who developed SSc six months before onset of disease manifestations (**B**) [66]. A total of 71% of the patients who developed dermatomyositis and 37% of the those who progressed to MCTD exhibited the "SD" pattern (**B**) [66].

In a series of patients with connective tissue disease and RP, 87.5% ($n = 14$) of the 16 participants with diffuse cutaneous SSc, and 61.6% ($n = 53$) of the 86 patients with limited cutaneous SSc, exhibited the "SD" pattern. Additionally, 13.8% of the patients with UCTD, 8.5% of those with SLE, and 26.9% of the ones with dermatomyositis and polymyositis exhibited the capillaroscopic pattern associated with SSc. In turn, none of the patients with rheumatoid arthritis (RA) or Sjögren's syndrome exhibited this pattern (**B**) [4]. When the "SD" pattern is found in these other diseases, it should always raise suspicion of SSc overlap syndrome.

Recommendation 8

Identification of the **"SD" pattern** on nailfold capillaroscopy is suggestive of systemic sclerosis. This pattern is also found in other connective tissue diseases, such as dermatomyositis and mixed connective tissue disease, and less frequently in systemic lupus erythematosus and undifferentiated connective tissue disease.

What CAPILLAROSCOPIC abnormalities are found in other autoimmune rheumatic diseases (systemic lupus erythematosus, rheumatoid arthritis, antiphospholipid syndrome, systemic vasculitis)?

Systemic lupus erythematosus

SLE is a multisystem, chronic inflammatory autoimmune disease that might be accompanied by microvascular damage. The findings on NFC have poor specificity for early diagnosis and prognostic assessment, as no specific pattern has been identified for this disease (B) [77, 78]. The main abnormal findings are increased capillary tortuosity, which occurs in more than 40% of patients, and an increased capillary length. Smaller proportions of patients might exhibit focal areas of capillary loss and increased visibility of the subpapillary venous plexus (**B**) [27, 78], (**C**) [79].

A retrospective analysis of 123 individuals diagnosed with SLE subjected to NFC found that the "major" capillary abnormalities (elongated loops, dilatation of the efferent side, increased tortuosity, and branching) occurred in 35.8% of the sample (**B**) [77]. A total of 28.5% of the patients exhibited a normal pattern on NFC, and 33.3% showed "minor" abnormalities (**B**) [77].

In another study with SLE patients, NFC findings such as increased capillary tortuosity, avascular areas and microhemorrhages, were more common among the cases with RP compared to those without it (**B**) [35].

Rheumatoid arthritis
The data on capillaroscopic findings among RA patients are scarce in the literature. In 1970, Redisch et al. reported that the most frequent findings in a series of RA patients were an increased capillary tortuosity, an increased capillary length, and a prominent subpapillary venous plexus (**C**) [80]. Another study of 32 RA patients reported capillary tortuosity and prominent subpapillary venous plexus, especially among the cases with positive antinuclear antibodies (**C**) [81]. In one study of 62 RA patients, the most frequent finding was a prominent subpapillary venous plexus, which was present in 69% of cases, and an increased capillary length (58%) (**C**) [82].

Antiphospholipid syndrome
Patients with antiphospholipid syndrome (APS) exhibit symmetric microhemorrhages (**B**) [83]. Morphological abnormalities are found in primary and secondary APS; the variation in the loop length is considerably more frequent in primary APS, while microhemorrhages are more evident in cases of APS secondary to SLE (**B**) [84].

Systemic vasculitis
A study which analyzed capillaroscopic abnormalities among patients with vasculitis (polyarteritis nodosa, Churg-Strauss syndrome, hypersensitivity vasculitis, and temporal arteritis) found discrete and isolated changes in 73% of the sample. Microhemorrhage was the most frequent finding among cases with active disease (**C**) [85]. Overall, the capillaroscopic findings were few and non-specific.

Behçet's disease
Some authors analyzed NFC findings of 128 patients with Behçet's disease. Discrete abnormalities were found in 40% of the sample, an increased capillary diameter in 26%, microhemorrhages in 16%, and capillary loss in 2% (**B**) [86].

Sjögren's syndrome
NFC was normal in more than half of patients diagnosed with Sjögren's syndrome without RP (**C**) [87]. Non-specific abnormalities, such as tortuous and irregular capillaries and increased visibility of the subpapillary venous plexus, were described in 29.5% of 61 individuals with primary Sjögren's syndrome (**B**) [88].

Recommendation 9
Overall, the capillaroscopic abnormalities found in other autoimmune rheumatic diseases, such as systemic lupus erythematosus, rheumatoid arthritis, antiphospholipid syndrome and systemic vasculitis, are non-specific.

Should NAILFOLD CAPILLAROSCOPY be repeated during the follow-up of patients with systemic sclerosis?
Several studies have consistently shown that devascularization and distortion of the capillary architecture—which characterize late microvascular injury among patients with SSc—are strong predictors of complications involving target organs, such as the skin, lungs, heart, gastrointestinal tract, and kidneys (**B**) [28, 89–91], (**C**) [92], (**D**) [93].

Some studies have reported results after treatment of SSc patients, including parameters such as blood flow, capillary permeability, and loop morphology. Thus, NFC might play a role in the monitoring of treatment (**B**) [94, 95]. However, this indication is still controversial, and studies with larger samples and longer durations of follow-up are needed.

Recommendation 10
Nailfold capillaroscopy plays a relevant role in the diagnosis of systemic sclerosis, as microvascular damage is an early marker of disease. It is also useful to assess the severity of disease. However, there is still no consensus on its role in the follow-up of SSc patients.

Are CAPILLAROSCOPY abnormalities associated with the risk of development of digital ulcers in patients with systemic sclerosis?
Digital ulcers (DU) are a common complication, affecting 30 to 50% of SSc patients [96, 97]. Although the understanding of the pathophysiology of DU has improved in recent years, the identification of patients at high risk of developing DU still poses a challenge. Some studies have described endothelial dysfunction biomarkers, and NFC findings as potential predictors of new DU (**B**) [98]. Avascular areas found on NFC might be related to an imbalance of angiogenic factors, and a higher risk of DU [99, 100].

A study that analyzed patients with SSc and RP found that individuals with DU predominantly exhibited the late pattern on NFC (neoangiogenesis, large avascular areas, and few dilated or giant capillaries) compared with those without DU. Among this latter group of patients, the capillaroscopic abnormalities corresponded to the active pattern (giant capillaries, microhemorrhages, and discrete avascular areas) (**B**) [89]. Corroborating these findings, a prospective observational study with 77 SSc patients found, on videocapillaroscopy with 200x magnification, that the development of DU during the 3-year follow-up was associated with the late pattern on NFC, particularly capillary disorganization, microhemorrhages, and avascular areas (**B**) [90]. Logistic regression analysis showed that this capillaroscopic pattern was the best independent predictor of both the first episode and recurrence of DU in the analyzed population (**B**) [90]. Reinforcing these findings, a study with 103 SSc patients subjected to videocapillaroscopy also reported a strong association between the late pattern abnormalities and DU (**B**) [28]. On the other side, an observational study with 36 SSc patients designed to investigate capillaroscopic patterns and their association with DU found the active "SD" pattern in all the patients with DU, but only in 47% of those without DU (**C**) [101].

Some authors have suggested quantitative risk scores for prognostic purposes of DU development (**A**) [102], (**B**) [103]. One score, the Capillaroscopic Skin Ulcer Risk Index (CSURI) is calculated by means of the equation D_xM/N^2, in which D is the maximum diameter of giant capillaries, M the number of giant capillaries, and N the number of capillaries in the distal row (**B**) [103–105]. In a multicenter study, CSURI exhibited 92.9 and 81.4% sensitivity and specificity, respectively, for the development of DU within three months of videocapillaroscopy, with an area under the receiver operating characteristic (ROC) curve of 0.884 (**B**) [104]. A limitation of this score is the mandatory presence of giant capillaries, which excludes the abnormalities corresponding to the late pattern.

Recommendation 11
In patients with systemic sclerosis microvascular abnormalities are frequently observed on capillaroscopy. Structural abnormalities, such as devascularization areas and distortion of the capillary bed architecture, characteristic of the late microvascular damage, are strong predictors of the occurrence of digital ulcers in this population of patients.

Is there a correlation between CAPILLAROSCOPIC findings and severity and prognosis among patients with systemic sclerosis?
Several studies have shown a positive correlation between the degree and extension of microvascular damage on NFC and the involvement of internal organs in SSc (**B**) [106–109].

The preliminary attempts to establish a correlation between NFC findings and clinical abnormalities among patients with SSc were initiated in the 1970s with the study by Maricq et al. (**C**) [54]. In that study, with

patients with SSc ($n = 28$) and dermatomyositis ($n = 3$), a positive correlation was found between the degree and extension of microvascular damage and involvement of many body systems (**C**) [54]. Although criticized by its small sample size, the results of the study suggest that the number of involved organs is associated with more severe capillaroscopic abnormalities. Another observational study conducted with patients with isolated RP and SSc analyzed the association between antinuclear antibodies, capillaroscopic patterns, and clinical findings. The results showed that patients with SSc and the "active" capillaroscopic pattern exhibited the highest levels of target-organ involvement, including the kidneys, muscles, and skin in particular (**C**) [30]. These patients were also at higher risk of developing hypertension and anemia. In turn, the individuals with the "slow" capillaroscopic pattern, i.e., with a predominance of dilated loops and few avascular areas, exhibited a lower frequency of visceral involvement (**C**) [30]. Corroborating the aforementioned findings, an observational study with 112 patients, 45 of whom had SSc, found that more severe abnormalities on NFC were associated with more extensive systemic involvement (**C**) [109].

A prospective observational study that independently analyzed two cohorts of SSc patients found that organ involvement was strongly associated with the pattern on NFC (**B**) [110]. However, conflicting results have also been reported, as some authors did not find a correlation between the systemic involvement and abnormalities on NFC (**B**) [111].

In a study conducted in Spain, progressive capillary loss on NFC was associated with greater disease severity and an increased risk of DU occurrence (**B**) [112]. A study performed in 2007 found that patients with the "late" capillaroscopic pattern (on nailfold videocapillaroscopy) were at higher risk of disease activity (OR = 3.50, 95% CI: 1.31 to 9.39) and DU occurrence (OR = 5.74, 95% CI: 2.08 to 15.89) (**B**) [28].

Other studies have shown that among patients with SSc, the degree of capillary loss on NFC differs between those with or without pulmonary hypertension (**B**) [106, 107]. A study found that SSc patients with severe capillaroscopic abnormalities exhibited a higher prevalence of ground-glass opacities on high-resolution computed tomography (**B**) [29]. Finally, a study conducted with SSc patients reported that the risk of death was higher among those with higher degrees of devascularization on NFC (**B**) [113]. Therefore, NFC might be used for the assessment of disease severity and to predict the occurrence of systemic complications among patients with SSc.

Recommendation 12
Nailfold capillaroscopy plays a relevant role in the diagnosis of systemic sclerosis. Despite being controversial,

the available evidence indicates a positive correlation between capillaroscopic abnormalities and the involvement of target organs.

Conclusions

Nailfold capillaroscopy is increasingly being used among rheumatologists. It is an important method for the investigation of RP and for the early diagnosis of SSc. In the present recommendations, the main indications, the technical equipments that should be used, and standardization on nomenclature, parameters, and the interpretation of NFC findings were proposed based on a systematic review of the literature and the experience of a panel of experts. Thus, the standardized indications and definitions will increase the reliability and quality of NFC performance among rheumatologists and clinicians.

Additional file

Additional file 1: Methodological details, expanded results and rationale of the formulated questions for the present recommendations [114–117].

Abbreviations

APS: Antiphospholipid syndrome; DU: Digital ulcers; MCTD: Mixed connective tissue disease; NFC: Nailfold capillaroscopy; NPV: Negative predictive value; PPV: Positive predictive value; RA: Rheumatoid arthritis; RP: Raynaud's phenomenon; SD: Scleroderma; SLE: Systemic lupus erythematosus; SSc: Systemic sclerosis; UCTD: Undifferentiated connective tissue disease

Acknowledgements

The authors wish to acknowledge the researchers Ricardo Simoes, Renata Buzzini, Wanderley Marques Bernardo, from the Brazilian Medical Association (Associação Médica Brasileira), Guidelines Project, who performed the systematic review that is presented in detail in the Additional file 1, funded by the Brazilian Society of Rheumatology.

Authors' contributions

All authors contributed to write and review the manuscript. All authors read and approved the final version of the manuscript.

Author details

[1]Rheumatology Division, Escola Paulista de Medicina, Universidade Federal de São Paulo (UNIFESP), Rua Botucatu 740, 3° andar, São Paulo, SP 04023-062, Brazil. [2]Rheumatology Service, Hospital Nossa Senhora da Conceição, Grupo Hospitalar Conceição, Porto Alegre, RS, Brazil. [3]Rheumatology Division, Hospital das Clinicas HCFMUSP, Faculdade de Medicina, Universidade de Sao Paulo, Sao Paulo, Brazil. [4]Rheumatology Service, Moinhos de Vento Hospital, Porto Alegre, Brazil. [5]Rheumatology Division, Universidade Federal do Rio de Janeiro, Rio de Janeiro, Brazil. [6]Departament of Medicine, Universidade Estadual do Ceará, Fortaleza, Brazil. [7]Rheumatology Service, Universidade Federal da Paraíba, João Pessoa, Brazil. [8]Rheumatology Service, Complexo Hospitalar da Santa Casa de Misericórdia de Porto Alegre, Universidade Federal de Ciências da Saúde de Porto Alegre, Porto Alegre, Brazil. [9]Faculdade de Ciências Médicas, Universidade Estadual de Campinas (UNICAMP), Campinas, SP, Brazil. [10]Rheumatology Division, Hospital de Clínicas, Universidade Federal do Paraná (UFPR), Curitiba, Brazil.

References

1. Cortes S, Cutolo M. Capillarosecopic patterns in rheumatic diseases. Acta Reumatol Port. 2007;32(1):29–36.
2. Wu PC, Huang MN, Kuo YM, Hsieh SC, Yu CL. Clinical applicability of quantitative nailfold capillaroscopy in differential diagnosis of connective tissue diseases with Raynaud's phenomenon. J Formos Med Assoc. 2013;112(8):482–8.
3. Damjanov N, Pavlov-Dolijanović S, Zlatanović M. Capillaroscopy as a prognostic tool for the development of connective tissue disease in patients with Raynaud's phenomenon. Reumatizam. 2010;57(2):119–20.
4. Nagy Z, Czirják L. Nailfold digital capillaroscopy in 447 patients with connective tissue disease and Raynaud's disease. J Eur Acad Dermatol Venereol. 2004;18(1):62–8.
5. Mannarino E, Pasqualini L, Fedeli F, Scricciolo V, Innocente S. Nailfold capillaroscopy in the screening and diagnosis of Raynaud's phenomenon. Angiology. 1994;45(1):37–42.
6. Smith V, Beeckman S, Herrick AL, Decuman S, Deschepper E, De Keyser F, et al. An EULAR study group pilot study on reliability of simple capillaroscopic definitions to describe capillary morphology in rheumatic diseases. Rheumatology (Oxford). 2016;55(5):883–90.
7. Maricq HR, Carpentier PH, Weinrich MC, Keil JE, Franco A, Drouet P, Ponçot OC, Maines MV. Geographic variation in the prevalence of Raynaud's phenomenon: Charleston, SC, USA, vs Tarentaise, Savoie, France. J Rheumatol. 1993;20(1):706.
8. Linnemann B, Erbe M. Raynaud's phenomenon - assessment and differential diagnoses. Vasa. 2015;44(3):166–77.
9. Maricq HR, Carpentier PH, Weinrich MC, Keil JE, Palesch Y, Biro C, VionnetFuasset M, Jiguet M, Valter I. Geographic variation in the prevalence of Raynaud's phenomenon: a 5 region comparison. J Rheumatol. 1997;24(5):879–89.
10. De Angelis R, Salaffi F, Grassi W. Raynaud's phenomenon: prevalence in an Italian population sample. Clin Rheumatol. 2006;25(4):506–10.
11. Block JA, Sequeira W. Raynaud's phenomenon. Lancet. 2001;357(9273):2042–8.
12. Cutolo M, Grassi W, Matucci CM. Raynaud's phenomenon and the role of capillaroscopy. Arthritis Rheum. 2003;48(11):3023–30.
13. Meli M, Gitzelmann G, Koppensteiner R, Amann-Vesti BR. Predictive value of nailfold capillaroscopy in patients with Raynaud's phenomenon. Clin Rheumatol. 2006;25(2):153–8.
14. Koenig M, Joyal F, Fritzler MJ, Roussin A, Abrahamowicz M, Boire G, et al. Autoantibodies and microvascular damage are independent predictive factors for the progression of Raynaud's phenomenon to systemic sclerosis: a twenty-year prospective study of 586 patients, with validation of proposed criteria for early systemic sclerosis. Arthritis Rheum. 2008;58(12):3902–12.
15. Luggen M, Belhorn L, Evans T, Fitzgerald O, Spencer-Green G. The evolution of Raynaud's phenomenon: a longterm prospective study. J Rheumatol. 1995;22(12):2226–32.
16. Hirschl M, Hirschl K, Lenz M, Katzenschlager R, Hutter HP, Kundi M. Transition from primary Raynaud's phenomenon to secondary Raynaud's phenomenon identified by diagnosis of an associated disease: results of ten years of prospective surveillance. Arthritis Rheum. 2006;54(6):1974–81.
17. Spencer-Green G. Outcomes in primary Raynaud phenomenon: a meta-analysis of the frequency, rates, and predictors of transition to secondary diseases. Arch Intern Med. 1998;158(6):595–600.
18. Kim SH, Kim HO, Jeong YG, Lee SY, Yoo WH, Choi TH, Lee SI. The diagnostic accuracy of power Doppler ultrasonography for differentiating secondary from primary Raynaud's phenomenon in undifferentiated connective tissue disease. Clin Rheumatol. 2008;27(6):783–6.
19. Ingegnoli F, Boracchi P, Gualtierotti R, Lubatti C, Meani L, Zahalkova L, et al. Prognostic model based on nailfold capillaroscopy for identifying Raynaud's phenomenon patients at high risk for the development of a scleroderma spectrum disorder: PRINCE (prognostic index for nailfold capillaroscopic examination). Arthritis Rheum. 2008;58(7):2174–82.
20. Guiducci S, Giacomelli R, Cerinic MM. Vascular complications of scleroderma. Autoimmun Rev. 2007;6(8):520–3.
21. Bussone G, Mouthon L. Interstitial lung disease in systemic sclerosis. Autoimmun Rev. 2011;10(5):248–55.
22. Tiev KP, Cabane J. Digestive tract involvement in systemic sclerosis. Autoimmun Rev. 2011;11(1):68–73.
23. Valentini G, Vettori S, Cuomo G, Iudici M, D'Abrosca V, Capocotta D, Del Gênio G, Santoriello C, Cozzolino D. Early systemic sclerosis: short-term disease evolution and factors predicting the development of new manifestations of organ involvement. Arthritis Res Ther. 2012;14(4):R188.

24. Cutolo M, Sulli A, Pizzorni C, Accardo S. Nailfold videocapillaroscopy assessment of microvascular damage in systemic sclerosis. J Rheumatol. 2000;27(1):155–60.

25. Grassi W, Medico PD, Izzo F, Cervini C. Microvascular involvement in systemic sclerosis: capillaroscopic findings. Semin Arthritis Rheum. 2001; 30(6):397–402.

26. Maricq HR, LeRoy EC, D'Angelo WA, Medsger TA Jr, Rodnan GP, Sharp GC, Wolfe JF. Diagnostic potential of in vivo capillary microscopy in scleroderma and related disorders. Arthritis Rheum. 1980;23(2):183–9.

27. Kabasakal Y, Elvins DM, Ring EF, McHugh NJ. Quantitative nailfold capillaroscopy findings in a population with connective tissue disease and in normal healthy controls. Ann Rheum Dis. 1996;55(8):507–12.

28. Caramaschi P, Canestrini S, Martinelli N, Volpe A, Pieropan S, Ferrari M, et al. Scleroderma patients nailfold videocapillaroscopic patterns are associated with disease subset and disease severity. Rheumatology (Oxford). 2007; 46(10):1566–9.

29. Bredemeier M, Xavier RM, Capobianco KG, Restelli VG, Rohde LE, Pinotti AF, et al. Nailfold capillary microscopy can suggest pulmonary disease activity in systemic sclerosis. J Rheumatol. 2004;31(2):286–94.

30. Chen ZY, Silver RM, Ainsworth SK, Dobson RL, Rust P, Maricq HR. Association between fluorescent antinuclear antibodies, capillary patterns, and clinical features in scleroderma spectrum disorders. Am J Med. 1984;77(5):812–22.

31. Leteurtre E, Hachulla E, Janin A, Hatron PY, Brouillard M, Devulder B. Vascular manifestations of dermatomyositis and polymyositis. Clinical, capillaroscopic and histological aspects. Rev Med Interne. 1994;15(12):800–7.

32. Manfredi A, Sebastiani M, Cassone G, Pipitone N, Giuggioli D, Colaci M, et al. Nailfold capillaroscopic changes in dermatomyositis and polymyositis. Clin Rheumatol. 2015;34(2):279–84.

33. Mugii N, Hasegawa M, Matsushita T, Hamaguchi Y, Horie S, Yahata T, et al. Association between nail-fold capillary findings and disease activity in dermatomyositis. Rheumatology (Oxford). 2011;50(6):1091–8.

34. Groen H, ter Borg EJ, Postma DS, Wouda AA, van der Mark TW, Kallenberg CG. Pulmonary function in systemic lupus erythematosus is related to distinct clinical, serologic, and nailfold capillary patterns. Am J Med. 1992; 93(6):619–27.

35. Pavlov-Dolijanovic S, Damjanov NS, Vujasinovic Stupar NZ, Marcetic DR, Sefik-Bukilica MN, Petrovic RR. Is there a difference in systemic lupus erythematosus with and without Raynaud's phenomenon? Rheumatol Int. 2013;33(4):859–65.

36. de Holanda Mafaldo Diógenes A, Bonfá E, Fuller R, Correia Caleiro MT. Capillaroscopy is a dynamic process in mixed connective tissue disease. Lupus. 2007;16(4):254–8.

37. Granier F, Vayssairat M, Priollet P, Housset E. Nailfold capillary microscopy in mixed connective tissue disease. Comparison with systemic sclerosis and systemic lupus erythematosus. Arthritis Rheum. 1986;29(2):189–95.

38. Ingegnoli F, Gualtierotti R, Lubatti C, Zahalkova L, Meani L, Boracchi P, et al. Feasibility of different capillaroscopic measures for identifying nailfold microvascular alterations. Semin Arthritis Rheum. 2009;38(4):289–95.

39. Sekiyama JY, Camargo CZ, Eduardo L, Andrade C, Kayser C. Reliability of widefield nailfold capillaroscopy and video capillaroscopy in the assessment of patients with Raynaud's phenomenon. Arthritis Care Res (Hoboken). 2013; 65(11):1853–61.

40. Wildt M, Wuttge DM, Hesselstrand R, Scheja A. Assessment of capillary density in systemic sclerosis with three different capillaroscopic methods. Clin Exp Rheumatol. 2012;30(2 Suppl 71):S50–4.

41. Beltrán E, Toll A, Pros A, Carbonell J, Pujol RM. Assessment of nailfold capillaroscopy by x 30 digital epiluminescence (dermoscopy) in patients with Raynaud phenomenon. Br J Dermatol. 2007;156(5):892–8.

42. Bergman R, Sharony L, Schapira D, Nahir MA, Balbir-Gurman A. The handheld dermatoscope as a nail-fold capillaroscopic instrument. Arch Dermatol. 2003;139(8):1027–30.

43. Baron M, Bell M, Bookman A, Buchignani M, Dunne J, Hudson M, et al. Office capillaroscopy in systemic sclerosis. Clin Rheumatol. 2007;26(8):1268–74.

44. Ingegnoli F, Gualtierotti R, Lubatti C, Bertolazzi C, Gutierrez M, Boracchi P, et al. Nailfold capillary patterns in healthy subjects: a real issue in capillaroscopy. Microvasc Res. 2013;90:90–5.

45. Andrade LE, Gabriel Júnior A, Assad RL, Ferrari AJ, Atra E. Panoramic nailfold capillaroscopy: a new reading method and normal range. Semin Arthritis Rheum. 1990;20(1):21–31.

46. Boulon C, Devos S, Mangin M, et al. Reproducibility of capillaroscopic classifications of systemic sclerosis: results from the SCLEROCAP study. Rheumatology (Oxford). 2017;56(10):1713–20.

47. Piotto DP, Sekiyama J, Kayser C, Yamada M, Len CA, Terreri MT. Nailfold videocapillaroscopy in healthy children and adolescents: description of normal patterns. Clin Exp Rheumatol. 2016;34(Suppl 100(5)):193–9.

48. Herrick AL, Moore T, Hollis S, Jayson MI. The influence of age on nailfold capillary dimensions in childhood. J Rheumatol. 2000;27(3):797–800.

49. Maricq HR, Maize JC. Nailfold capillary abnormalities. Clin Rheum Dis. 1982; 8(2):455–78.

50. Jones BF, Oral M, Morris CW, Ring EF. A proposed taxonomy for nailfold capillaries based on their morphology. IEEE Trans Med Imaging. 2001;20(4):33341.

51. Hoerth C, Kundi M, Katzenschlager R, Hirschl M. Qualitative and quantitative assessment of nailfold capillaries by capillaroscopy in healthy volunteers. Vasa. 2012;41(1):19–26.

52. Lo LC, Lin KC, Hsu YN, Chen TP, Chiang JY, Chen YF, et al. Pseudo three-dimensional vision-based nail-fold morphological and hemodynamic analysis. Comput Biol Med. 2012;42(9):873–84.

53. Anderson ME, Allen PD, Moore T, Hillier V, Taylor CJ, Herrick AL. Computerized nailfold video capillaroscopy -- a new tool for assessment of Raynaud's phenomenon. J Rheumatol. 2005;32(5):841–8.

54. Maricq HR, Spencer-Green G, LeRoy EC. Skin capillary abnormalities as indicators of organ involvement in scleroderma (systemic sclerosis), Raynaud's syndrome and dermatomyositis. Am J Med. 1976;61(6):862–70.

55. Sulli A, Secchi ME, Pizzorni C, Cutolo M. Scoring the nailfold microvascular changes during the capillaroscopic analysis in systemic sclerosis patients. Ann Rheum Dis. 2008;67:885–7.

56. Etehad Tavakol M, Fatemi A, Karbalaie A, Emrani Z, Erlandsson BE. Nailfold Capillaroscopy in rheumatic diseases: which parameters should be evaluated? Biomed Res Int. 2015;2015:974530.

57. Zufferey P, Depairon M, Chamot AM, Monti M. Prognostic significance of nailfold capillary microscopy in patients with Raynaud's phenomenon and scleroderma-pattern abnormalities. A six-year follow-up study. Clin Rheumatol. 1992;11(4):536–41.

58. Cutolo M, Pizzorni C, Sulli A. Nailfold video-capillaroscopy in systemic sclerosis. Z Rheumatol. 2004;63(6):457–62.

59. Chojnowski MM, Felis-Giemza A, Olesińska M. Capillaroscopy - a role in modern rheumatology. Reumatologia. 2016;54(2):67–72.

60. Carpentier PH, Maricq HR. Microvasculature in systemic sclerosis. Rheum Dis Clin N Am. 1990;16(1):75–91.

61. Bollinger A, Jäger K, Siegenthaler W. Microangiopathy of progressive systemic sclerosis. Evaluation by dynamic fluorescence videomicroscopy. Arch Intern Med. 1986;146(8):1541–5.

62. Thompson RP, Harper FE, Maize JC, Ainsworth SK, LeRoy EC, Maricq HR. Nailfold biopsy in scleroderma and related disorders. Correlation of histologic, capillaroscopic, and clinical data. Arthritis Rheum. 1984;27(1):97–103.

63. Houtman PM, Kallenberg CG, Fidler V, Wouda AA. Diagnostic significance of nailfold capillary patterns in patients with Raynaud's phenomenon. An analysis of patterns discriminating patients with and without connective tissue disease. J Rheumatol. 1986;13(3):556–63.

64. Le JH, Cho KI. Association between endothelial function and microvascular changes in patients with secondary Raynaud's phenomenon. Clin Rheumatol. 2014;33(11):1627–33.

65. De Angelis R, Cerioni A, Del Medico P, Blasetti P. Raynaud's phenomenon in undifferentiated connective tissue disease (UCTD). Clin Rheumatol. 2005; 24(2):145–51.

66. Pavlov-Dolijanovic S, Damjanov NS, Stojanovic RM, Vujasinovic Stupar NZ, Stanisavljevic DM. Scleroderma pattern of nailfold capillary changes as predictive value for the development of a connective tissue disease: a follow-up study of 3,029 patients with primary Raynaud's phenomenon. Rheumatol Int. 2012;32(10):303945.

67. Ingegnoli F, Boracchi P, Gualtierotti R, Biganzoli EM, Zeni S, Lubatti C, Fantini F. Improving outcome prediction of systemic sclerosis from isolated Raynaud's phenomenon: role of autoantibodies and nail-fold capillaroscopy. Rheumatology (Oxford). 2010;49(4):797–805.

68. LeRoy EC, Medsger TA Jr. Raynaud's phenomenon: a proposal for classification. Clin Exp Rheumatol. 1992;10(5):485–8.

69. Maverakis E, Patel F, Kronenberg DG, Chung L, Fiorentino D, Allanore Y, et al. International consensus criteria for the diagnosis of Raynaud's phenomenon. J Autoimmun. 2014;48-49:60–5.

70. van den Hoogen F, Khanna D, Fransen J, Johnson SR, Baron M, Tyndall A, et al. 2013 classification criteria for systemic sclerosis: an American College of Rheumatology/European league against rheumatism collaborative initiative. Arthritis Rheum. 2013;65(11):2737–47.

71. Valentini G, Marcoccia A, Cuomo G, Iudici M, Vettori S. The concept of early systemic sclerosis following 2013 ACR\EULAR criteria for the classification of systemic sclerosis. Curr Rheumatol Rev. 2014;10(1):38–44.

72. Bellando-Randone S, Matucci-Cerinic M. From Raynaud's phenomenon to very early diagnosis of systemic sclerosis- the VEDOSS approach. Curr Rheumatol Rev. 2013;9(4):245–8.

73. Camargo CZ, Sekiyama JY, Arismendi MI, Kayser C. Microvascular abnormalities in patients with early systemic sclerosis: less severe morphological changes than in patients with definite disease. Scand J Rheumatol. 2015;44(1):48–55.

74. Ingegnoli F, Ardoino I, Boracchi P, Cutolo M. EUSTAR co-authors. Nailfold capillaroscopy in systemic sclerosis: data from the EULAR scleroderma trials and research (EUSTAR) database. Microvasc Res. 2013;89:122–8.

75. Cutolo M, Sulli A, Smith V. Assessing microvascular changes in systemic sclerosis diagnosis and management. Nat Rev Rheumatol. 2010;6(10):578–87.

76. Bissell LA, Abignano G, Emery P, Del Galdo F, Buch MH. Absence of scleroderma pattern at nail fold capillaroscopy valuable in the exclusion of scleroderma in unselected patients with Raynaud's phenomenon. BMC Musculoskelet Disord. 2016;17(1):342.

77. Ingegnoli F, Zeni S, Meani L, Soldi A, Lurati A, Fantini F. Evaluation of nailfold videocapillaroscopic abnormalities in patients with systemic lupus erythematosus. J Clin Rheumatol. 2005;11(6):295–8.

78. Riccieri V, Spadaro A, Ceccarelli F, Scrivo R, Germano V, Valesini G. Nailfold capillaroscopy changes in systemic lupus erythematosus: correlations with disease activity and autoantibody profile. Lupus. 2005; 14(7):521–5.

79. Kuryliszyn-Moskal A, Ciolkiewicz M, Klimiuk PA, Sierakowski S. Clinical significance of nailfold capillaroscopy in systemic lupus erythematosus: correlation with endothelial cell activation markers and disease activity. Scand J Rheumatol. 2009;38(1):38–45.

80. Redisch W, Messina EJ, Hughes G, McEwen C. Capillaroscopic observations in rheumatic diseases. Ann Rheum Dis. 1970;29(3):244–53.

81. Altomonte L, Zoli A, Galossi A, Mirone L, Tulli A, Martone FR, Morini P, Laraia P, Magarò M. Microvascular capillaroscopic abnormalities in rheumatoid arthritis patients. Clin Exp Rheumatol. 1995;13(1):83–6.

82. Lambova SN, Müller-Ladner U. Capillaroscopic pattern in inflammatory arthritis. Microvasc Res. 2012;83(3):318–22.

83. Aslanidis S, Pyrpasopoulou A, Doumas M, Triantafyllou A, Chatzimichailidou S, Zamboulis C. Association of capillaroscopic microhaemorrhages with clinical and immunological antiphospholipid syndrome. Clin Exp Rheumatol. 2011;29(2):307–9.

84. Candela M, Pansoni A, De Carolis ST, Pomponio G, Corvetta A, Gabrielli A, Danieli G. Nailfold capillary microscopy in patients with antiphospholipid syndrome. Recenti Prog Med. 1998;89(9):444–9.

85. Sendino Revuelta A, Barbado Hernández FJ, Torrijos Eslava A, González Anglada I, Peña Sánchez de Rivera JM, Vázquez Rodríguez JJ. Capillaroscopy in vasculitis. An Med Interna. 1991;8(5):217–20.

86. Movasat A, Shahram F, Carreira PE, Nadji A, Akhlaghi M, Naderi N, Davatchi F. Nailfold capillaroscopy in Behçet's disease, analysis of 128 patients. Clin Rheumatol. 2009;28(5):603–5.

87. Tektonidou M, Kaskani E, Skopouli FN, Moutsopoulos HM. Microvascular abnormalities in Sjögren's syndrome: nailfold capillaroscopy. Rheumatology (Oxford). 1999;38(9):826–30.

88. Capobianco KG, Xavier RM, Bredemeier M, Restelli VG, Brenol JC. Nailfold capillaroscopic findings in primary Sjögren's syndrome: clinical and serological correlations. Clin Exp Rheumatol. 2005;23(6):789–94.

89. Silva I, Loureiro T, Teixeira A, Almeida I, Mansilha A, Vasconcelos C, et al. Digital ulcers in systemic sclerosis: role of flow-mediated dilatation and capillaroscopy as risk assessment tools. Eur J Dermatol. 2015;25(5):444–51.

90. Silva I, Teixeira A, Oliveira J, Almeida I, Almeida R, Águas A, Vasconcelos C. Endothelial dysfunction and Nailfold Videocapillaroscopy pattern as predictors of digital ulcers in systemic sclerosis: a cohort study and review of the literature. Clin Rev Allergy Immunol. 2015;49(2):240–52.

91. Clements PJ, Lachenbruch PA, Furst DE, Maxwell M, Danovitch G, Paulus HE. Abnormalities of renal physiology in systemic sclerosis. A prospective study with 10-year followup. Arthritis Rheum. 1994;37(1):67–74.

92. Kinsella MB, Smith EA, Miller KS, LeRoy EC, Silver RM. Spontaneous production of fibronectin by alveolar macrophages in patients with scleroderma. Arthritis Rheum. 1989;32(5):577–83.

93. Clements PJ, Furst DE. Heart involvement in systemic sclerosis. Clin Dermatol. 1994;12(2):267–75.

94. Grassi W, Core P, Carlino G, Cervini C. Acute effects of single dose nifedipine on cold-induced changes of microvascular dynamics in systemic sclerosis. Br J Rheumatol. 1994;33(12):1154–61.

95. Filaci G, Cutolo M, Scudeletti M, Castagneto C, Derchi L, Gianrossi R, Ropolo F, Zentilin P, Sulli A, Murdaca G, Ghio M, Indiveri F, Puppo F. Cyclosporin a and iloprost treatment of systemic sclerosis: clinical results and interleukin-6 serum changes after 12 months of therapy. Rheumatology (Oxford). 1999;38(10):992–6.

96. Amanzi L, Braschi F, Fiori G, Galluccio F, Miniati I, Guiducci S, et al. Digital ulcers in scleroderma: staging, characteristics and sub-setting through observation of 1614 digital lesions. Rheumatology (Oxford). 2010;49(7):1374–82.

97. Ferri C, Valentini G, Cozzi F, Sebastiani M, Michelassi C, La Montagna G, et al. Systemic Sclerosis Study Group of the Italian Society of Rheumatology (SIR-GSSSc). Systemic sclerosis: demographic, clinical, and serologic features and survival in 1,012 Italian patients. Medicine (Baltimore). 2002;81(2):139–53.

98. Silva I, Almeida C, Teixeira A, Oliveira J, Vasconcelos C. Impaired angiogenesis as a feature of digital ulcers in systemic sclerosis. Clin Rheumatol. 2016;35(7):1743–51.

99. Avouac J, Vallucci M, Smith V, Senet P, Ruiz B, Sulli A, et al. Correlations between angiogenic factors and capillaroscopic patterns in systemic sclerosis. Arthritis Res Ther. 2013;15(2):R55.

100. Farouk HM, Hamza SH, El Bakry SA, Youssef SS, Aly IM, Moustafa AA, Assaf NY, El Dakrony AH. Dysregulation of angiogenic homeostasis in systemic sclerosis. Int J Rheum Dis. 2013;16(4):448–54.

101. Lambova S, Müller-Ladner U. Capillaroscopic findings in systemic sclerosis - are they associated with disease duration and presence of digital ulcers? Discov Med. 2011;12(66):413–8.

102. Silva I, Almeida J, Vasconcelos C. A PRISMA-driven systematic review for predictive risk factors of digital ulcers in systemic sclerosis patients. Autoimmun Rev. 2015;14(2):140–52.

103. Sebastiani M, Manfredi A, Colaci M, D'amico R, Malagoli V, Giuggioli D, Ferri C. Capillaroscopic skin ulcer risk index: a new prognostic tool for digital skin ulcer development in systemic sclerosis patients. Arthritis Rheum. 2009; 61(5):688–94.

104. Sebastiani M, Manfredi A, Vukatana G, Moscatelli S, Riato L, Bocci M, Iudici M, Principato A, Mazzuca S, Del Medico P, De Angelis R, D'Amico R, Vicini R, Colaci M, Ferri C. Predictive role of capillaroscopic skin ulcer risk index in systemic sclerosis: a multicentre validation study. Ann Rheum Dis. 2012;71(1):67–70.

105. Sebastiani M, Manfredi A, Colaci M, Giuggioli D, La Sala R, Elkhaldi N, Antonelli A, Ferri C. Correlation of a quantitative videocapillaroscopic score with the development of digital skin ulcers in scleroderma patients. Reumatismo. 2008;60(3):199–205.

106. Hofstee HM, Vonk Noordegraaf A, Voskuyl AE, Dijkmans BA, Postmus PE, et al. Nailfold capillary density is associated with the presence and severity of pulmonary arterial hypertension in systemic sclerosis. Ann Rheum Dis. 2009; 68(2):191–5.

107. Ohtsuka T, Hasegawa A, Nakano A, Yamakage A, Yamaguchi M, Miyachi Y. Nailfold capillary abnormality and pulmonary hypertension in systemic sclerosis. Int J Dermatol. 1997;36(2):116–22.

108. Bredemeier M, Xavier RM, Capobianco KG, Restelli VG, Rohde LE, et al. Capilaroscopia periungueal pode sugerir atividade de doença pulmonar na esclerose sistêmica. Rev Bras Reumatol. 2004;44(1):19–30.

109. Joyal F, Choquette D, Roussin A, Levington C, Senécal JL. Evaluation of the severity of systemic sclerosis by nailfold capillary microscopy in 112 patients. Angiology. 1992;43(3 Pt 1):203–10.

110. Smith V, Riccieri V, Pizzorni C, Decuman S, Deschepper E, Bonroy C, Sulli A, Piette Y, De Keyser F, Cutolo M. Nailfold capillaroscopy for prediction of novel future severe organ involvement in systemic sclerosis. J Rheumatol. 2013;40(12):2023–8.

111. Lovy M, MacCarter D, Steigerwald JC. Relationship between nailfold capillary abnormalities and organ involvement in systemic sclerosis. Arthritis Rheum. 1985;28(5):496–501.

112. Tolosa-Vilella C, Morera-Morales ML, Simeón-Aznar CP, Marí-Alfonso B, Colunga-Arguelles D, Callejas Rubio JL, et al. RESCLE Investigators, Autoimmune Diseases Study Group (GEAS). Digital ulcers and cutaneous subsets of systemic sclerosis: Clinical, immunological, nailfold capillaroscopy, and survival differences in the Spanish RESCLE Registry. Semin Arthritis Rheum. 2016;46(2):200–8.

113. Kayser C, Sekiyama JY, Próspero LC, Camargo CZ, Andrade LE. Nailfold capillaroscopy abnormalities as predictors of mortality in patients with systemic sclerosis. Clin Exp Rheumatol. 2013;31(2 Suppl 76):103–8.

114. Jadad AR, Moore RA, Carroll D, Jenkinson C, Reynolds DJ, Gavaghan DJ, et al. Assessing the quality of reports of randomized clinical trials: is blinding necessary? Control Clin Trials. 1996;17:1–12.

115. Goldet G, Howick J. Understanding GRADE: an introduction. J Evid Based Med. 2013;6:50–4.

116. Wells G, Shea B, O'Connell D, Robertson J, Peterson J, Welch V, et al. The Newcastle-Ottawa Scale (NOS) for assessing the quality of nonrandomised studies in meta-analyses.

117. Levels of Evidence and Grades of Recommendations - Oxford Centre for Evidence Based Medicine. http://www.cebm.net/index.aspx?o=5653.

25

Platelet/lymphocyte ratio and mean platelet volume in patients with granulomatosis with polyangiitis

Hamit Kucuk[1], Duygu Tecer[2]* (iD), Berna Goker[1], Ozkan Varan[1], Hakan Babaoglu[1], Serdar Can Guven[2], Mehmet Akif Ozturk[1], Seminur Haznedaroglu[1] and Abdurrahman Tufan[1]

Abstract

Background: Granulomatosis with polyangiitis (GPA) is a granulomatous necrotizing vasculitis with high morbidity and mortality. Anti-neutrophil cytoplasmic antibody is a valuable diagnostic marker, however its titer lacks predictive value for the severity of organ involvement. Platelet to lymphocyte ratio (PLR) and mean platelet volume (MPV) has been regarded as a potential marker in assessing systemic inflammation. We aimed to explore the value of PLR and MPV in the assessment of disease activity and manifestations of disease in GPA.

Methods: 56 newly diagnosed GPA patients and 53 age-sex matched healthy controls were included in this retrospective and cross-sectional study with comparative group. Complete blood count was performed with Backman Coulter automatic analyzer, erythrocyte sedimentation rate (ESR) with Westergen method and C-reactive protein (CRP) levels with nephelometry. The PLR was calculated as the ratio of platelet and lymphocyte counts.

Result: Compared to control group, ESR, CRP and PLR were significantly higher and MPV significantly lower in GPA patients. In patients group, PLR was positively correlated with ESR and CRP ($r = 0.39$, $p = 0.005$ and $r = 0.51$, $p < 0.001$, respectively). MPV was negatively correlated with ESR and CRP ($r = -0.31$, $p = 0.028$ and $r = -0.34$ $p = 0.014$, respectively). Patients with renal involvement had significantly higher PLR than patients without renal involvement (median:265.98, IQR:208.79 vs median:180.34 IQR:129.37, $p = 0.02$). PLR was negatively correlated with glomerular filtration rate ($r = -0.27$, $p = 0.009$). A cut-off level of 204 for PLR had 65.6% sensitivity and 62.5 specificity to predict renal involvement.

Conclusion: PLR exhibit favorable diagnostic performance in predicting renal involvement in patients with GPA.

Keywords: Granulomatosis with polyangiitis, Platelet to lymphocyte ratio, Mean platelet volume, Biomarker, Activity

Background

Granulomatosis with polyangiitis (GPA), formerly known as Wegener's granulomatosis (WG) is an autoimmune vasculitis characterized by granulomatous inflammation with necrotizing vasculitis affecting small to medium sized vessels [1]. The main autoantibody associated with the disease is the cytoplasmic antineutrophil cytoplasmic antibodies (c-ANCA), usually directed against the enzyme proteinase-3 (PR-3) [2]. Due to involvement of vital organs, GPA has significant morbidity and mortality. Renal involvement observed as rapidly progressive glomerulonephritis may lead to end-stage renal failure. Other potentially fatal common manifestations are alveolar and gastrointestinal hemorrhage and myocarditis. With the advanced treatment regimens, the disease has become more of a chronic relapsing–remitting pattern. Relapses occur in 50% or more of patients during the long-term follow-up [3]. One of the major challenges in the management of GPA is lack of reliable markers for activity and predicting relapse to guide therapy. Moreover, association between initial presentation features and subsequent relapses are controversial [4]. Because of ANCA titres and conventional inflammation markers such as C-reactive protein (CRP) and erythrocyte

* Correspondence: duygu-tecer@hotmail.com
[2]Faculty of Medicine, Department of Physical Medicine & Rehabilitation, Division of Rheumatology, Gazi University, Ankara, Turkey
Full list of author information is available at the end of the article

sedimentation rate (ESR) have limited value, new biomarkers are needed for the assessment of disease activity, and to predict relapse [5–7].

Platelet to lymphocyte ratio (PLR) is absolute count of platelets divided by the absolute count of lymphocytes derived from routine complete blood count (CBC). PLR was emerged as a marker of inflammation and used in combination with other inflammatory markers to determine severity of inflammation in many diseases. In recent years, utility of PLR was evaluated in numerous studies including cancers, cardiovascular diseases, rheumatic disease [8–11]. As novel markers of inflammation, we aim to investigate utility of PLR and mean platelet volume (MPV) in the assessment of disease activity and manifestations of disease in patients with GPA.

Methods

This study was planned as the retrospective and cross-sectional study with comparative group. 56 patients with GPA who were diagnosed between 2012 and 2017 were included. All patients met the Chapel Hill Consensus Conference Nomenclature/Criteria for Vasculitis and/or the American College of Rheumatology (ACR) criteria for GPA [12, 13]. 53 age and sex-matched healthy subjects were served as control group. Subjects in either group with one of the following concomitant diseases/situations were excluded: 1) acute or chronic infections; 2) concomitant inflammatory diseases 3) metabolic diseases including diabetes mellitus, thyroid dysfunction, liver disease and 4) any kind of malignancy.

Demographic, clinical and laboratory data were retrieved from medical records. Disease activity was assessed with Birmingham Vasculitis Activity Score for WG vasculitis (BVAS/WG) [14]. Blood collection and calculation of BVAS/WG were held at the same time. All blood samples were collected from newly diagnosed patients. Complete blood count (CBC) was performed with Backman Coulter automatic analyzer within 2 h of blood collection. ESR and CRP levels were determined with Westergen method and nephelometry respectively. The PLR was calculated as the ratio of platelet and lymphocyte counts of the same CBC. Renal involvement was diagnosed if patient had at least one of the following findings: a. active, biopsy proven, pauci-immune glomerulonephritis, b. active urinary sediment, c. rise in serum creatinine > 30% or > 25% decline in creatinine clearance which was attributed to active AAV in the kidney. The study protocol was approved by the Local Research Ethics Committee. A written informed consent form was signed by the all participants. Study was conducted in accordance with the ethical principles as described by the declaration of Helsinki.

Statistical analysis

Statistical Package for Social Science (SPSS) version of 16.0 was used for the analyzes (SPSS Inc., Chicago, IL). The variables were analyzed using visual (histograms, probability plots) and analytical methods (Kolmogorov-Smirnov) for the distribution of normality. All demographic and quantitative data were presented as means ± SD or percentages (%). Comparison of categorical data was performed by chi-square tests. Mann-Whitney U-test was used to compare independent samples which did not have a normal distribution. A p-value < 0.05 were considered statistically significant. Spearman test was used for the assessment of correlations between variables. Sensitivity, specificity and cut off values are determined by using ROC curve and diagram. Comparison of ROC curves were used for comparing predictive performances of RDW, ESR and CRP variables to detect renal involvement.

Results

Fifty-six patients with GPA and 53 healthy controls were included. Clinical characteristics and laboratory findings of the study groups are shown in Table 1. The patients were predominantly male (58.9%) with a mean age of 48.14 ± 14.09 years. C-ANCA was positive in 51 (91.07%) of patients and p-ANCA was positive in 8 (16.07%) of patients. Mean BVAS/WG was 13.54 ± 4.94 at diagnosis. Clinical manifestations at diagnosis was as follow, general manifestation 51 (91.07%), ear nose throat involvement 33 (58.93%), pulmonary involvement 37 (66.1%), renal involvement 32 (57.1%), cutaneous involvement 25 (44.64%), ocular 17 (30.36%), gastrointestinal tract 5 (8.93%).

ESR, CRP and PLR were significantly higher in patients with GPA than controls. MPV was significantly lower in patients with GPA compared to healthy controls. In patients group, PLR positively correlated with ESR and CRP ($r = 0.39$, $p = 0.005$ and $r = 0.51$, $p < 0.001$, respectively). In contrast, MPV negatively correlated with ESR and CRP ($r = - 0.31$, $p = 0.03$ and $r = - 0.34$, $p = 0.014$, respectively). There were no significant correlations between PLR, MPV and BVAS/WG.

Patients with renal involvement had remarkably higher PLR than patients without renal involvement (median: 265.98, IQR: 208.79 vs median: 180.34 IQR:129.37, $p = 0.02$). Moreover, PLR negatively correlated with glomerular filtration rate ($r = - 0.27$, $p = 0.009$). Patients with renal involvement tended to have lower MPV, but this difference did not reach statistical significance (median: 7.60, IQR:1.17 vs median 7.75, IQR:1.46, $p = 0.786$). Receiver operating characteristic curve of PLR, ESR and CRP for differentiating renal involvement is presented in Fig. 1. Area Under Curves (AUCs) for PLR, CRP and ESR were 0.703 (95% confidence interval [CI], 0.558–0.849, $p = 0.016$), 0.577 (95% CI: 0.416–0.738, $p = 0.362$), 0.508 (95% CI: 0.337–0.678, $p = 0.929$), respectively. A cut-off level of 204 for PLR had 65.6% sensitivity and 62.5 specificity (positive predictive value 70%, negative

Table 1 Clinical characteristics and laboratory findings of the study population

	GPA patients	Controls	p
Age mean ± SD (years)	48.14 ± 14.09	46.77 ± 14.14	0.614
Males (n)	33 (58.9%)	26 (49.1%)	0.301
WBC (× 10³/mL)	11.600 (3.240; 35.490; 6.907)	7.040 (4.100; 11.870; 2.413)	< 0.001
Neutrophils (× 10³/mL)	8.230 (1.300; 33.420; 6.830)	4000 (2.300; 11.870; 1.525)	< 0.001
Lymphocytes (× 10³/mL)	1.665 (0.300; 5.550; 0.951)	2.320 (1.270; 4.090; 0.690)	< 0.001
Platelets (× 10³/mL)	308.000 (82.600; 1126.000; 191.500)	224.600 (136.000; 373.900; 73.600)	< 0.001
ESR (mm/H)	47.5 (3; 131; 60)	8 (1; 34; 7.50)	< 0.001
CRP (mg/L)	34 (1.27; 300; 99.14)	3.1 (1.16; 7.40; 2.07)	< 0.001
MPV	7.54 (6.08; 10.38; 1.29)	8.62 (6.88; 13.10; 1.41)	< 0.001
PLR	212.65 (29.86; 1638.33; 159.62)	101.43 (58.37; 210.63; 35.44)	< 0.001
Creatinine (mg/dL)	0.912 (0.45; 19.90; 1)	0.79 (0.53; 1.12; 0.24)	0.002
GFR	83.50 (2.70; 141.0; 75.25)	99.70 (65.30; 130.70; 21.30)	0.003

Values are presented as median (min; max; interquartile range). *GPA* Granulomatosis with polyangiitis, *WBC* white blood cell, *ESR* erythrocyte sedimentation rate, *CRP* C-reactive protein, *MPV* mean platelet volume, *PLR* platelet/lymphocyte ratio, *GFR* glomerular filtration ratio

predictive value 57.7%) for renal involvement (Fig. 2). Patients with alveolar hemorrhage tended to have higher PLR and lower MPV but this difference did not reach statistical significance (277.34 ± 181.95 vs 240.61 ± 252.43 $p = 0.382$ for PLR, 7.69 ± 0.66 vs 7.83 ± 1.08, $p = 0.809$ for MPV, respectively).

Discussion

Significant progress has been made in the understanding of pathogenesis and treatment of GPA, but there is still unmet need for biomarkers for predicting specific organ involvement, disease activity, relapse and long term prognosis. Identification of such markers may guide the

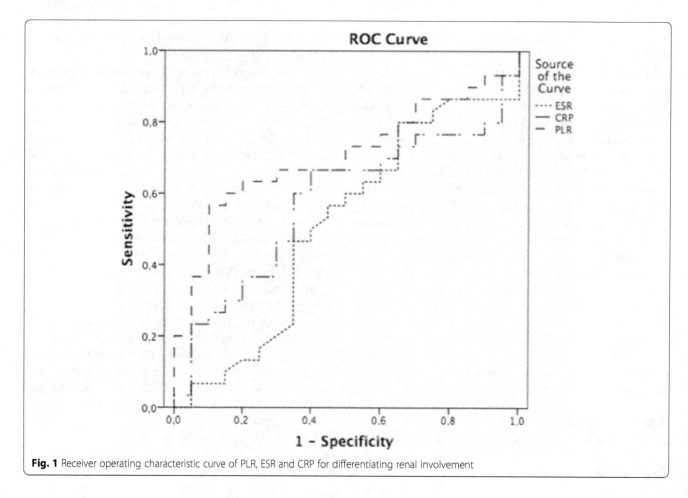

Fig. 1 Receiver operating characteristic curve of PLR, ESR and CRP for differentiating renal involvement

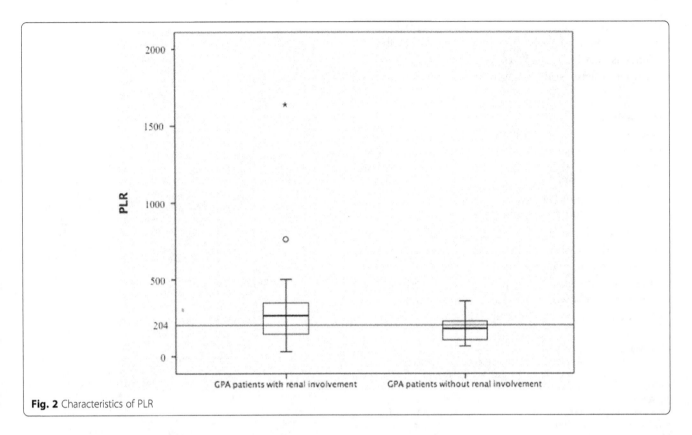

Fig. 2 Characteristics of PLR

therapy and help to determine those patients at high risk of relapse. Available markers, including ANCA titers, and commonly used inflammatory markers, ESR and CRP, are not adequate. Although these markers substantially elevated in active stages of disease their values are not correlated with disease activity and lack of prognostic information and prediction of relapses.

Systemic inflammation is associated with alterations in circulating peripheral blood cells quantity and composition. Normochromic anemia, thrombocytosis, neutrophilia and lymphocytopenia usually accompanies many inflammatory conditions [15]. In acute inflammation number and volume of platelets increase. Therefore, these features of circulating blood cell components can be used for the assessment of inflammatory activity [16, 17]. One of these, PLR has emerged as a marker of activity and as a prognostic marker in many diseases.

In our study, we found that PLR is significantly elevated in patients with GPA and correlated with other commonly used acute phase reactants. There is no correlation between PLR and BVAS/WG indicating that PLR might not reflect overall activity of disease. However, those patients with renal involvement had remarkably higher levels and PLR was significantly correlated with GFR. Therefore, we suggest that PLR might be a marker for renal activity of GPA.

In recent years, utility of PLR was evaluated in numerous studies. It has been reported to be elevated in patients with chronic renal failure (CRF) and is associated with increased mortality among the end stage CRF patients [18, 19]. Another striking evidence is correlation between PLR and disease activity of dermatomyositis which is widely accepted as a vasculitic process [20]. In addition, previous studies show that PLR is positively correlated with inflammatory indices such as CRP and ESR, and PLR is also associated with disease activity in psoriasis, RA and systemic lupus erythematosus [21–24]. Systemic lupus erythematosus (SLE) patients with nephritis had higher PLR levels than those without nephritis [24].

MPV was significantly lower in patients with GPA compared to healty control and negatively correlated witih ESR and CRP. There was no correlation between BVAS/WG, GFR and MPV. MPV values have previously been studied in various inflammatory conditions, such as familial mediterranean fever, rheumatoid arthritis, ankylosing spondylitis, inflammatory bowel disease, juvenile SLE, psoriasis, systemic sclerosis and acute rheumatic fever [16, 25–31]. But the results are contradictory. It would seem that the size of circulating platelets is dependent on the intensity of systemic inflammation. Low-grade inflammatory conditions are associated with high levels of MPV and high-grade inflammatory diseases are associated with low levels of MPV [32, 33].

Herein, we presented 56 patients with GPA and tried to analyze the relation between PLR, MPV and disease activity. These costs may change from country to country, but the cost-effectiveness of these new parameters is valid worldwide. We have some limitations in our study.

First, our study is cross sectional and long term prognosis of patients are largely unknown. Second, number of
patients is relatively small. Hence, our results must be
confirmed in large scale longitudinal prospective studies.

Conclusions

Patients with GPA had significantly higher PLR and
lower MPV compared to healthy controls. We have
demonstrated a significant correlation between ESR,
CRP, MPV and PLR. GPA patients with renal involvement had higher PLR levels than those without renal involvement and PLR was significantly correlated with
GFR. Newer biomarkers detected in urine or blood
could greatly assist with diagnosis, disease activity assessment, and prognosis of patients with GPA; however,
at present there is a need for prospective and longitudinal studies followed by validation in different groups
of GPA patients to confirm their clinical value [34].

Abbreviation
ACR: American College of Rheumatology; ANCA: Antineutrophil cytoplasmic
antibodies; BVAS/WG: Birmingham Vasculitis Activity Score for WG vasculitis;
CBC: Complete blood count; CRP: C-reactive protein; ESR: Erythrocyte
sedimentation rate; GPA: Granulomatosis with polyangiitis; IQR: Inter-quartile
range; MPV: Mean platelet volume; PLR: Platelet to lymphocyte ratio; PR-
3: Proteinase-3; SD: Standard deviation; SPSS: Statistical Package for Social
Science; WG: Wegener's granulomatosis

Acknowledgements
None

Authors' contributions
All of the authors declare that they have all participated in the design, execution,
and analysis of the paper, and that they have approved the final version.

Author details
[1]Faculty of Medicine, Department of Internal Medicine, Division of
Rheumatology, Gazi University, Ankara, Turkey. [2]Faculty of Medicine,
Department of Physical Medicine & Rehabilitation, Division of Rheumatology,
Gazi University, Ankara, Turkey.

References
1. Pagnoux C. Updates in ANCA-associated vasculitis. Eur J Rheumatol. 2016;
   3(3):122–33.
2. van der Woude FJ, Rasmussen N, Lobatto S, Wiik A, Permin H, van Es LA,
   et al. Autoantibodies against neutrophils and monocytes: tool for diagnosis
   and marker of disease activity in Wegener's granulomatosis. Lancet. 1985;
   1(8426):425–9.
3. Weiner M, Segelmark M. The clinical presentation and therapy of diseases
   related to anti-neutrophil cytoplasmic antibodies (ANCA). Autoimmun Rev.
   2016;15(10):978–82.
4. Pagnoux C, Hogan SL, Chin H, Jennette JC, Falk RJ, Guillevin L, et al.
   Predictors of treatment resistance and relapse in antineutrophil cytoplasmic
   antibody-associated small-vessel vasculitis: comparison of two independent
   cohorts. Arthritis Rheum. 2008;58(9):2908–18.
5. Verstockt B, Bossuyt X, Vanderschueren S, Blockmans D. There is no benefit
   in routinely monitoring ANCA titres in patients with granulomatosis with
   polyangiitis. Clin Exp Rheumatol. 2015;33(2 Suppl 89):S-72 6.
6. Tomasson G, Grayson PC, Mahr AD, Lavalley M, Merkel PA. Value of ANCA
   measurements during remission to predict a relapse of ANCA-associated
   vasculitis--a meta-analysis. Rheumatology (Oxford). 2012;51(1):100–9.
7. Thai LH, Charles P, Resche-Rigon M, Desseaux K, Guillevin L. Are anti-
   proteinase-3 ANCA a useful marker of granulomatosis with polyangiitis
   (Wegener's) relapses? Results of a retrospective study on 126 patients.
   Autoimmun Rev. 2014;13(3):313–8.
8. Zhang M, Huang XZ, Song YX, Gao P, Sun JX, Wang ZN. High platelet-to-
   lymphocyte ratio predicts poor prognosis and Clinicopathological
   characteristics in patients with breast Cancer: a meta-analysis. Biomed Res
   Int. 2017;2017:9503025.
9. Idil Soylu A, Arikan Cortcu S, Uzunkaya F, Atalay YO, Bekci T, Gungor L, et al. The
   correlation of the platelet-to-lymphocyte ratio with the severity of stenosis and
   stroke in patients with carotid arterial disease. Vascular. 2017;25(3):299–306.
10. Prodromidou A, Andreakos P, Kazakos C, Vlachos DE, Perrea D, Pergialiotis V.
    The diagnostic efficacy of platelet-to-lymphocyte ratio and neutrophil-to-
    lymphocyte ratio in ovarian cancer. Inflamm Res. 2017;66(6):467–75.
11. Zhu Y, Si W, Sun Q, Qin B, Zhao W, Yang J. Platelet-lymphocyte ratio acts as
    an indicator of poor prognosis in patients with breast cancer. Oncotarget.
    2017;8(1):1023–30.
12. Jennette JC, Falk RJ, Andrassy K, Bacon PA, Churg J, Gross WL, et al.
    Nomenclature of systemic vasculitides. Proposal of an international
    consensus conference. Arthritis Rheum. 1994;37(2):187–92.
13. Leavitt RY, Fauci AS, Bloch DA, Michel BA, Hunder GG, Arend WP, et al. The
    American College of Rheumatology 1990 criteria for the classification of
    Wegener's granulomatosis. Arthritis Rheum. 1990;33(8):1101–7.
14. Stone JH, Hoffman GS, Merkel PA, Min YI, Uhlfelder ML, Hellmann DB, et al. A
    disease-specific activity index for Wegener's granulomatosis: modification of
    the Birmingham Vasculitis activity score. International network for the study of
    the systemic Vasculitides (INSSYS). Arthritis Rheum. 2001;44(4):912–20.
15. Gabay C, Kushner I. Acute-phase proteins and other systemic responses to
    inflammation. N Engl J Med. 1999;340(6):448–54.
16. Kisacik B, Tufan A, Kalyoncu U, Karadag O, Akdogan A, Ozturk MA, et al.
    Mean platelet volume (MPV) as an inflammatory marker in ankylosing
    spondylitis and rheumatoid arthritis. Joint Bone Spine. 2008;75(3):291–4.
17. Kucuk H, Goker B, Varan O, Dumludag B, Haznedaroglu S, Ozturk MA, et al.
    Predictive value of neutrophil/lymphocyte ratio in renal prognosis of
    patients with granulomatosis with polyangiitis. Ren Fail. 2017;39(1):273–6.
18. Ahbap E, Sakaci T, Kara E, Sahutoglu T, Koc Y, Basturk T, et al. Neutrophil-to-
    lymphocyte ratio and platelet-to-lymphocyte ratio in evaluation of
    inflammation in end-stage renal disease. Clin Nephrol. 2016;85(4):199–208.
19. Yaprak M, Turan MN, Dayanan R, Akin S, Degirmen E, Yildirim M, et al. Platelet-
    to-lymphocyte ratio predicts mortality better than neutrophil-to-lymphocyte
    ratio in hemodialysis patients. Int Urol Nephrol. 2016;48(8):1343–8.
20. Yang W, Wang X, Zhang W, Ying H, Xu Y, Zhang J, et al. Neutrophil-
    lymphocyte ratio and platelet-lymphocyte ratio are 2 new inflammatory
    markers associated with pulmonary involvement and disease activity in
    patients with dermatomyositis. Clin Chim Acta. 2017;465:11–6.
21. Kim DS, Shin D, Lee MS, Kim HJ, Kim DY, Kim SM, et al. Assessments of neutrophil
    to lymphocyte ratio and platelet to lymphocyte ratio in Korean patients with
    psoriasis vulgaris and psoriatic arthritis. J Dermatol. 2016;43(3):305–10.
22. Asahina A, Kubo N, Umezawa Y, Honda H, Yanaba K, Nakagawa H.
    Neutrophil-lymphocyte ratio, platelet-lymphocyte ratio and mean platelet
    volume in Japanese patients with psoriasis and psoriatic arthritis: response
    to therapy with biologics. J Dermatol. 2017;44(10):1112–21.
23. Fu H, Qin B, Hu Z, Ma N, Yang M, Wei T, et al. Neutrophil- and platelet-to-
    lymphocyte ratios are correlated with disease activity in rheumatoid
    arthritis. Clin Lab. 2015;61(3–4):269–73.
24. Qin B, Ma N, Tang Q, Wei T, Yang M, Fu H, et al. Neutrophil to lymphocyte
    ratio (NLR) and platelet to lymphocyte ratio (PLR) were useful markers in
    assessment of inflammatory response and disease activity in SLE patients.
    Mod Rheumatol. 2016;26(3):372–6.
25. Yavuz S, Ece A. Mean platelet volume as an indicator of disease activity in
    juvenile SLE. Clin Rheumatol. 2014;33(5):637–41.
26. Ozdemir R, Karadeniz C, Doksoz O, Celegen M, Yozgat Y, Guven B, et al. Are
    mean platelet volume and platelet distribution width useful parameters in
    children with acute rheumatic carditis? Pediatr Cardiol. 2014;35(1):53–6.
27. Karabudak O, Ulusoy RE, Erikci AA, Solmazgul E, Dogan B, Harmanyeri Y.
    Inflammation and hypercoagulable state in adult psoriatic men. Acta Derm
    Venereol. 2008;88(4):337 40.

28. Abanonu GB, Daskin A, Akdogan MF, Uyar S, Demirtunc R. Mean platelet volume and beta-thromboglobulin levels in familial Mediterranean fever: effect of colchicine use? Eur J Intern Med. 2012;23(7):661–4.

29. Ozturk ZA, Dag MS, Kuyumcu ME, Cam H, Yesil Y, Yilmaz N, et al. Could platelet indices be new biomarkers for inflammatory bowel diseases? Eur Rev Med Pharmacol Sci. 2013;17(3):334–41.

30. Soydinc S, Turkbeyler IH, Pehlivan Y, Soylu G, Goktepe MF, Bilici M, et al. Mean platelet volume seems to be a valuable marker in patients with systemic sclerosis. Inflammation. 2014;37(1):100–6.

31. Tecer D, Sezgin M, Kanik A, Incel NA, Cimen OB, Bicer A, et al. Can mean platelet volume and red blood cell distribution width show disease activity in rheumatoid arthritis? Biomark Med. 2016;10(9):967–74.

32. Balta I, Balta S, Koryurek OM, Demirkol S, Celik T, Akbay G, et al. Mean platelet volume is associated with aortic arterial stiffness in patients with Behcet's disease without significant cardiovascular involvement. J Eur Acad Dermatol Venereol. 2014;28(10):1388–93.

33. Gasparyan AY, Ayvazyan L, Mikhailidis DP, Kitas GD. Mean platelet volume: a link between thrombosis and inflammation? Curr Pharm Des. 2011;17(1):47–58.

34. Vega LE, Espinoza LR. Predictors of poor outcome in ANCA-associated Vasculitis (AAV). Curr Rheumatol Rep. 2016;18(12):70.

26

Within and between-days repeatability and variability of plantar pressure measurement during walking in children, adults and older adults

Pedro S. Franco[1,2], Cristiane F. Moro[1], Mariane M. Figueiredo[1], Renato R. Azevedo[1,2], Fernando G. Ceccon[1,2] and Felipe P. Carpes[1,2]* (iD)

Abstract

Background: Previous studies discussed the repeatability and variability in plantar pressure measurement, but a few considered different age groups. Here we determine within and between-days repeatability and variability of plantar pressure measurement during gait in participants from different age groups.

Method: Plantar pressure was recorded in children, young adults and older adults walking at preferred speed in four non-consecutive days within one week. Data from 10 steps from each foot in each day were analyzed considering the different regions of the foot. Mean and peak plantar pressure and data variability were compared between the steps, foot regions and days.

Results: To describe mean and peak pressure during gait in children and adults a single measurement can be enough, but elderly will requires more attention especially concerning peak values. Variability in mean pressure did not differ between age groups, but peak pressure variability differed across foot regions and age groups.

Conclusion: One single observation can be used to describe plantar pressure during gait in children and adults. When the interest concerns older people, it might be pertinent to consider more than one day of assessment, especially when looking at peak pressure.

Keywords: Kinetics, Foot, Gait, Aging, Peak pressure

Background

Plantar pressure analysis concerns the quantification and interpretation of the force applied to the ground and its distribution over the foot plantar surface area. Among the different ways for its quantification is the use of pressure mat systems that allows not only quantification of the pressure distribution but also analysis of the specific foot regions [1–4]. Instrumentation, foot region, and number of steps are factors influencing repeatability and variability of plantar pressure measurement [1–4]. The number of steps required for characterization of

plantar pressure during gait is a source of discussion in the literature [5]. Three steps are commonly assumed in clinical analysis of gait [6], and three to five steps are assumed to be enough to record plantar pressure in adults aged 20 to 35 years old [7].

Plantar pressure variability is also a topic of interest because most of clinical decisions are based in single-day measurement. Considering data from three [4], four [4] and five [1] different days, mean pressure, peak pressure, peak force, and force-time integral showed good repeatability. However, participants of different ages were considered in each of these studies [1, 2, 4]. There is a lack of evidences concerning differences between age groups, which are especially important for studies interested in influence of age on plantar pressure.

* Correspondence: carpes@unipampa.edu.br
[1]Applied Neuromechanics Research Group, Federal University of Pampa,Uruguaiana, BR 472 km 592, Po box 118, Uruguaiana, RS ZIP 97500-970, Brazil
[2]Graduated Program in Physical Education, Federal University of Santa Maria, Santa Maria, Brazil

There are gait characteristics that influence plantar pressure in people of different ages. In children, it includes changes in body mass and contact area of the foot [8] as well the establishment of a heel-strike landing pattern [9, 10]. Children also experience increase in peak pressure, ground reaction forces and foot length that influence center of pressure displacement [11]. Among young adults, magnitudes of pressure become stable and patterns of higher peak pressures in the rearfoot and hallux are observed [12–14]. Among older adults, a change in foot landing pattern may occur and pressure and reaction forces in the rearfoot decrease with a longer contact time [12]. These illustrate the differences between age groups that may influence plantar pressure measurements. Therefore, in this study we determine within and between-days repeatability and variability of plantar pressure measurement in people from different age groups.

Methods

Participants and experimental design

This research was conducted in agreement with the declaration of Helsinki and was approved by the local institution ethics committee. All participants and the parents (for the case of children) signed a consent term. To be included participants should be able to walk independently, be free of lower extremity injuries that limit locomotion and should be able to visit the laboratory on days previously scheduled. Those subjects that missed one evaluation session were excluded from the data analysis. Sixty participants (20 children, 20 young adults, and 20 elderly) from the local community started participation in the study. During the development of the study (see the flowchart; Fig. 1) some participants missed sessions and were excluded. In the end, 37 subjects completed all the procedures, which included 12 children, 13 adults, and 12 older adults. Participants completed four sessions of assessment in non-consecutive days within a period of 7 days for measurement of plantar pressure during walking at preferred speed.

Data acquisition

Plantar pressure was recorded during barefoot walking at preferred gait speed. Participants were requested to walk as they walk in streets. Data were acquired at 400 Hz using a pressure mat system (Matscan, Tekscan Inc., Boston, MA, US) placed halfway in a 9 m walkway. The mat had 5 mm thickness, detection area of 435.9 × 368.8 mm, comprising 2288 resistive sensors (1.4 sensors / cm²). The system was calibrated before every evaluation for each individual using the individual body mass. Ten steps were randomly recorded for each foot, and data from right foot were considered in the analyses. Gait speed was determined using a chronometer. The evaluation session was

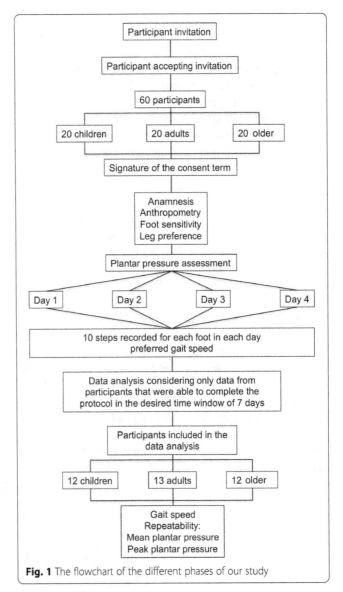

Fig. 1 The flowchart of the different phases of our study

repeated in four non-consecutives days within a period of up to 7 days.

Plantar pressure was analyzed considering the forefoot (FF), midfoot (MF) and rearfoot (RF) regions defined using a software (Research Foot 6.64, Tekscan Inc., Boston, MA, USA) and anatomical aspects determining that the rearfoot comprised 31% of the foot length, the midfoot comprised 19% of the foot length, and the forefoot comprised 50% of the foot length [15]. Data were averaged for each foot region and normalized to the total foot pressure to minimize effects body mass and foot size that differ among the participants [16]. Variables of interested in our study were mean pressure, computed by the average pressure over active sensors, and peak pressure, defined as the highest value observed among the selected active sensors [17]. Data variability was determined by the coefficient of variation that is the ratio between standard deviation and mean values.

Statistical analyses

Data are present considering mean (standard deviation). All data were checked for normality with Shapiro-Wilk test. ANOVA one-way with Tukey post-hoc was used to compare steps and to compare foot regions within a same day of assessment. Similar approach was used to compare the different days of assessment and the different groups. All analyses considered a significance level of 0.05 using a commercial statistical package.

Results

Groups of study included 12 children [8 women; 10 (1) years old, 44 (16) kg, 1.43 (0.1) m, for age, body mass and height, respectively], 13 adults [7 women; 38 (6) years old, 71 (15) kg, 1.65 (0.1) m], and 12 older adults [7 women; 74 (3) years old, 70 (14) kg, 1.59 (0.1) m]. Preferred gait speed in children was 1.21 (0.1) m/s, in adults was 1.56 (0.2) m/s, and in older adults was 0.89 (0.10) m/s. Mean pressure did not differ between the steps in both adults and older adults in within-day comparisons (Fig. 2). Among children, mean pressure differed between some of the steps only for the fourth day (F $_{(9)}$ = 4.389; P = 0.03; Fig. 2). Peak pressure did not differ between the steps in adults and older adults (Fig. 3). Peak pressure in children differed between some of the steps only in the rearfoot for the fourth day (F $_{(9)}$ = 2.688; P = 0.04, Fig. 3).

Regardless of the day of measurement, when comparing the foot regions, adults showed lower peak pressure in the midfoot compared to forefoot and rearfoot (Fig. 4). In children, peak pressure was smaller in the midfoot than forefoot and rearfoot, while forefoot and rearfoot showed similar values. Among older adults, peak pressures were higher in the forefoot and differed between the three regions of the foot (Fig. 4).

To compare pressure between the days we considered the average of mean and peak pressures from each day of measurement (Fig. 4). Mean and peak pressure in children did not differ between the days. Among adults, mean pressure in the midfoot was higher for the fourth day [F $_{(3)}$ = 5.190; P = 0.027], while peak pressure was similar for the different days. In older adults, mean pressure did not differ between the days, but peak pressure differed between all the days [F $_{(3)}$ = 4.717; P = 0.008].

Data on pressure variability were also considered in our analyses (see Table 1 for variability of mean and peak pressure). Mean pressure variability did not differ between the days of measurement in foot regions of children, adults and older adults. However, when mean pressure variability was compared between the foot regions, regardless of the day of measurement, higher variability in the midfoot, and similar variability in the rearfoot and forefoot were observed in children (F $_{(2)}$ = 36.10; P < 0.001), adults (F $_{(2)}$ = 174.1; P < 0.001), and older adults (F $_{(2)}$ = 125.4; P < 0.001). When groups were

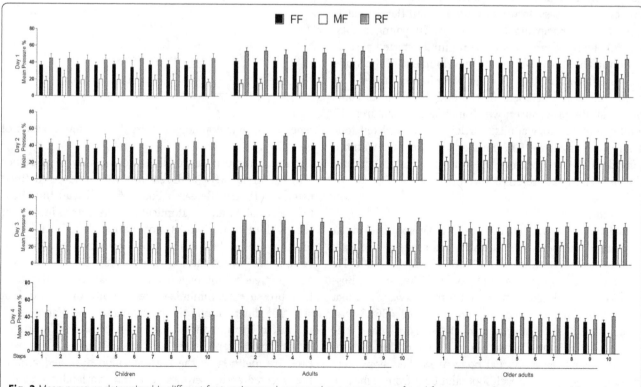

Fig. 2 Mean pressure determined in different foot regions and expressed as a percentage of total foot pressure. Data are presented for each step and group in the four days of measurement. * indicates difference between the steps

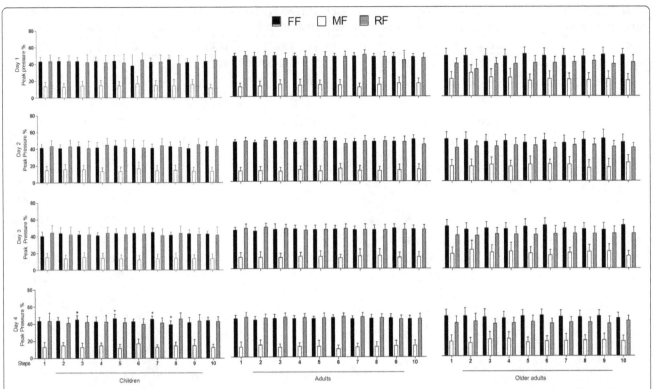

Fig. 3 Peak pressure determined in different foot regions and expressed as a percentage of total foot pressure. Data are presented for each step and group in the four days of measurement. * indicates difference between the steps

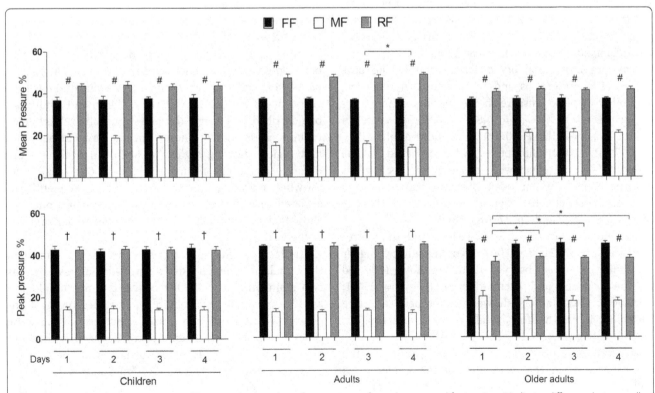

Fig. 4 Mean and peak pressure compared between the four days of measurement for each group and foot region. # indicates difference between all foot regions. † indicate difference in the rearfoot (RF) and forefoot (FF) compared to midfoot (MF) * indicates difference between the days

Table 1 Coefficient of variation determined for each day, foot region and group, considering data of mean and peak pressure. Data are expressed in percentage (%) considering mean and standard deviation data from each foot region. FF: forefoot; MF: midfoot; FR: rearfoot

Variable	Group	Foot region	Day 1 (%)	Day 2 (%)	Day 3 (%)	Day 4 (%)
Mean pressure variability	Children	FF	13.6 (7.6)	12.2 (5.8)	9.1 (3.9)	7.8 (4.0)
		MF	29.5 (5.9)*	27.0 (5.7)*	26.6 (6.1)*	24.6 (12.3)*
		RF	14.3 (2.7)	13.5 (2.5)	14.3 (5.0	11.3 (3.0)
	Adults	FF	10.2 (1.3)	9.3 (1.8)	9.7 (2.0	10.5 (2.2)
		MF	38.4 (8.0)*#	29.9 (5.1)*#	34.1 (7.8)*#	34.1 (7.4)*#
		RF	11.8 (5.0)	9.1 (3.2)	10.4 (4.4)	9.8 (1.4)
	Older adults	FF	14.2 (2.8)	15.9 (3.4)	12.7 (1.7)	12.8 (2.6)
		MF	26.1 (3.9)*	29.5 (10.1)*	25.6 (6.0)*	23.1 (4.7)*
		RF	10.7 (2.5)	10.7 (3.0)	12.4 (3.0)	10.0 (1.8)
Peak pressure variability	Children	FF	14.9 (7.3)$	13.5 (3.7)$	11.3 (2.7)$	10.6 (2.5)$
		MF	41.2 (6.3)*	37.7 (4.0)*	36.8 (4.0)*	32.7 (9.8)*
		RF	20.4 (2.8)+	18.4 (2.1)+	19.5 (2.1)+	16.0 (2.9)+
	Adults	FF	7.9 (1.4)$+	6.8 (1.7)$+	9.9 (1.8)$+	8.4 (1.6)$+
		MF	43.7 (6.9) *	38.8 (5.5) *	42.6 (7.7) *	43.2 (7.8) *
		RF	13.4 (4.5)	10.2 (2.8)	11.9 (1.7)	10.4 (1.4)
	Older adults	FF	17.0 (1.4)$+	18.0 (1.8)$+	15.0 (1.9)$+	16.0 (2.3)$+
		MF	40.8 (4.8)*	44.2 (9.7)*	41.5 (5.1)*	36.3 (4.8)*
		RF	19.3 (5.6)	16.7 (3.8)	19.6 (2.7)	17.1 (3.1)

* different of FF and RF (P < 0.05); $ different of RF and MF (P < 0.05); # different of children and older adults (P < 0.05); + identify days that differed between them (P < 0.05)

compared, the only difference relies on the mean pressure variability in the midfoot that showed an effect for age (F $_{(2)}$ = 8.88; P = 0.002), being higher in adults compared to older adults. Mean pressure variability in other foot regions did not differ between groups.

Peak pressure variability differed between the days in the different groups and foot regions. In children, variability of peak pressure in the rearfoot differed between the days (F $_{(3)}$ = 4.84; P = 0.015), while in adults (F $_{(3)}$ = 5.37; P = 0.011) and older adults (F $_{(3)}$ = 8.12; P = 0.002) differences were observed in the forefoot. No differences were observed in foot regions not mentioned. When peak pressure variability was compared between the regions, regardless of the day of assessment, children showed higher variability in the midfoot, followed by the rearfoot and then forefoot (F $_{(2)}$ = 67.21; P < 0.001). Among adults, higher variability also was observed in the midfoot, followed by the rearfoot and then forefoot (F $_{(2)}$ = 177.1; P < 0.001). Older adults showed higher peak pressure variability in the midfoot, while rearfoot and forefoot did not differ (F $_{(2)}$ = 177.1; P < 0.001).

We compared peak pressure variability between the groups and found that variability in the forefoot was higher in adults and older adults, which differed of children (F $_{(2)}$ = 11.26; P = 0.006). An age effect was also observed for rearfoot peak pressure variability (F $_{(2)}$ = 6.21;

P = 0.010), which was higher in children compared to adults and older adults.

Discussion

In this study we set out to determine within and between-days repeatability of plantar pressure in participants from different age groups. Our main findings suggest that plantar pressure in the children and adults can be described by a single-day assessment, but elderly may require assessments in more than one day. Furthermore, foot region showing higher variability in peak pressure differs between age groups. It might be of special interest when analyzing peak pressure, which is frequently associated with sites of foot injuries. Additionally, our data show that measurement of plantar pressure variability is influenced by age and foot region.

The lack of difference between the steps for most of the variables obtained from a single-day assessment has two main implications. One concerns a methodological aspect, in which repeatability of the measurement increases as the number of records increases [18]. In the other hand, the lack of differences in the magnitude of pressure may reflect repeated loading over the foot regions. Is has been suggested that foot injuries depend on the magnitude of load, especially in the rearfoot [19] and the head of the metatarsals [20]. We observed that plantar pressure differed between some of the steps of children in the last day of assessment. However, differences were between a few particular steps and it is possible that after the repeated days of testing children were impatience and it might have affected their gait pattern. Despite of differences observed only in the last day, other possible explanation is the higher within-trials variability in spatial gait parameters, which is know to be higher among children [21].

Differences in mean plantar pressure between the foot regions were similar in children and adults (see Fig. 4). Children and adults showed smaller peak pressure in the midfoot and similar peak pressure in the rearfoot and forefoot. In the older adults higher peak pressure occurred in the forefoot, followed by rearfoot and midfoot. Higher peak of pressure in the forefoot in older adults may rely on altered foot sensitivity in the midfoot and rearfoot. According to a previous research [22], the forward shift in plantar pressure (away from the insensitive heel) constitutes a strategy of older adults to maintain balance. This hypothesis is reinforced by the results of variability in the peak pressure, which was higher in the forefoot of older adults and may be a strategy of older adults to promote propulsion during weight bearing [22].

Assuming that pressure did not differ between steps within each day, we compared the mean values between the fours days of measurement. Children and adults presented similar peak pressure in different days, but in older adults peak values differed between all the days. Children gait suffer continuous adaptations until the adulthood, and therefore some patterns of gait change very fast [23]. However, after reaching the adult age, patterns can be much more stable [14]. We observed that peak pressure varied between the days in older adults. One could argue that variability in the gait speed could determine the variability in peak pressure in older adults. However, gait speed variability in the older adults was 11.23%, which is similar to the 12.80% observed in adults whom showed no differences in the peak pressure between the days. It is possible that variability in the peak pressure rely on tissue characteristics for impact absorption in the elderly, especially stiffness observed in the rearfoot and midfoot [24, 25]. This hypothesis may find support on the higher variability in pressure observed among older adults in comparison to the other groups and the apparent higher dependence on forefoot sensitivity during weight bearing tasks [22].

The age group showed influence on pressure across the regions of the foot. Children and young adults showed similar patterns of plantar pressure distribution with pressure varying between the regions but higher in the rearfoot. In the older adult loading on midfoot was larger than in children and adults. The change in midfoot pressure may rely on increased stiffness in forefoot (hallux and metatarsal I, III and V) as result of aging

[25]. The higher variability in the peak pressure in forefoot among older adults can also be related to the change in foot landing pattern leading to longer contact time during support phase of gait [12].

Our study has inherent limitations. We opted for participants walking at preferred speed. Walking speed may affect plantar pressure and to minimize its effects we considered pressure data normalized to the foot total pressure. Participants were evaluated barefoot, which do not permit to infer on shod walking.

Conclusion

Plantar pressure in children and adults is consistent within and between-days. In other hand, plantar pressure in older adults requires measurements in different days to determine the plantar pressure, especially peak values.

Acknowledgements

PSF, RRA and FGC were supported by student fellowships from CAPES. FAPERGS granted this research to FPC (grant number 1013100).

Authors' contributions

Experiment design: PSF and FPC.
Data collection and analysis: PSF, CFM, MMF, RAR, FGC.
Manuscript draft and critical review: PSF, CFM, MMF, RAR, FGC and FPC.
Approval of the final version: PSF, CFM, MMF, RAR, FGC and FPC.

References

1. Gurney JK, Kersting UG, Rosenbaum D. Between-day reliability of repeated plantar pressure distribution measurements in a normal population. Gait & posture. 2008;27:706–9.
2. Franco PS, Silva CB, Rocha ES, Carpes FP. Variability and repeatability analysis of plantar pressure during gait in older people. Rev Bras Reumatol. 2015;55: 427–33.
3. Deepashini H, Omar B, Paungmali A, Amaramalar N, Ohnmar H, Leonard J. An insight into the plantar pressure distribution of the foot in clinical practice: narrative review. Polish Annals of Medicine. 2014;21:51–6.
4. Cousins SD, Morrison SC, Drechsler WI. The reliability of plantar pressure assessment during barefoot level walking in children aged 7-11 years. J Foot Ankle Res. 2012;5
5. Zammit GV, Menz HB, Munteanu SE. Reliability of the TekScan MatScan(R) system for the measurement of plantar forces and pressures during barefoot level walking in healthy adults. J Foot Ankle Res. 2010;3:11.
6. Bus SA, de Lange A. A comparison of the 1-step, 2-step, and 3-step protocols for obtaining barefoot plantar pressure data in the diabetic neuropathic foot. Clin Biomech (Bristol, Avon). 2005;20:892–9.
7. McPoil TG, Cornwall MW, Dupuis L, Cornwell M. Variability of plantar pressure data. A comparison of the two-step and midgait methods. J Am Podiatr Med Assoc. 1999;89:495–501.
8. Hennig EM, Staats A, Rosenbaum D. Plantar pressure distribution patterns of young school children in comparison to adults. Foot & ankle international. 1994;15:35–40.
9. Hennig EM, Rosenbaum D. Pressure distribution patterns under the feet of children in comparison with adults. Foot & ankle. 1991;11:306–11.
10. Bosch K, Gerss J, Rosenbaum D. Preliminary normative values for foot loading parameters of the developing child. Gait & posture. 2007;26:238–47.
11. Bosch K, Gerss J, Rosenbaum D. Development of healthy children's feet—nine-year results of a longitudinal investigation of plantar loading patterns. Gait & posture. 2010;32:564–71.
12. Scott G, Menz HB, Newcombe L. Age-related differences in foot structure and function. Gait & posture. 2007;26:68–75.
13. Menz HB, Zammit GV, Munteanu SE, Scott G. Plantarflexion strength of the toes: age and gender differences and evaluation of a clinical screening test. Foot & ankle international. 2006;27:1103–8.

14. Bosch K, Nagel A, Weigend L, Rosenbaum D. From "first" to "last" steps in life–pressure patterns of three generations. Clin Biomech (Bristol, Avon). 2009;24:676–81.
15. Burns J, Crosbie J, Hunt A, Ouvrier R. The effect of pes cavus on foot pain and plantar pressure. Clin Biomech (Bristol, Avon). 2005;20:877–82.
16. Fernandez-Seguin LM, Diaz Mancha JA, Sanchez Rodriguez R, Escamilla Martinez E, Gomez Martin B, Ramos Ortega J. Comparison of plantar pressures and contact area between normal and cavus foot. Gait & posture. 2014;39:789–92.
17. Shu L, Hua T, Wang YY, Li QA, Feng DD, Tao XM. In-shoe plantar pressure measurement and analysis system based on fabric pressure sensing Array. Ieee T Inf Technol B. 2010;14:767–75.
18. Hughes J, Pratt L, Linge K, Clark P, Klenerman L. Reliability of pressure measurements: the EM ED F system. Clin Biomech (Bristol, Avon). 1991;6:14–8.
19. Wong DW, Niu W, Wang Y, Zhang M. Finite element analysis of foot and ankle impact injury: risk evaluation of calcaneus and talus fracture. PLoS One. 2016;11:e0154435.
20. Zwitser EW, Breederveld RS. Fractures of the fifth metatarsal; diagnosis and treatment. Injury. 2010;41:555–62.
21. Stolze H, Kuhtz-Buschbeck JP, Mondwurf C, Johnk K, Friege L. Retest reliability of spatiotemporal gait parameters in children and adults. Gait & posture. 1998;7:125–30.
22. Machado AS, Bombach GD, Duysens J, Carpes FP. Differences in foot sensitivity and plantar pressure between young adults and elderly. Arch Gerontol Geriatr. 2016;63:67–71.
23. Guffey K, Regier M, Mancinelli C, Pergami P. Gait parameters associated with balance in healthy 2- to 4-year-old children. Gait & posture. 2016;43:165–9.
24. Hsu CC, Tsai WC, Chen CP, et al. Effects of aging on the plantar soft tissue properties under the metatarsal heads at different impact velocities. Ultrasound Med Biol. 2005;31:1423–9.
25. Kwan RL, Zheng YP, Cheing GL. The effect of aging on the biomechanical properties of plantar soft tissues. Clin Biomech. 2010;25:601–5.

27

Assessment of gesture behavior and knowledge on low back pain among nurses

Hisa Costa Morimoto[1], Anamaria Jones[1] and Jamil Natour[1,2]*

Abstract

Background: Low back pain is particularly problematic among nursing professionals. Education is part of the rehabilitation process for low back pain and has been heavily studied. In parallel, gestural behaviors play an important role during the evaluation of the low back pain, especially while performing the activities of daily living. The aim of the present study was to evaluate gesture behavior and knowledge on LBP among nurses with and without LBP and correlate these factors with pain, physical functioning and quality of life.

Methods: An observational, controlled, cross-sectional study was carried out in 120 female nurses: 60 with LBP and 60 without LBP. The two groups were matched for age. The measures used for the evaluation were the Gesture Behavior Test, LBP Knowledge Questionnaire, Numerical Pain Scale for LBP, Roland Morris Disability Questionnaire and the Short Form-36 (SF-36) to assess quality of life.

Results: Mean age in both groups was 31 years. In the group with LBP, the mean Numerical Pain Scale score was 5.6 cm and the mean score on the Roland Morris questionnaire was 2.7. No statistically differences between groups were found regarding the scores of the LBP Knowledge Questionnaire or Gesture Behavior Test ($p = 0.531$ and $p = 0.292$, respectively). Statistically lower scores were found in the group with LBP for the following SF-36 domains: physical functioning ($p < 0.001$), physical role ($p = 0.015$), pain ($p = 0.001$), general health perceptions ($p = 0.015$), vitality ($p < 0.001$) and mental health ($p = 0.001$).

Conclusions: No differences were found when comparing nurses with or without LBP regarding gesture behavior or knowledge on LBP. Nurses with LBP showed a decrease in some domains of quality of life.

Keywords: Low back pain, Nurses, Behavior and patient's knowledge

Background

Low back pain is one of the most painful disorders, it is also a common cause of morbidity and is associated with significant social and economic impact worldwide. Epidemiological studies indicate that the prevalence of low back pain in the general population is between 60 and 80% [1, 2]. The literature reports that 90% of adults will experience back pain at least once in their lives [1, 3].

Low back pain is particularly problematic among nursing professionals in terms of absenteeism and litigation processes; it is also an important source of morbidity in this population. Its prevalence seems to be higher among nurses and nurses' aids than in the rest of the population, ranging between 56 and 90% respectively. Emotional stress, physical and psychosocial factors at work are crucial to the onset of low back pain [4–6].

Flexion, twisting, weight transfer and sudden movements were related to low back pain [7]. Similar findings were observed in another study, considering hoisting associated with spinal twisting, previous injury and excess of weight as risk factors for low back pain in nurses [8].

In 2008, researchers conducted a cross-sectional study of nurses with an average age of 26 years, in which they assessed the risk of developing low back pain due to occupational exposure in new nurses and students [9]. They concluded that over the course of one year in the profession, the risk of experiencing an increase in back pain was 90%, suggesting that the act of transferring patients in bed was detrimental and that preventive strategies should be aimed at this population.

Education is part of the rehabilitation process for low back pain and has been heavily studied. In parallel, gestural behaviors play an important role during the evaluation of the low back pain, especially while performing the activities of daily living (ADLs). Assessment

---

* Correspondence: jnatour@unifesp.br
[1]Rheumatology Division, Universidade Federal de São Paulo, São Paulo, Brazil
[2]Disciplina de Reumatologia, Rua Botucatu, 740, Sao Paulo, SP 04023-090, Brazil

instruments, such as the low back pain knowledge questionnaire (LKQ) and the gestural behavior test (GBT), were created and validated to expand the ways to evaluate the patient in a more specific manner [10, 11]. Because gestural behavior and knowledge of the disease are important variables in the management of low back pain, the aim of the present study was to evaluate the gestural and knowledge of low back pain in nurses with low back pain and compare with nurses without low back pain, as there are no studies in the literature for this purpose.

Methods

Sample

A hundred twenty nurses from the Hospital Sao Paulo - Universidade Federal de São Paulo / Escola Paulista de Medicina (UNIFESP / EPM) were included: 60 nurses with low back pain and 60 nurses who served as controls without back pain. The nurses in the control group were matched by age with the low back pain group. The study was approved by the Ethics and Research Committee of the University.

Sample size was calculated using GBT as the main parameter, with a standard deviation of 5 points.11 For the determination of a minimal difference of 3 points between groups among healthcare professionals, a 5% α error and a power of 90% were established. The calculation determinate a minimal sample of 60 nurses per group.

The low back pain group included nurses in activity, aged between 22 and 60 years, working in different hospital sectors (wards, emergency room and/or intensive care units) with a minimum workload of 6 h/day who experienced back pain on most days during the last three months, with a report of pain greater than 3 cm on a numerical pain scale (NPS) 0–10 cm. The control group included nurses with the same features but without back pain.

Nurses in situations of dispute, with prior surgery of the spine and/or a current pregnancy, were excluded from the study.

Outcomes

The participants completed an evaluation form with demographic (age, marital status, body mass index), clinical and professional information (disease duration and time since graduation), information's regarding smoking habits and life style and applied assessment tools to specify the level of low back pain. Almost all questionnaires were self-applied, only the GBT evaluation, was done by evaluator not blinded.

The assessment instruments used included the following:

* Gesture Behavior Test (GBT): this test evaluates the gestural behavior of patients with chronic non- specific low back pain. It consists of five functional tasks:

  ○ Task 1: getting out of bed after sleeping;
  ○ Task 2: sweep under the bed;
  ○ Task 3: lift and carry a garbage disposal;
  ○ Task 4: simulate tying shoelaces without help;
  ○ Task 5: organize objects with various weights on shelves of various heights.

Each task is characterized by an instruction, allowing several standardized scoring criteria. The score ranges from 0 to 32, with a higher score indicating a better gestural behavior [11].

* Low Back Pain Knowledge Questionnaire (LKQ): this instrument assesses knowledge about back pain. Composed of 16 questions, divided into the following categories: general aspects, concepts and treatment. The score ranges from 0 to 24 points, with a higher score denoting a better knowledge of low back pain [10].
* Numerical Pain Scale (NPS): this instrument subjectively assesses pain. The nurse quantifies the intensity of low back pain following a line of 0–10 cm, 0 being no pain and 10 being unbearable pain [12].
* Roland Morris Disability Questionnaire (RM): this instrument assesses the functional disability in patients with low back pain. It consists of 24 questions of self - response (yes or no), and the score ranges from zero (no disability) to 24 points (severe disability) [13].
* Short Form - 36 (SF-36): generic questionnaire that assesses quality of life, with 36 items about general health that fall into eight domains: physical functioning, role limitations due to physical health, bodily pain, general health, vitality, social health, emotional health and mental health. The score for each domain ranges from 0 to 100, and higher scores indicate a better quality of life [14].

Statistical analysis

The statistical program SPSS 19.0 was used. The level of significance was set to 0.05.

Descriptive statistics were presented by the frequency and percentage for categorical data and the mean with standard deviation for quantitative data. The Kolmogorov-Smirnov test was applied to assess the normality of the variables. To evaluate the homogeneity of the sample at baseline, chi-square tests, Student t-tests and Mann-Whitney tests were performed. The Spearman correlation test was used to assess the quantitative variables [15, 16].

Results

Table 1 summarizes the mean and standard deviation (SD) of the sociodemographic data, demonstrating the homogeneity of the sample for these parameters. The mean age of total sample was 31.6 years. The groups were similar in terms of age, body mass index (BMI),

Table 1 Sample characteristics

	LBP group N = 60	Control group N = 60	P intergrupo
Age (years)	31,7 ± 7,8	31,6 ± 7,5	0,979[b]
BMI (kg/m^2)	24,6 ± 4,9	23,5 ± 3,2	0,518[b]
Marital status	–	–	0,727[a]
Single	39 (65%)	41 (68,3%)	–
Maried	19 (31,7%)	16 (26,7%)	–
Divorced	2 (3,3%)	3 (5,0%)	–
Time since graduation (years)	7,2 ± 6,9	6,6 ± 6,0	0,983[b]
Disease duration (years)	4,2 ± 2,6	–	–
NPS (cm)	5,6 ± 1,7	–	–
Roland Morris	2,7 ± 2,5	–	–

Data presented as mean ± standard deviation or percentage (%)
BMI body mass index, *NPS* numeric pain scale, *p* significance value in the comparison between groups
[a]chi-square test
[b]Mann-Whitney

marital status and training time. The mean duration of symptoms in the low back pain group was 4.2 years. Table 1 also shows the NPS and RM scores of the low back pain group.

According to the lifestyle evaluation of the nurses, the groups were homogeneous regarding inactivity ($p = 0.838$) and smoking ($p = 0.679$). The proportions are presented in Table 2.

With respect to the variables of GBT and LKQ, we found no significant differences between the groups ($p = 0.292$ and $p = 0.531$, respectively). The means and standard deviation scores are presented in Table 3.

In the quality of life assessment using the SF-36, there were significant differences between the groups in the following domains: physical functioning ($p = 0.001$), role limitations due to physical health ($p = 0.015$), pain ($p < 0.001$), general health ($p = 0.015$), vitality ($p < 0.001$) and mental health ($p = 0.001$). There were no significant differences between the groups in the areas of social and emotional health (Table 4).

In Table 5 shows the statistically significant correlations between the SF-36 domains, LKQ and GBT scores in the

Table 2 Ratio of sedentary and smoking among nurses

	LBP group N = 60	Control group N = 60	P intergrupo
Sedentary	–	–	0,838
Yes	44 (73,3%)	43 (71,7%)	–
No	16 (26,7%)	17 (28,3%)	–
Smoking	–	–	0,679
Yes	4 (6,7%)	2 (3,3%)	–
No	56 (93,3%)	58 (96,7%)	–

Data presented as n and percentage (%) using the Chi-square test
p significance value in the comparison between groups

Table 3 Scores of the Gestural Behavior Test (GBT) and Low Back Pain Knowledge Questionnaire (LKQ)

	LBP group N = 60	Control group N = 60	P intergrupo
GBT	17,7 ± 3,9	18,5 ± 4,3	0,292
LKQ	–	–	–
General aspects	8,2 ± 1,0	8,0 ± 0,8	0,217
Concept	3,1 ± 1,1	3,1 ± 0,9	0,867
Treatment	8,0 ± 1,8	8,0 ± 1,7	0,781
Total	19,2 ± 3,1	19,1 ± 2,5	0,531

Data presented as mean ± standard deviation using the Mann-Whitney test
GBT gestural behavior test, *LKQ* low back pain knowledge questionnaire, *p* significance value in the comparison between groups

control and low back pain groups. No correlations were found between the RM, LKQ and GBT questionnaires.

Discussion

LBP is the most prevalent and costly musculoskeletal disorder worldwide. Studies in nurses with low back pain have reported strong associations among work environment, lifestyle and postural factors [17].

The aim of this study was to evaluate the gestures and knowledge of disease in nurses because the literature indicates that these variables are relevant in the perpetuation and management of low back pain.

Our study evaluated only nurses and not nurses aids. It is known that in Brazil, these professionals have distinct and unique roles, commonly involving activities that require constant movement of the lumbar spine, such as caring for patients in bed and performing transfers. However, a regulation imposed by the Board of Nursing describes the full range of functions for nursing professionals, which includes being exposed to physical and biomechanical factors that can trigger back pain. Therefore, to avoid bias, we chose to only evaluate nurses because each group has a professional profile and distinct function. The study evaluated nurses' aids and nurses within a single group [18].

d'Ericco et al. in 2013, investigated the prevalence of back pain and the association with absenteeism in nurses and concluded that the prevalence was 58.2%, being 55.9% to chronic low back pain and 61.9% to acute low back pain. Relative to the nurses' aids, the prevalence was higher (67.5% among the nurses and 36.4% among the nurses' aids) [19].

Our sample included only women to ensure a homogeneous sample by gender, as male hospital nurses represent a minority. Some of the other studies previously in the literature also opted for a heterogeneous sample by gender [20–22].

The average age of the nurses assessed was 31.7 years. These data are similar to Yip and Jaromi et al. studies

Table 4 Evaluation of the SF-36 demonstrated as mean and standard deviation

	LBP group N = 60	Control group N = 60	P intergrupo
Physical functioning	82,1 ± 16,6	91,8 ± 9,1	< 0,001[a]
Role limitations due to physical health	72,5 ± 32,1	84,2 ± 26,4	0,015[a]
Bodily pain	56,4 ± 16,2	74,0 ± 21,8	< 0,001[a]
General health	74,7 ± 15,6	81,4 ± 14,6	0,015[a]
Vitality	52,1 ± 17,5	64,3 ± 16,0	< 0,001[a]
Social Health	74,8 ± 20,9	80,0 ± 18,7	0,179
Emotional health	72,8 ± 35,0	75,0 ± 30,5	0,970
Mental health	66,5 ± 16,7	75,5 ± 13,1	0,001[a]

Data presented as mean ± standard deviation using the Mann-Whitney test
p significance value in the comparison between groups
[a]Value statistically significant

and are consistent with the literature, which places the age group with the highest incidence of low back pain between 18 and 65 years [23, 24]. A study by Sikiru & Hanifa [22], showed that the prevalence of back pain increased with age. The group < 35 years showed a prevalence of 6.3%; the group 36–45 years showed a prevalence of 27%; and the group > 46 years showed a prevalence of 66.7%.

Other variables, such as physical inactivity and smoking, were also collected to characterize the sample. Physical inactivity and smoking, in association with other variables, have been reported as important factors for increasing the risk of low back pain [25]. In this study, 73% of the nurses were sedentary. In contrast, only 6% of the sample were smokers. In Vieira et al. [21] study, the nurses were less sedentary (55%) but included more smokers (35%). Yip found no significant correlation between inactivity and low back pain in nurses.

The GBT was the instrument chosen to assess the gestural behavior of the nurses. This test was initially created to evaluate the gestures of patients with chronic nonspecific low back pain who have participated in an educational program that typically consists of information on joint protection and energy conservation, as well as advice on spinal anatomy, conservative treatment, medication and disease management.

Importantly, the literature does not describe a specific test for evaluating the gestural behavior of nurses. The GBT does not evaluate gestures performed during the work activities of a nurse but rather those performed while simulating the activities of daily living. We believe that the behaviors that nurses adopt in their day-to-day will also adapt to their work environment.

Although this is a cross-sectional study and does not propose an educational intervention for nurses, it is interesting to evaluate the gestural behavior of this

Table 5 Correlations between of SF-36 domains, the Gestural Behavior Test (GBT) and Low Back Pain Knowledge Questionnaire (LKQ) scores in the control and low back pain groups

SF-36	LKQ -GA	LKQ -Concept	LKQ -Treatment	LKQ - Total	GBT
Control group					
Bodily Pain	NS	0.270 (0.037)	NS	NS	NS
Global health	NS	NS	NS	NS	0.290 (0.024)
Vitality	NS	NS	NS	NS	0.290 (0.049)
LBP group					
Physical functioning	NS	0.258 (0.047)	NS	NS	NS
Bodily pain	0.227 (0.032)	NS	NS	NS	NS
General health	NS	0.312 (0.015)	NS	NS	NS
Social Health	NS	0.269 (0.038)	NS	NS	NS
Emotional health	NS	NS	0.268 (0.038)	NS	NS
Mental health	NS	NS	NS	0.256 (0.048)	NS

Correlations presented were statistically significant (p < 0.05)
LKQ low back pain knowledge questionnaire, GA general aspects, LKQ low back pain knowledge questionnaire, LBP low back pain, NS non significant

population because the relationship between physical factors and low back pain has been heavily discussed in the literature, and to date, no other study has used this instrument.

Regarding the assessment of knowledge of the disease, the only specific questionnaire addressing low back pain in the literature is the LKQ. This is the first study to evaluate the knowledge of low back pain in nurses using the LKQ.

Sikiru & Hanifa evaluated the knowledge of joint protection of the spine in 300 nurses with low back pain using a no validated questionnaire formulated by the authors themselves [22]. They observed that 80 nurses (26.6%) exhibited knowledge about joint protection, whereas 220 (73.3%) had no knowledge on this topic. There was a significant correlation between the knowledge of joint protection of the spine with the incidence of low back pain. In this study, it would be appropriate to use the LKQ that include issues regarding joint protection and energy conservation.

Pain and disability are important variables in the characterization of low back pain. There are many instruments that assess pain and functional disability in low back pain. For pain assessment, the NPS was chosen because of its easy application and improved understanding, and the RM was used to assess functional disability due to its status as a questionnaire widely used in the literature. The nurses presented an average pain level of 5.6 cm (SD = 1.7) and showed no severe disability according to the RM questionnaire. In a study by Lin et al. in 2012, nurses were evaluated using the Visual Analogue Scale (VAS) 0–100 mm, and the average pain level was 41.6 mm [26]. With respect to functional disability, we cannot compare our data with those in the literature because we did not find any studies that evaluated low back pain in nurses and utilized the RM.

The quality of life, assessed using the SF-36, was worse in terms of functional capacity, role limitations due to physical health, bodily pain, general health, vitality and mental health in the low back pain group compared to the control group. Carugno et al. showed similar results to those of our study [27]. The authors used the mental health domain of SF-36 to evaluate 751 nurses and found that nurses with musculoskeletal disorders, including back pain, presented worse mental health. No studies that correlated the SF-36 with the instruments used in our study were found.

Regarding knowledge of disease and gestural behavior, we found no statistical differences between the groups. Regarding the GBT, the total average score in the two groups was 19 points, with a maximum score of 32 points. In a study by Furtado et al., the average score among all patients with low back pain was 16.3, whereas rehabilitation professionals without back pain had a mean score of 26 points. Despite the smaller scores within the general population, these results are similar to those of nurses, indicating a low level of knowledge in this area even among health professionals [11].

Regarding the assessment using the LKQ, the mean score for nurses was 19 points, in a total score of 24 points. Maciel et al. [10] showed that the mean total score of patients with chronic low back pain was 9 points, far below the results observed for our sample.

Based on these results, we believe that both nurses with low back pain and the control group have a good level of knowledge about the important aspects of low back pain but do not use this knowledge in their day-to-day lives, resulting in behaviors that include inappropriate gestures. This line of thought further strengthens the importance and necessity of adopting a behavioral approach during the treatment of chronic nonspecific low back pain that includes disease management, adherence to therapy and conservative treatment, thereby improving both mental and physical behaviors.

Although the nurses showed no difference between gestural behavior and knowledge of the disease, we found positive (weak and moderate) correlations between some SF-36 domains with GBT and LKQ. These data reflect that the two variables are directly related to the quality of life, mainly in the physical aspects and vice versa.

We found no correlation between pain and disability using the GBT and LKQ. Similarly, a study by Furtado et al. [11], found no correlation between pain and GBT. However, our data showed a correlation between RM and GBT. The authors believe that the disability caused by chronic low back pain leads the patient to adopt copping towards protecting and not overloading the spine. It is likely that our results did not agree with those of the study by Furtado et al. because nurses with LBP have only low disability, according to the assessment by RM.

This study has some limitations, among them the small sample, the lack of men in the sample and also the lack of blind evaluator.

We believe that no difference was found between the groups in GBT and LKQ, because the nurses in the low back pain group did not show an important disability. As shown in the results, according to the RM, the nurses were classified as having mild disability. A possible explanation for RM results may be the level of knowledge of the sample, because it is a health professional and because of the classification of low back pain. The study chose to evaluate nurses with chronic low back pain. Perhaps in the acute phase, the results would be different from those presented in the present study. It is important to note that GBT is not specific to assess the disease's impairment. We believe that RM is more sensitive to evaluate this variable.

As seen in the literature, there are few studies evaluating the variables evaluated in our study. Therefore, it is necessary that new controlled studies be carried out in order to deepen the use of these instruments and to corroborate the results of the present study; epidemiological studies with large samples to evaluate the prevalence of low back pain in nurses; and other studies with educational intervention.

Conclusion

Nurses with back pain do not show differences in behavior or in gestural knowledge about back pain when compared to nurses without low back pain. However, nurses with low back pain show less quality of life.

Authors' contributions

All authors contributed to conception and design of the study, analysis and interpretation of data, drafting the article and revising it critically for important intellectual content and final approval of the version to be submitted. HCM and AJ contributed with the data acquisition too.

References

1. Deyo RA, Weinstein JN. Primary care - low back pain. N Engl J Med. 2001; 344(5):363–70.
2. Jaromi M, Nemeth A, Kranicz J, Laczko T, Betlehem J. Treatment and ergonomics training of work-related lower back pain and body posture problems for nurses. J Clin Nurs. 2012;21(11–12):1776–84.
3. Frymoyer JW, Pope MH, Constanza MC, Osen JC, Goggin JE, Wilder DJ. Epidemiologic studies of low back pain. Spine. 1980;5:419–23.
4. Maul I, Laubli T, Klipstein A, Krueger H. Course of low back pain among nurses: a longitudinal study across eight years. Occup Environ Med. 2003;60:497–503.
5. Smedley J, Trevelyan F, Inskip H, Bucle P, Cooper C, Coggon D. Impact of ergonomic intervention on back pain among nurses. Scand J Work Environ Health. 2003;29(2):117–23.
6. Eriksen W, Bruusgaard D, Knardahl S. Work factors as predictors of intense a disabling low back pain; a prospective study of nurses' aides. Occup Environ Med. 2004;61:398–404.
7. Punnet L, Fine LJ, Keyserling WM, Hersen GD, Chaffin DB. Back disorders and nonneutral trunk postures of automobile assembly workers. Scand J of Work, Environ Health. 1991;17(5):337–46.
8. Fuortes LJ, Shi Y, Zhang M, Zwerling C, Schootman M. Epidemiology of back injury in university hospital nurses from review of workers compensation records and a case-control survey. J Occup Med. 1994; 36:1022–6.
9. Mitchell T, O'Sullivan PB, Burnett AF, Straker I, Rudd C. Low back pain chacteristics from undergraduate student to working nurse in Australia: a cross-sectional survey. Int J Nurs Stud. 2008;45(11):1636–44.
10. Maciel SC, Jennings F, Jones A, Natour J. The development and validation of a low back pain knowledge questionnaire – LKQ. Clinics. 2009;64(12):1167–75.
11. Furtado R, Jones A, Furtado RNV, Jennings F, Natour J. Validation of the Brazilian portuguese version of the gesture behavior test for patients with non-specific chronic low back pain. Clinics. 2009;64(2):83–90.
12. Ferraz MB, Oliveira LM, Araujo PM, Atra E, Tugwell P. Crosscultural reability of physicalability dimension of the health assessment questionaire. J Rheumatol. 1990a;17(6):813–7.
13. Nusbaum L, Natour J, Ferraz MB, Goldenberg J. Translation, adaptation and validation of the Roland-Morris questionnaire – Brazil Roland-Morris. Braz J Med Biol Res. 2001;34(2):203–10.
14. Ciconelli RM, Ferraz MB, Santos W, Meinão I, Quaresma MR. Tradução para a língua portuguesa e validação do questionário genérico de avaliação de qualidade de vida SF-36 (Brasil SF-36). Rev Bras Reumatol. 1999;39(3):143–50.
15. Zar JH. Biostatistical analysis. Upper Saddle River: Prentice Hall; 1999.
16. Brunner E, Langer F. Nonparametric análisis of ordered categorical data in designs with longitudinal observations and small sample sizes. Biom J. 2000; 42(6):663–75.
17. Woolf AD, Pfleger B. Burden of major musculoskeletal conditions. Bull World Health Organ. 2003;81(9):646–56.
18. Hartvigsen J, Lauritzen S, Lings S, Lauritzen T. Intensive education combined with low tech ergonomic intervention does not prevent low back pain in nurses. Occup Environ Med. 2005;62:13–7.
19. d'Errico A, Viotti S, Baratti A, Mottura B, Barocelli AP, Tagna M, et al. Low back pain and associated presenteeism among hospital nursing staff. J Ocupp Health. 2013;55(4):276–83.
20. Yip VY. New low back pain in nurses: work activies, work stress and sedentary lifestyle. J Adv Nurs. 2004;46(4):430–40.
21. Vieira ER, Kumar S, Coury HJCG, Narayan Y. Low back problems and possible improvements in nursing jobs. J Adv Nurs. 2006;55(1):79–89.
22. Sikiru L, Hanifa S. Prevalence and risk factors of low back pain among nurses in a typical Nigerian hospital. Afr Health Sci. 2010;10(1):26–30.
23. Leclaire R, Esdaile JM, Suissa S, Rossignol M, Proulx R, Dupuis M. Back school in a first episode of compensated acute low back pain: a clinical trial to assess efficacy and prevent relapse. Arch Phys Med Rehabil. 1996;77(7):673–9.
24. Glomsrod B, Loon JH, Soukup MG, Bo K, Larsen S. (2001). Active back school. Prophylactic management for low back pain: three year follow-up of a randomized controlled trial. J Rehab Med. 2001;33:26–30.
25. Bejia I, Younes M, Jamila HB, Khalfallah T, Bem Salem K, Touzi M, et al. Prevalence and factors associated to low back pain among hospital staff. Joint Bone Spine. 2005;72(3):254–9.
26. Lin PH, Tsai YA, Chen WC, Huang SF. Prevalence, characteristics, and work-related risk factors of low back pain among hospital nurses in Taiwan: a cross-sectional survey. Int J Occup Med Environ Health. 2012;25(1):41–50.
27. Carugno M, Pesatori AC, Ferrario MM, Ferrari AL, Silva FJ, Martins AC, et al. Physical and psychosocial risk factors for musculoskeletal disorders in Brazilian and Italian nurses. Cad Saude Publica. 2012;28(9):1632–42.

Permissions

List of Contributors

Liete Zwir, Melissa Fraga, Monique Sanches, Carmen Hoyuela and Claudio Len
Universidade Federal de São Paulo (UNIFESP), Rua Guilherme Moura, São Paulo 95, Brazil

Melek Kechida, Rim Klii, Sonia Hammami and Ines Khochtali
Internal Medicine and Endocrinology Department, Fattouma Bourguiba University Hospital, 1st June Avenue, 5000 Monastir, Tunisia

Sana Salah
Physical Medicine and Rehabilitaion Department, Fattouma Bourguiba University Hospital, Monastir, Tunisia

Rim Kahloun
Ophtalmology Department, Fattouma Bourguiba University Hospital, Monastir, Tunisia

Renata Miossi
Hospital das Clinicas HCFMUSP, Faculdade de Medicina, Universidade de Sao Paulo, São Paulo, SP, Brazil
Division of Rheumatology, Hospital das Clinicas HCFMUSP, Faculdade de Medicina, Universidade de Sao Paulo, Sao Paulo, Brazil
Division of Rheumatology, Faculdade de Medicina FMUSP, Universidade de Sao Paulo, Av. Dr. Arnaldo, 455, 3 andar, sala 3150 - Cerqueira César, CEP 01246-903 Sao Paulo, Brazil
Rheumatology Division, Hospital das Clinicas HCFMUSP, Faculdade de Medicina, Universidade de Sao Paulo, Sao Paulo, Brazil

Daniel Brito de Araújo
Universidade Federal de Pelotas (UFP), Pelotas, RS, Brazil

Verônica Silva Vilela
Universidade do Estado do Rio de Janeiro (UERJ), Rio de Janeiro, RJ, Brazil

Mailze Campos Bezerra
Hospital Geral de Fortaleza (HGF), Fortaleza, CE, Brazil

Bernardo Matos da Cunha
Rede Sarah de Hospitais de Reabilitação, Brasília, Brazil

Gecilmara Salviato Pileggi
SBR. Faculdade de Ciências da Saúde de Barretos - FACISB, Barretos, São Paulo, Brazil

School of Medical Science Barretos- FACISB, Avenue Masonic Lodge Renovadora 68, No. 100 – Airport Neighborhood, Barretos/SP 14785-002, Brazil

Alexandre Wagner De Souza
SBR. Escola Paulista de Medicina, Universidade Federal de São Paulo, São Paulo, Brazil

Aline Rocha
Pós graduanda do programa de Medicina Baseada em Evidências, Universidade Federal do Estado de São Paulo (UNIFESP), São Paulo, Brazil

Ana Karla Guedes de Melo
SBR. Hospital Universitário Lauro Wanderley, Universidade Federal da Paraíba (UFPB), João Pessoa, Brazil

Caroline Araujo M. da Fonte
SBR. Hospital Getulio Vargas, Recife, Brazil

Cecilia Bortoletto
SBD. Faculdade de Medicina do ABC, Santo Andre, Brazil

Claiton Viegas Brenol
SBR. Hospital de Clínicas de Porto Alegre, Universidade Federal do Rio Grande do Sul, Porto Alegre, Brazil

Claudia Diniz Lopes Marques
SBR. Hospital das Clínicas, Universidade Federal de Pernambuco, Recife, Brazil

Cyrla Zaltman
GEDIIB. Presidente do GEDIIB 2017-2019, Universidade Federal do Rio de Janeiro, Rio de Janeiro, Brazil

Eduardo Ferreira Borba
SBR. Hospital das Clinicas, Faculdade de Medicina, Universidade de Sao Paulo, Sao Paulo, Brazil

Enio Ribeiro Reis
SBR. Diretor médico do Centro de infusão do Hospital Humanitas, Varginha, Brazil

Eutilia Andrade Medeiros Freire and Evandro Mendes Klumb
SBR. Unidade Docente Assistencial de Reumatologia, Universidade do Estado do Rio de Janeiro, Rio de Janeiro, Brazil

Georges Basile Christopoulos
SBR. Presidente da Sociedade Brasileira de Reumatologia, Maceio-AL, Brazil

Ieda Maria M. Laurindo
SBR. Escola de Medicina da Universidade Nove de Julho, São Paulo, Brazil

Isabella Ballalai
SBIm. Vice-Presidente da Sociedade Brasileira de Imunizações (SBIm), SBiM, Rio de Janeiro, Brazil

Izaias Pereira Da Costa
SBR. Professor da Faculdade de Medicina da Universidade Federal do Mato Grosso do Sul, Cuiabá, Brazil

Lessandra Michelin
SBI. Professora na faculdade de Medicina, Universidade de Caxias do Sul, Caxias do Sul, Brazil

Lilian David de Azevêdo Valadares
SBR. Reumatologista. Hospital Getulio Vargas, Recife, Brazil

Liliana Andrade Chebli
GEDIIB, Faculdade de Medicina da Universidade Federal de Juiz de Fora, Juiz de Fora, Brazil

Marcus Lacerda
SMBT. Instituto Leônidas e Maria Deane (Fiocruz - Amazônia), Fundação de Medicina Tropical Dr. Heitor Vieira Dourado (FMT-HVD), Maceio-AL, Brazil

Maria Amazile Ferreira Toscano
SBR. Medica reguladora da Secretaria Estadual da Saúde de Santa Catarina, Florianópolis, Brazil

Michel Alexandre Yazbek
SBR. Escola de Medicina, Universidade Estadual de Campinas, Campinas, Brazil

Rejane Maria R. De Abreu Vieira
SBR. Hospital Geral de Fortaleza e Universidade de Fortaleza, Fortaleza, Brazil

Renata Magalhães
SBD. Faculdade de Medicina da Universidade Estadual de Campinas, Campinas, Brazil

Renato Kfouri
SBIm. Presidente do Departamento de Imunizações da Sociedade Brasileira de Pediatria (SBP), Maceio-AL, Brazil

Rosana Richtmann
SBI. Instituto de Infectologia Emilio Ribas, Maceio-AL, Brazil

Selma Da Costa Silva Merenlender
SBR. Presidente da SRRJ. Chefe do Serviço de Reumatologia do Hospital Estadual Eduardo Rabelo RJ, Rio de Janeiro, Brazil

Valeria Valim
SBR. Faculdade de Medicina, Universidade Federal do Espírito Santo, Vitória, Brazil

Marcos Renato De Assis
SBR. Escola Médica de Marilia, Marilia, Brazil

Sergio Candido Kowalski
SBR. Universidade federal do Paraná, Curitiba, Brazil

Virginia Fernandes Moça Trevisani
SBR. Universidade Federal de São Paulo (UNIFESP), São Paulo; Universidade Santo Amaro (UNISA), Sao Paulo, Brazil

Jozélio Freire de Carvalho and Roberto Paulo Correia de Araujo
SOS Vida, Rheumatology Unit, Salvador, Bahia, Brazil
Institute of Health Sciences, Universidade Federal da Bahia (Federal University of Bahia), Salvador, Bahia, Brazil

Maria Natividade Pereira dos Santos, Joyce Meyre Vieira de Oliveira, Andrea Nogueira S. Lanty Silva and Juliana Bahia Cardozo
SOS Vida, Rheumatology Unit, Salvador, Bahia, Brazil

Glaucia Santin and Valderilio Feijó Azevedo
Edumed Educação em Saúde, Rua Bispo Dom José, 2495, Curitiba, Paraná 80440-080, Brazil
Universidade Federal do Paraná, Rua General Carneiro 181, Curitiba, Paraná 80060-900, Brazil

Mariana Moreira Magnabosco da Silva, Vinicius Augusto Villarreal, Leane Dhara Dalle Laste, Eduardo de Freitas Montin and Luis Eduardo Ribeiro Betiol
Universidade Federal do Paraná, Rua General Carneiro 181, Curitiba, Paraná 80060-900, Brazil

Júlio Cesar Bertacini de Moraes
Division of Rheumatology, Hospital das Clinicas HCFMUSP, Faculdade de Medicina, Universidade de Sao Paulo, Sao Paulo, Brazil

Eloisa Bonfá
Division of Rheumatology, Faculdade de Medicina FMUSP, Universidade de Sao Paulo, Sao Paulo, Brazil

Manar Amanouil Said, Liana Soido Teixeira e Silva, Aline Maria de Oliveira Rocha, Gustavo Guimarães Barreto Alves, Daniela Gerent Petry Piotto and Claudio Arnaldo Len
Division of Pediatric Rheumatology, Department of Pediatrics, Federal University Sao Paulo (Unifesp), Rua Borges Lagoa, 802, Sao Paulo, Brazil

Maria Teresa Terreri
Division of Pediatric Rheumatology, Department of Pediatrics, Federal University Sao Paulo (Unifesp), Rua Borges Lagoa, 802, Sao Paulo, Brazil
Rheumatology Division, Medicine Department of Escola Paulista de Medicina (EPM), Universidade Federal de São Paulo (UNIFESP), São Paulo, Brazil
Universidade Federal de São Paulo (UNIFESP), Rua Guilherme Moura, São Paulo 95, Brazil

Gustavo Guimarães Moreira Balbi
Serviço de Reumatologia, Hospital Universitário, Universidade Federal de Juiz de Fora (UFJF), Av. Eugênio do Nascimento, s/n - Dom Bosco, Juiz de Fora, MG 36038-330, Brazil

Marcelo de Souza Pacheco and Adriana Danowski
Serviço de Reumatologia, Hospital Federal dos Servidores do Estado (HFSE), Rio de Janeiro, RJ, Brazil

Odirlei Andre Monticielo
Serviço de Reumatologia, Departamento de Medicina Interna, Hospital de Clínicas de Porto Alegre (HCPA), Universidade Federal do Rio Grande do Sul (UFGRS), Porto Alegre, RS, Brazil

Andreas Funke
Serviço de Reumatologia, Hospital de Clínicas, Universidade Federal do Paraná (UFPR), Curitiba, PR, Brazil

Mittermayer Barreto Santiago
Serviço de Reumatologia, Universidade Federal da Bahia (HUPES) e Escola Baiana de Medicina e Saúde Pública, Salvador, BA, Brazil

Henrique Luiz Staub
Serviço de Reumatologia, Escola de Medicina, Pontifícia Universidade Católica do Rio Grande do Sul (PUCRS), Porto Alegre, RS, Brazil

Jozelia Rêgo
Serviço de Reumatologia, Faculdade de Medicina, Universidade Federal de Goiás (UFG), Goiânia, GO, Brazil

Danieli Castro Oliveira de Andrade
Disciplinade Reumatologia, Faculdade de Medicina, Universidade de São Paulo (USP), São Paulo, SP, Brazil

Nilton Salles Rosa Neto, Judith Campos de Barros Bento and Rosa Maria Rodrigues Pereira
Rheumatology Division, Faculdade de Medicina da Universidade de São, Paulo, São Paulo, Brazil

Ricardo Santos Simões and Wanderley Marques Bernardo
Hospital das Clinicas HCFMUSP, Faculdade de Medicina, Universidade de Sao Paulo, São Paulo, SP, Brazil

Fernando Henrique Carlos de Souza
Hospital das Clinicas HCFMUSP, Faculdade de Medicina, Universidade de Sao Paulo, São Paulo, SP, Brazil
Division of Rheumatology, Faculdade de Medicina FMUSP, Universidade de Sao Paulo, Av. Dr. Arnaldo, 455, 3 andar, sala 3150 - Cerqueira César, CEP 01246-903 Sao Paulo, Brazil

Thais Amanda Frank
Programa Diretrizes da Associação Médica Brasileira (AMB), Brasília, Brazil

Maria da Conceição Costa and Claudio A. Len
Rheumatology Division, Medicine Department of Escola Paulista de Medicina (EPM), Universidade Federal de São Paulo (UNIFESP), São Paulo, Brazil

Hilda A. V. Oliveira
Rheumatology Unit of Pediatrics Department of Escola Paulista de Medicina (EPM), Universidade Federal de São Paulo (UNIFESP), Rua Borges Lagoa, 802, São Paulo, SP 04038.001, Brazil

Jamil Natour
Rheumatology Division, Universidade Federal de São Paulo, São Paulo, Brazil
Disciplina de Reumatologia, Rua Botucatu, 740, Sao Paulo, SP 04023-090, Brazil
Rheumatology Unit of Pediatrics Department of Escola Paulista de Medicina (EPM), Universidade Federal de São Paulo (UNIFESP), Rua Borges Lagoa, 802, São Paulo, SP 04038.001, Brazil

Pablo Arturo Olivo Pallo and Samuel Katsuyuki Shinjo
Division of Rheumatology, Faculdade de Medicina FMUSP, Universidade de Sao Paulo, Av. Dr. Arnaldo, 455, 3 andar, sala 3150 - Cerqueira César, CEP 01246-903 Sao Paulo, Brazil

Diego Sales de Oliveira and Rafael Giovani Misse
Division of Rheumatology, Faculdade de Medicina FMUSP, Universidade de Sao Paulo, Av. Dr. Arnaldo, 455, 3° andar, sala 3150 - Cerqueira César, Sao Paulo 01246-903, Brazil

Fernanda Rodrigues Lima
Division of Rheumatology, Hospital das Clinicas HCFMUSP, Faculdade de Medicina, Universidade de Sao Paulo, Sao Paulo, Brazil

Edgard Torres dos Reis Neto and Marcelo de Medeiros Pinheiro
Disciplina de Reumatologia, Escola Paulista de Medicina, Universidade Federal de São Paulo, São Paulo, Brazil
Rheumatology Division, Universidade Federal de São Paulo/Escola Paulista de Medicina (Unifesp/EPM), Rua Leandro Dupré, 204, conj. 74, Vila Clementino, São Paulo, São Paulo-SP CEP 04025-010, Brazil

Emília Inoue Sato
Disciplina de Reumatologia, Escola Paulista de Medicina, Universidade Federal de São Paulo, São Paulo, Brazil

Gilda Aparecida Ferreira
Serviço de Reumatologia do Hospital das Clínicas da Universidade Federal de Minas Gerais, Belo Horizonte, Brazil

Adriana Maria Kakehasi
SBR. Faculdade de Medicina, Universidade Federal de Minas Gerais, Belo Horizonte, Brazil
Serviço de Reumatologia do Hospital das Clínicas da Universidade Federal de Minas Gerais, Belo Horizonte, Brazil

Cláudia Diniz Lopes Marques
Serviço de Reumatologia do Hospital das Clínicas da Universidade Federal de Pernambuco, Recife, Brazil

Ana Paula Monteiro Gomides Reis
Hospital Universitário - UnB/EBSERH, Brasília, Brazil

Licia Maria Henrique Da Mota
SBR. Serviço de Reumatologia do Hospital Universitário de Brasília, Universidade de Brasília, Brasília, Brazil
Hospital Universitário - UnB/EBSERH, Brasília, Brazil

Eduardo dos Santos Paiva
Serviço de Reumatologia do Hospital das Clínicas da Universidade Federal do Paraná, Curitiba, Brazil

Gecilmara Cristina Salviato Pileggi
Instituto de Ensino e Pesquisa (IEP), Hospital Amor, Barretos, Brazil

Ricardo Machado Xavier
Serviço de Reumatologia do Hospital de Clínicas de Porto Alegre da Universidade Federal do Rio Grande do Sul, Porto Alegre, Brazil

José Roberto Provenza
Pontifícia Universidade Católica de Campinas, Campinas, Brazil

Ali Şahin, Mehmet Emin Derin, Fatih Albayrak and Burak Karakaş
Department of Internal Medicine – Rheumatology, Faculty of Medicine, Cumhuriyet University, Unit Sivas Cumhuriyet, 58140 Sivas, Turkey

Yalçın Karagöz
Department of Biostatistic, Medical Faculty, Sivas Cumhuriyet University, Sivas, Turkey

Sandra Lúcia Euzébio Ribeiro, Luiz Fernando de Souza Passos and Helena Lúcia Alves Pereira
Department of Clinical Medicine, Federal University of Amazonas, Faculty of Health Sciences, Rua Afonso Pena, 1053, Praça 14, Manaus, AM, Brazil

Antonio Luiz Boechat and Maria Cristina Dos-Santos
Department of Parasitology, Federal University of Amazonas, Immunochemistry Laboratory, Av General Rodrigo Otavio, 6200 Coroado I, Manaus, AM, Brazil

Neusa Pereira Silva and Emilia Ionue Sato
Division of Rheumatology, Escola Paulista de Medicina, Federal University of São Paulo, São Paulo, Brazil

Maria das Graças Souza Cunha
Alfredo da Matta Foundation, Manaus, Amazonas, Brazil

Rebeka Paulo Santos and Edgard Torres dos Reis-Neto
Division of Rheumatology, Universidade Federal de São Paulo, São Paulo, SP, Brazil

Marcelo Medeiros Pinheiro
Division of Rheumatology, Universidade Federal de São Paulo, São Paulo, SP, Brazil
Disciplina de Reumatologia, Escola Paulista de Medicina – Universidade Federal de São Paulo, Rua Leandro, Dupré, 204, conjunto 74, Vila Clementino, São Paulo, SP 04025-010, Brazil

Bruna Aurora Nunes Cavalcante Castro and Vera Lucia Szejnfeld
Rheumatology Division, Universidade Federal de São Paulo/Escola Paulista de Medicina (Unifesp/EPM), Rua Leandro Dupré, 204, conj. 74, Vila Clementino, São Paulo, São Paulo-SP CEP 04025-010, Brazil

Jacob Szejnfeld
Radiology Department, Universidade Federal de São Paulo/Escola Paulista de Medicina (Unifesp/EPM), São Paulo, Brazil

Valdecir Marvulle
Statistics Department, Universidade Federal de São Paulo/Escola Paulista de Medicina (Unifesp/EPM), São Paulo, Brazil

Juleimar Soares Coelho de Amorim
Ciências da Reabilitação, Instituto Federal de Educação, Ciência e Tecnologia do Rio de Janeiro – IFRJ, Rio de Janeiro, RJ, Brasil Colina, Manhuaçu, Brazil

Renata Cristine Leite and Renata Brizola
Centro Universitário Filadélfia – UNIFIL, Londrina, PR, Brasil

Cristhiane Yumi Yonamine
Saúde Coletiva, Centro Universitário Filadélfia – UNIFIL, Londrina, PR, Brasil

Thâmara Cristiane Alves Batista Morita
Faculdade de Medicina FMUSP, Universidade de Sao Paulo, Sao Paulo, SP, Brazil
Private practice, Aracaju, SE, Brazil

Gabriela Franco Sturzeneker Trés and Ilana Halpern
Faculdade de Medicina FMUSP, Universidade de Sao Paulo, Sao Paulo, SP, Brazil

Maria Salomé Cajas García
Instituto Dermatológico Professor Rubem David Azulay, Rio de Janeiro, RJ, Brazil

Paulo Ricardo Criado
Faculdade de Medicina FMUSP, Universidade de Sao Paulo, Sao Paulo, SP, Brazil
Faculdade de Medicina do ABC FMABC, Santo Andre, SP, Brazil

Jozelio Freire de Carvalho
Instituto de Ciências da Saúde, Universidade Federal da Bahia (UFBA), Salvador, BA, Brazil

Latika Gupta, Durga Prasanna Misra, Sakir Ahmed, Avinash Jain, Abhishek Zanwar, Able Lawrence, Vikas Agarwal, Amita Aggarwal and Ramnath Misra
Department of Clinical Immunology and Rheumatology, Sanjay Gandhi Postgraduate Institute of Medical Sciences, Lucknow 226014, India

E. Cunha
Undergraduate student, Faculty of Medicine, University of São Paulo, São Paulo, SP, Brazil

C. Sobrado and V. Guzela
Discipline of Colorectal Surgery, Hospital das Clínicas/ Faculdade de Medicina (HC-FMUSP), University of São Paulo, São Paulo, SP, Brazil

D. Andrade
Discipline of Rheumatology, Hospital das Clínicas/ Faculdade de Medicina (HC-FMUSP), University of São Paulo, Av. Dr. Arnaldo 455, Third Floor, Room 3109, São Paulo 01246903, Brazil

G. G. M. Balbi
Discipline of Rheumatology, Hospital das Clínicas/ Faculdade de Medicina (HC-FMUSP), University of São Paulo, Av. Dr. Arnaldo 455, Third Floor, Room 3109, São Paulo 01246903, Brazil
Discipline of Rheumatology, Hospital Universitário, Federal University of Juiz de Fora, Juiz de Fora, MG, Brazil

Cristiane Kayser
Rheumatology Division, Escola Paulista de Medicina, Universidade Federal de São Paulo (UNIFESP), Rua Botucatu 740, 3° andar, São Paulo, SP 04023-062, Brazil

Markus Bredemeier
Rheumatology Service, Hospital Nossa Senhora da Conceição, Grupo Hospitalar Conceição, Porto Alegre, RS, Brazil

Maria Teresa Caleiro
Rheumatology Division, Hospital das Clinicas HCFMUSP, Faculdade de Medicina, Universidade de Sao Paulo, Sao Paulo, Brazil

Karina Capobianco
Rheumatology Service, Moinhos de Vento Hospital, Porto Alegre, Brazil

Tatiana Melo Fernandes
Rheumatology Division, Universidade Federal do Rio de Janeiro, Rio de Janeiro, Brazil

Sheila Márcia de Araújo Fontenele
Departament of Medicine, Universidade Estadual do Ceará, Fortaleza, Brazil

Eutilia Freire
Rheumatology Service, Universidade Federal da Paraíba, João Pessoa, Brazil

Lilian Lonzetti
Rheumatology Service, Complexo Hospitalar da Santa Casa de Misericórdia de Porto Alegre, Universidade Federal de Ciências da Saúde de Porto Alegre, Porto Alegre, Brazil

Juliana Sekiyama
Faculdade de Ciências Médicas, Universidade Estadual de Campinas (UNICAMP), Campinas, SP, Brazil

Carolina de Souza Müller
Rheumatology Division, Hospital de Clínicas, Universidade Federal do Paraná (UFPR), Curitiba, Brazil

Hamit Kucuk, Berna Goker, Ozkan Varan, Hakan Babaoglu, Mehmet Akif Ozturk, Seminur Haznedaroglu and Abdurrahman Tufan
Faculty of Medicine, Department of Internal Medicine, Division of Rheumatology, Gazi University, Ankara, Turkey

Duygu Tecer and Serdar Can Guven
Faculty of Medicine, Department of Physical Medicine & Rehabilitation, Division of Rheumatology, Gazi University, Ankara, Turkey

Cristiane F. Moro and Mariane M. Figueiredo
Applied Neuromechanics Research Group, Federal University of Pampa,Uruguaiana, BR 472 km 592, Uruguaiana, RS, Brazil

Pedro S. Franco, Renato R. Azevedo, Fernando G. Ceccon and Felipe P. Carpes
Applied Neuromechanics Research Group, Federal University of Pampa,Uruguaiana, BR 472 km 592, Uruguaiana, RS, Brazil
Graduated Program in Physical Education, Federal University of Santa Maria, Santa Maria, Brazil

Hisa Costa Morimoto and Anamaria Jones
Rheumatology Division, Universidade Federal de São Paulo, São Paulo, Brazil

Index

Printed in the USA
CPSIA information can be obtained
at www.ICGtesting.com
JSHW060010020124
54623JS00006B/118